Neurological Care and the COVID-19 Pandemic

Neurological Care and the COVID-19 Pandemic

EDITED BY

AHMAD RIAD RAMADAN

Neurologist,
Stroke and Neurocritical Care,
Henry Ford Neuroscience Institute,
Henry Ford Hospital, Detroit, MI, United States

GAMALELDIN OSMAN

Mayo Clinic Comprehensive Epilepsy Center,
Neurology Department,
Rochester, MN, United States

Epilepsy fellow at Mayo Clinic Hospital,
Assistant Professor of Neurology,
Mayo School of Medicine,
Rochester, MN, United States

ELSEVIER

Elsevier
Radarweg 29, PO Box 211, 1000 AE Amsterdam, Netherlands
The Boulevard, Langford Lane, Kidlington, Oxford OX5 1GB, United Kingdom
50 Hampshire Street, 5th Floor, Cambridge, MA 02139, United States

Notices

Knowledge and best practice in this field are constantly changing. As new research and experience broaden
our understanding, changes in research methods, professional practices, or medical treatment may become
necessary.

Practitioners and researchers must always rely on their own experience and knowledge in evaluating and
using any information, methods, compounds, or experiments described herein. In using such information or
methods they should be mindful of their own safety and the safety of others, including parties for whom they
have a professional responsibility.

To the fullest extent of the law, neither the Publisher nor the authors, contributors, or editors, assume any
liability for any injury and/or damage to persons or property as a matter of products liability, negligence or
otherwise, or from any use or operation of any methods, products, instructions, or ideas contained in the
material herein.

Library of Congress Cataloging-in-Publication Data
A catalog record for this book is available from the Library of Congress

British Library Cataloguing-in-Publication Data
A catalogue record for this book is available from the British Library

ISBN: 978-0-323-82691-4

For information on all Elsevier publications
visit our website at https://www.elsevier.com/books-and-journals

Publisher: Nikki Levy
Acquisitions Editor: Melanie Tucker
Editorial Project Manager: Kristi Anderson
Production Project Manager: Sreejith Viswanathan
Cover designer: Alan Studholme

Typeset by STRAIVE, India

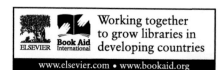

To COVID-19 victims and frontline workers all over the world:
past, present, and future.

Contents

Contributors

Alex Abou Chebl
Comprehensive Stroke Center; Department of Neurology, Henry Ford Hospital, Detroit, MI, United States

Hassan Aboul Nour
Department of Neurology, Henry Ford Hospital, Detroit, MI, United States

Ashhar Ali
Department of Neurology, Henry Ford Hospital; Department of Neurology, Wayne State University School of Medicine, Detroit, MI, United States

Owais Khadem Alsrouji
Comprehensive Stroke Center; Department of Neurology, Henry Ford Hospital, Detroit, MI, United States

Gregory L. Barkley
Department of Neurology, Henry Ford Hospital; Department of Neurology, Wayne State University, School of Medicine, Detroit, MI, United States

Helena Bulka
Department of Neurology, Henry Ford Hospital, Detroit, MI, United States

Mirela Cerghet
Department of Neurology, Henry Ford Hospital; Wayne State University, School of Medicine, Detroit, MI, United States

Jules E.C. Constantinou
Department of Neurology, Henry Ford Health System; Wayne State University School of Medicine, Detroit, MI, United States

Omar A. Danoun
Department of Neurology, Henry Ford Health System, Detroit, MI, United States

Elissa Fory
Department of Neurology, The Icahn School of Medicine at Mount Sinai, New York, NY, United States

Shailendra Giri
Department of Neurology, Henry Ford Hospital, Detroit, MI, United States

Kavita M. Grover
Wayne State University, Henry Ford Hospital, Detroit, MI, United States

Angelos Katramados
Department of Neurology, Henry Ford Hospital; Department of Neurology, Wayne State University, School of Medicine, Detroit, MI, United States

Hannah Kopinsky
Department of Neurology, Henry Ford Hospital; Wayne State University School of Medicine, Detroit, MI, United States

Shelley Lee
Department of Neurology, Henry Ford Health System, Detroit, MI, United States

Peter A. LeWitt
Department of Neurology, Henry Ford Hospital; Department of Neurology, Wayne State University, Detroit, MI, United States

Tessa M. LeWitt
Department of Neurology, Henry Ford Hospital; Wayne State University School of Medicine, Detroit, MI, United States

Chandan Mehta
Department of Neurology, Henry Ford Hospital, Detroit, MI, United States

Anza B. Memon
Department of Neurology, Henry Ford Hospital; Wayne State University School of Medicine, Detroit, MI, United States

Panayiotis D. Mitsias
Comprehensive Stroke Center; Department of Neurology, Henry Ford Hospital; School of Medicine, Wayne State University, Detroit, MI, United States; School of Medicine, University of Crete; Department of Neurology, University General Hospital, Heraklion, Greece

Ghada A. Mohamed
Department of Neurology, Henry Ford Health System, Detroit, MI, United States

Ali Mohamud
Department of Neurology, Henry Ford Hospital, Detroit, MI, United States

Daniel Newman
Wayne State University, Henry Ford Hospital, Detroit, MI, United States

Gamaleldin Osman
Mayo Clinic Comprehensive Epilepsy Center, Neurology Department; Epilepsy fellow at Mayo Clinic Hospital, Assistant Professor of Neurology, Mayo School of Medicine, Rochester, MN, United States

Jacob Pawloski
Department of Neurosurgery, Henry Ford Hospital, Detroit, MI, United States

Ahmad Riad Ramadan
Neurologist, Stroke and Neurocritical Care, Henry Ford Neuroscience Institute, Henry Ford Hospital, Detroit, MI, United States

Mohammed F. Rehman
Departments of Neurology and Neurosurgery, Henry Ford Hospital, Detroit, MI, United States

James M. Snyder
Departments of Neurology and Neurosurgery; Hermelin Brain Tumor Center, Henry Ford Hospital, Detroit, MI, United States

Naganand Sripathi
Wayne State University, Henry Ford Hospital, Detroit, MI, United States

Natalie Stec
Department of Neurology, Henry Ford Hospital, Detroit, MI, United States

Aarushi Suneja
Department of Neurology, Cleveland Clinic, Cleveland, OH, United States

Ritika Suri
Department of Neurology, Henry Ford Hospital, Detroit, MI, United States

Quinton J. Tafoya
Department of Pharmacy, Veterans Affairs, San Antonio, TX, United States

George Vourakis
School of Medicine, University of Crete; Department of Neurology, University General Hospital, Heraklion, Greece

Vibhangini S. Wasade
Department of Neurology, Henry Ford Health System, Detroit, MI, United States

Victoria Watson
Department of Neurosurgery, Southern Illinois University, Springfield, IL, United States

Insha Zahoor
Department of Neurology, Henry Ford Hospital, Detroit, MI, United States

Editors Biography

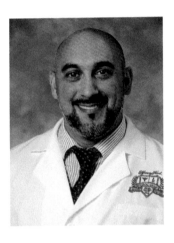

Dr. Ahmad Riad Ramadan is a board-certified neurologist with subspecialty training in vascular neurology (UT Houston) and neurocritical care (Johns Hopkins University). He is the program director for the Neurocritical Care Fellowship at Henry Ford Hospital in Detroit, Michigan. His research focuses are in the areas of vascular neurology, neuroinflammation, and the interaction between the microbiome and the nervous system in acute brain injuries. He currently chairs the scientific advisory board for the Neurology Department at Henry Ford Hospital and has led several research initiatives surrounding COVID-19. He is an advocate for diversity, equity, and inclusion (DEI) in medicine and particularly enjoys medical education and mentorship.

Ahmad Riad Ramadan, MD
Senior Staff Neurologist

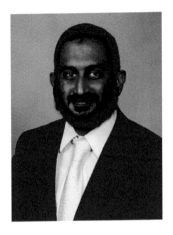

Dr. Gamaleldin Osman is a board-certified neurologist with subspeciality training in epilepsy (Mayo Clinic). He is currently an epilepsy fellow at Mayo Clinic Hospital in Rochester, Minnesota. He cochaired the COVID-19 Scientific Advisory Board for the neurology department at Henry Ford Hospital and has participated in research projects on the EEG findings in COVID-19 and the response of the health-care systems to the COVID-19 epidemic.

Preface

Not a soul has been spared or left indifferent by this strange virus that saw the light over a year ago and has since cast a net of darkness over the planet. One way or another, the novel coronavirus has permeated our daily lives. We all know someone who has lost either their loved ones or livelihood to it, been sick with it, or constrained by it. One surge after the other, we had to rethink ways to protect ourselves from getting infected or spreading the disease, innovate to continue conducting business, and transform education to meet the learning needs of our children. One of the most formidable adaptations has been the reshaping of health-care delivery. This pandemic will always be remembered as the one that truly put frontline workers at the front of the line, risking their lives to save others. Hospitals and medical centers all around the world had to swiftly and constantly reorganize themselves to address the dizzying surges of patients affected by the virus while continuing to care for those bearing other ailments.

This book is the collaborative work of a group of physicians, residents, and pharmacist aimed at delivering the latest and most up-to-date knowledge surrounding the various ways the novel coronavirus affects the nervous system. It is articulated around the many neurological manifestations of coronavirus disease 2019 and the impact the pandemic has had on the care of patients who suffer from neurological conditions. The state of knowledge surrounding the disease is in constant flux and, soon, some of the data presented in this book will be outdated, surpassed, nuanced, or perhaps even negated. With this in mind, we hope that the content of this work will bring some clarity and shed some light on the neurological ramifications of a new disease which, in so many ways, remains intriguingly nebulous.

Ahmad Riad Ramadan
Gamaleldin Osman

CHAPTER 1

Fears and Hopes

AHMAD RIAD RAMADAN[a] • GAMALELDIN OSMAN[b,c]
[a]Neurologist, Stroke and Neurocritical Care, Henry Ford Neuroscience Institute, Henry Ford Hospital, Detroit, MI, United States, [b]Mayo Clinic Comprehensive Epilepsy Center, Neurology Department, Rochester, MN, United States, [c]Epilepsy fellow at Mayo Clinic Hospital, Assistant Professor of Neurology, Mayo School of Medicine, Rochester, MN, United States

A NOVEL VIRUS SEES THE DAY

China awoke on December 31, 2019 to the first public message from the Wuhan Municipal Health Commission alerting its residents of a cluster of 27 cases of viral pneumonia of unknown etiology that had emerged in Wuhan, capital of the Hubei province and home to over 11 million people.[1] The news reached the US Centers for Disease Control and Prevention (CDC) later that day. Four days later, the genomic sequence of the new respiratory virus was established by the Chinese National Institute of Viral Disease Control and Prevention (NIVDC), which isolated the pathogen from patients in Wuhan and named it novel coronavirus, or 2019-nCoV. The sequence was posted on the NIH genetic sequence database, GenBank, on January 13, 2020.[2] On that day, the first case outside of China was confirmed in Thailand, and a week later the United States in turn reported its first case.[3, 4] On February 11, the International Committee on Taxonomy of Viruses (ICTV) rebaptized the virus SARS-CoV-2 due to the similarity of its genetic sequence with the virus responsible for the 2003 Severe Acute Respiratory Syndrome (SARS) outbreak. That same day, the World Health Organization (WHO) named the disease produced by SARS-CoV-2, COVID-19, an acronym which stands for Coronavirus Disease 2019.[5] By mid-February 2020, the global death toll had surpassed the one thousand mark, exceeding the fatalities caused by the SARS and Middle East Respiratory Syndrome (MERS) epidemics (774 and 866 lives, respectively; Fig. 1.1).[6] The WHO eventually declared the outbreak a global pandemic on March 11, 2020, 6 weeks after its designation of "public health emergency of international concern."[7]

ORIGINS AND ZOONOTIC TRANSMISSION OF SARS-COV-2

Coronaviruses belong to the *Coronaviridae* family of single-stranded RNA viruses. They owe their name to their characteristic appearance under electron microscopy: a viral envelope with petal-like spike projections, akin to the solar corona. Coronaviruses are divided into four main genera based on their genomic characteristics: *Alphacoronavirus, Betacoronavirus, Gammacoronavirus*, and *Deltacoronavirus*. The first two genera are known to infect mammals (including humans), while the last two predominantly infect birds along with pigs. There are currently seven known human coronaviruses that have been recognized since the 1960s. Three of them, MERS-CoV, SARS-CoV, and the novel SARS-CoV-2, are beta-coronaviruses and are credited with large outbreaks and the ability to produce severe respiratory and extrapulmonary symptoms. The other four, HCoV-NL63 and HCoV-229E of the *Alphacoronavirus* genus, and HCoV-OC43 and HCoVHKU1 of the *Betacoronavirus* genus, however, usually only cause a mild upper respiratory tract illness.

Phylogenetic genomic analyses of isolated SARS-CoV-2 virions confirm the zoonotic nature of viral transmission to humans. These analyses have revealed a high degree of similarity with the genomes of horseshoe bat coronaviruses, making bats of the *Rhinolophus* genus the most likely primary reservoir for the novel coronavirus. Specifically, SARS-CoV-2 shares 96.2% of its genomic identity with the BatCoV-RaTG13 strain,[8, 9] and 87%–88% with the bat-SL-CoVZC45 and bat-SL-CoVZXC21 strains.[10] There is less similarity with the genome of SARS-CoV (79%) and even less with that of MERS-CoV (50%).[10] Interestingly, while the whole genome of SARS-CoV-2 is closest to that of bat coronaviruses, the receptor-binding domain (RBD) of the spike protein responsible for the docking of the virion particle to the angiotensin-converting enzyme 2 (ACE2) receptor on human cells (Chapter 2) is closest to that of a SARS-like coronavirus isolated from dead Malayan pangolins smuggled into the Guangdong province of China.[9, 11] One of the posited putative mechanisms for the origin and zoonotic transfer to humans of SARS-CoV-2 is therefore the genetic recombination of bat and pangolin

Neurological Care and the COVID-19 Pandemic. https://doi.org/10.1016/B978-0-323-82691-4.00007-8

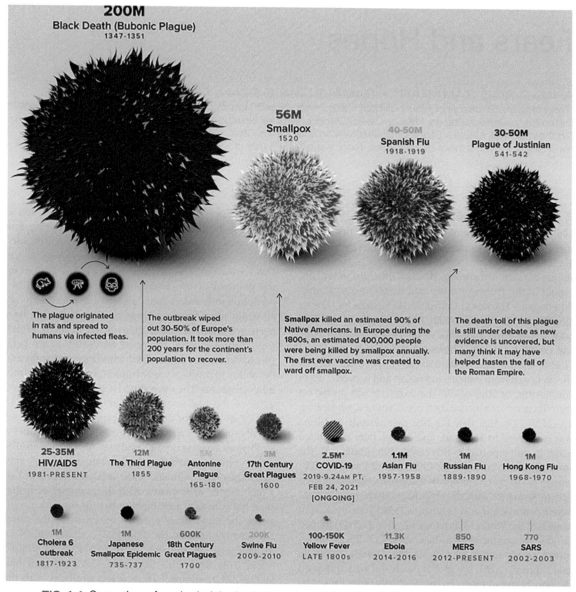

FIG. 1.1 Comparison of pandemics' death tolls throughout history. (Modified from LePan N. *Visualizing the History of Pandemics*. Visual Capitalist. https://www.visualcapitalist.com/history-of-pandemics-deadliest/; 2021 Accessed March 5, 2021.)

coronaviruses within an animal host that has yet to be fully identified, followed by a "jump" to humans which then acquired enough adaptations to enable a human-to-human transmission. Although beyond the scope of this manual, the theory of laboratory manipulations being at the origin of the emergence of SARS-CoV-2 is disputed and believed to be largely improbable.[12]

At the start of the outbreak in China, the Huanan Seafood Wholesale Market in Wuhan came under the lens of policy officials and scientists for being the location where the SARS-CoV-2 outbreak may have originated as a majority of the initial cases were traced back to exposure to the market. The "wet" part of the market where wildlife is commonly traded has been under particular scrutiny as mounting phylogenetic data identified pangolins and bats as likely reservoirs and intermediate hosts of the virus. To this day, the claim that the Wuhan market is at the origin of the outbreak remains significantly contested since many initial cases could not be traced back to the market and, reportedly, no animal samples tested positive for the virus.[13, 14]

As of late 2020, the rise of so-called "variants" has been a source of concern for scientists and public officials worldwide. These viral mutants are problematic because, compared to the "wild-type" SARS-CoV-2 virus, they are transmitted more efficiently, evade currently established diagnostic tests, are more resistant to available treatments, make developed vaccines less effective, and can produce more severe disease. Variants that fulfill the above criteria of enhanced transmissibility and virulence are referred to as "variants of concern," or VOC. Five such VOCs have been detected in the United States and are the object of close monitoring by the CDC and other federal agencies.[15] At the end of February 2021, the most rampant variant in the United States was the B.1.429 variant, initially detected in California and making up about 8% of all SARS-CoV-2 lineages in the country.[15, 16] Another variant, B.1.427, also discovered in California, represents 3.3% of all lineages found in the United States. Both variants have a 20% increased transmissibility and have a moderate impact on the efficacy of therapeutics and reduced neutralization by antibodies produced during the previous infection or vaccination.[15, 16] A close third is the "United Kingdom" or B.1.1.7 variant which accounts for 2.6% of lineages in the United States. Although it is more transmissible than other VOCs (~50%), it appears to have only a minimal impact on the efficacy of therapeutics and convalescent or postvaccination antibody neutralization. Finally, the "South African" B.1.351 and "Brazilian/Japanese" P.1 variants only account for 0.1%–0.2% of all lineages found in the United States at the time of writing.[15, 16]

A PANDEMIC OF UNPRECEDENTED MAGNITUDE

What started in January 2020 as an outbreak seemingly confined to a single region in China spread with astounding velocity to all continents, vehicled by the free movement of people, powered by the engines of globalization. While it took over 3 months to reach the first 100,000 cases, the global doubling time, i.e., the period of time it takes for the number of cases to double worldwide, came down to only 6 days at the end of March 2020. The first million cases were reached on April 2, 2020. The month of June saw a spectacular acceleration of the global caseload, with one million increments occurring every 7–8 days. For most societies, the summer of 2020 (July to September) came as a period of relative lull with regard to the spread of the virus allowing communities to reopen businesses and governments to loosen restrictions. This slowing of viral activity was, however, short-lived and, from October 2020 to January 2021, a sharp increase in cases and fatalities spiked across the world as people were drawn closer together indoors due to holiday celebrations and colder temperatures in the Northern Hemisphere. With much anticipation, the eyes of the world were turned to the progress made in the development of vaccines, approval for their emergency use, and mass vaccination campaigns. December 2020 marks the beginning of vaccination rollouts, starting in the United Kingdom and quickly spreading across the world. At the time of writing, as the world slowly gets immunized, the curves have started to show a decline in the rates of deaths and new cases, amid concerns of rising deadly variants. By the beginning of March 2021, over a year after it first emerged, SARS-CoV-2 had claimed 2.53 million lives, infected a known 114 million cases, and led the governments of more than half of the world population to enforce some form of confinement. The following section presents a timeline of the pandemic worldwide, highlighting important dates and events related to viral transmission, drug/vaccine development, and lockdowns.[17–19]

January 2020

- January 1: Chinese health authorities order the closure of the Huanan Seafood Wholesale Market in Wuhan to carry out investigations and disinfection.
- January 13: China reports the first death attributed to COVID-19.
- January 20: Human-to-human transmission is confirmed by the China National Health Commission. The United States confirms its first case of a man from Washington state who had recently returned from a trip to Wuhan.
- January 23: Wuhan, accompanied by other Chinese cities, shuts down all public transportation and goes into an official lockdown as countries around the globe start restricting flights from and to China.
- January 24: France reports its first cases of COVID-19, the first in the European Union (EU).
- January 26: The Chinese Center for Disease Control and Prevention (CCDC) starts to develop vaccines against SARS-CoV-2.

February 2020

- February 2: First death outside of China is reported in the Philippines.
- February 3: China begins a clinical trial of Gilead's remdesivir on patients with COVID-19. The drug was previously investigated during the Ebola outbreak.
- February 5: The Diamond Princess cruise ship docks in the port of Yokohama, Japan, with several passengers suspected of having contracted COVID-19. The ship remained in quarantine until March 1, its passengers gradually repatriated to their countries of origin. The ship outbreak eventually totaled 712 confirmed cases and 13 deaths.
- February 22-March: The period stretching from the third week of February into March was marked by a rapid spread of the infection across Western Europe which became a new epicenter of the outbreak. Northern Italy led the number of cases and fatalities, closely followed by France, Spain, and Germany, rapidly overwhelming the health-care system in these countries.
- February 26: Brazil confirms its first case of COVID-19, the first in South America. By this day, every continent with the exception of Antarctica has had confirmed COVID-19 cases.
- February 29: The United States reports its first death from the virus, but earlier fatalities may have occurred in retrospect.

March 2020

- March 11: The WHO declares the COVID-19 outbreak a pandemic.[20]
- March 15: The first stay-at-home order in the United States is issued by Puerto Rico, followed by most US states in the next 2 weeks.
- March 17: The EU, which now has "more reported cases and deaths than the rest of the world combined, apart from China," officially closes its borders to nonessential international travel. The travel restriction, initially set to last 30 days, was extended twice and has been undergoing gradual lifting with select countries since July 1, based on epidemiological, social, and economic considerations.
- March 18: The WHO launches the Solidarity trial which aims at comparing several treatments against COVID-19: remdesivir, chloroquine, hydroxychloroquine, lopinavir/ritonavir, and interferon-beta. Participating countries are Argentina, Bahrain, Canada, France, Iran, Norway, South Africa, Spain, Switzerland, and Thailand.
- March 26: The United States now has more COVID-19 cases than any other country in the globe. This trend continues through at least August 2020.

April 2020

- April 2: The number of COVID-19 cases around the world exceeds the million mark. More than 50,000 people have died from the virus worldwide.
- April 18: Use of hospital resources (ventilators, ICU, and all hospital beds) in the United States reaches its peak during the first wave of the pandemic.[21]
- April 28: The number of cases surpasses one million in the United States and the death toll in the country exceeds that incurred during the Vietnam war.

May 2020

- May 4: An old sample from a patient admitted to a French hospital in December with pneumonia was retested and confirmed the presence of the virus, retrodating the first known case of COVID-19 in Europe to December 27, 2019.[22]
- May 12: Russia now ranks second in caseload worldwide behind the United States.
- May 18: The biotechnology company, Moderna, releases preliminary phase 1 data on the safety and tolerability of its vaccine, mRNA-1273. This is the first human vaccine developed for COVID-19. Interim results of safety and immunogenicity will eventually be published in the *New England Journal of Medicine* on July 14.[23]
- May 22: Brazil outranks Russia in COVID-19 caseload and becomes the country with the second highest number of cases globally. Africa reaches the 100,000 mark in the number of cases.

June 2020

- June 15: The FDA revokes its Emergency Use Authorization (EUA) on the use of hydroxychloroquine as a treatment of COVID-19, following several studies reporting inefficacy.[24]
- June 16: Preliminary data from the UK's RECOVERY trial shows that the corticosteroid dexamethasone reduced the 28-day mortality rate by 35% among patients receiving invasive mechanical ventilation and by 20% in those requiring supplemental oxygen but not mechanically ventilated. The study is eventually published in the *New England Journal of Medicine* on July 17. The drug constitutes the first treatment shown to reduce mortality from COVID-19 in hospitalized patients.[25]
- June 28: Confirmed COVID-19 cases surpass 10 million and the death toll exceeds 500,000 globally.

July 2020

- July 1: The EU lifts its international travel restrictions with 15 countries but maintains its travel ban with the United States, Russia, and Brazil.
- July 20: The University of Oxford, United Kingdom, publishes in *The Lancet* the preliminary phase 1 trial results of its chimpanzee adenovirus-vectored vaccine, ChAdOx1 nCoV-19. The vaccine is found to be safe, well tolerated, and produces the desired immune response.[26]

August 2020

- August 24: The first case of reinfection is reported by the University of Hong Kong.

September 2020

- September 4: Early trial of Russia's Sputnik V vaccine is published in The Lancet.[27]

October 2020

- October 5: The RECOVERY Collaborative Group publishes the lack of benefit of lopinavir-ritonavir in patients hospitalized with COVID-19.[28]

November 2020

- November 9: Pfizer's mRNA vaccine, BNT162b2, showed more than 90% effectiveness in an interim analysis of the company's ongoing trial.[29]
- November 16: Moderna, in turn, announces that their mRNA vaccine is 94.5% effective in preventing COVID-19 in exposed patients.[30]
- November 23: Oxford-Astra Zeneca's ChAdOx1 nCoV-19 vaccine is found to be 62% effective.[31]

December 2020

- December 2: The United Kingdom is the first country to approve the Pfizer vaccine, followed 9 days later by the United States, which starts the vaccination rollout on December 14. The FDA grants EUA to Moderna's vaccine on December 18.

ECONOMIC IMPACTS AND RESPONSES

Not only has COVID-19 had dramatic effects on health and death, but it has also significantly affected economies and trade around the world. The pandemic is viewed as the worst global recession since the Great Depression in the 1930s, projected by the International Monetary Fund (IMF) to surpass the Great Recession of 2008–09.[32] COVID-19 emerged against the backdrop of an already stunted global economic growth in 2018–19, compounded by the trade war between the United States and China, and Brexit in Europe. The crisis began with supply chain interruptions and widespread shortages as plants in China and other parts of Asia started closing down. Early in the pandemic, panic buying of a variety of goods such as hand sanitizers, face masks, toilet papers and disinfectant wipes led to gouging of prices. As the epidemic became a pandemic and countries around the world went into lockdowns to curb the spread of the virus, the crisis shifted to a demand one.[33] Multiple sectors have been impacted, with the services sector being perhaps the hardest hit. The tourism, restaurant, aviation and automotive, arts and entertainment, energy (specifically oil), and retail industries have particularly suffered as a result of drastic declines in demand (Fig. 1.2).[33]

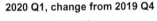

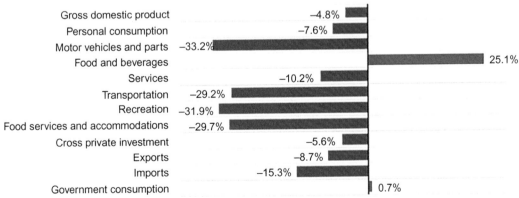

2020 Q1, change from 2019 Q4

Gross domestic product	−4.8%
Personal consumption	−7.6%
Motor vehicles and parts	−33.2%
Food and beverages	25.1%
Services	−10.2%
Transportation	−29.2%
Recreation	−31.9%
Food services and accommodations	−29.7%
Cross private investment	−5.6%
Exports	−8.7%
Imports	−15.3%
Government consumption	0.7%

FIG. 1.2 Change in US GDP by major industrial sector, Q4 2019 through Q1 2020. (Modified from Jackson J, Weiss M, Schwarzenberg A, Nelson R, Sutter K, Sutherland M. *Global Economic Effects of COVID-19*. Congressional Research Service. https://fas.org/sgp/crs/row/R46270.pdf; 2020 Accessed June 30, 2020.)

Consequently, unemployment has risen to soaring levels, pushing governments to respond in various ways, such as by providing economic recovery and stimulus packages (Fig. 1.3).[33, 34] For instance, in the United States, the national unemployment rate peaked at an unprecedented 14.5% in April 2020, up from 3.5% in February 2020. This is higher than the peak unemployment rate of 10.0% registered during the 2009 financial crisis in the country (Fig. 1.4).[35] By mid-July 2020, 52.7 Americans had filed for unemployment

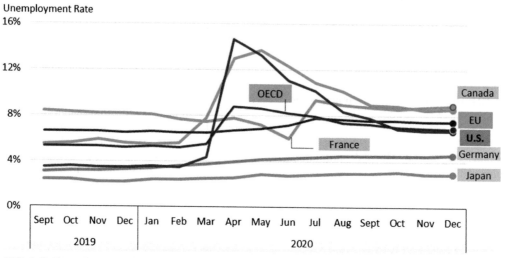

FIG. 1.3 Unemployment rate among major Organization for Economic Cooperation and Development (OECD) countries, Q4 2019 through Q4 2020. (Modified from Jackson J, Weiss M, Schwarzenberg A, Nelson R, Sutter K, Sutherland M. *Global Economic Effects of COVID-19*. Congressional Research Service. https://fas.org/sgp/crs/row/R46270.pdf; 2021 Accessed March 2, 2021.)

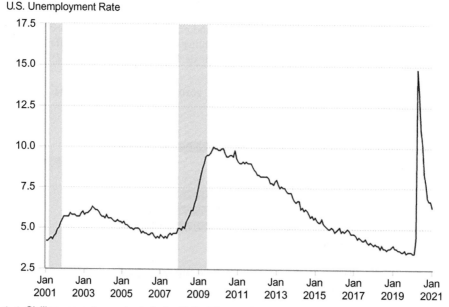

FIG. 1.4 Civilian unemployment rate in the United States, 2000–20. (Modified from *US Bureau of Labor Statistics*. https://www.bls.gov/charts/employment-situation/civilian-unemployment-rate.htm; 2020 Accessed March 2, 2021.)

insurance, a third of the US labor force, over a period of only 18 weeks.[36] Similarly, over 30 million people in France, Germany, Italy, Spain, and the United Kingdom have applied for wage assistance from their respective countries,[37] while an estimated 29 million people in Latin America risk slipping under the poverty line as a result of COVID-19.[38]

Governments around the world have responded to the economic downturn through various fiscal measures including tax cuts and deferrals to individuals and businesses, income supplementation, and expansion of unemployment insurance. The IMF estimates that a total of $11 trillion has been spent on economic recovery worldwide.[39] In the United States, for example, the Coronavirus Aid, Relief, and Economic Security Act, also known as the CARES Act, is a bipartisan economic stimulus bill signed into law by President Donald Trump on March 27, 2020 and constitutes the largest economic stimulus package in US history.[40] The final version of the bill amounted to $2.2 trillion, or 10% of the country's gross domestic product (GDP).[41] Members of the EU, on the other hand, had not had a coordinated effort until July 2020 when the European Commission met to approve a stimulus package totaling €1.82 trillion (about $2.14 trillion).[33, 42] On July 17, the United Nation released its third updated appeal of the Global Humanitarian Response Plan (GHRP) to the COVID-19 pandemic, stating that a $10.3 million envelope would need to be disbursed to 63 vulnerable countries to prevent a humanitarian disaster.[43]

TRANSMISSIBILITY AND SOCIAL POLICIES

What makes the SARS-CoV-2 pandemic different from prior pandemics and why have so many referred to it as unprecedented? Mankind has seen scores of epidemics and pandemics, some more deadly and more disseminated than others (Fig. 1.1).[6] *Yersinia pestis*, Black Death of the 14th century AD, for instance, claimed half of Europe's population and continued to sprout outbreaks for nearly four centuries. In more recent history, the Spanish flu pandemic of 1918–19 infected around 500 million people, a third of the world population, and killed 50 million people worldwide, numbers much higher than those spawned by SARS-CoV-2 at this stage. COVID-19, therefore, does not hold the record of pandemics for either highest infectivity or fatality rates. Its unprecedented nature comes from the economic fallout and drastic responses seen across the globe to try to contain its spread locally and internationally.

Despite similar zoonosis, transmission route, pathogenesis, and significant genomic overlap, COVID-19 differs substantially from SARS. The 2003 SARS outbreak did not reach pandemic status and disappeared after infecting 8096 and killing 774 people in 29 countries. SARS was effectively eradicated in 8 months, whereas COVID-19 cases remain on the rise in many countries a year following its emergence. How can two viruses with such similar genetic profiles result in two very disparate outcomes? To answer this question and understand the resulting health and economic ramifications of SARS-CoV-2, we must familiarize ourselves with the transmissibility characteristics of the virus which makes this pathogen particularly infectious.

- Transmissibility is more commonly measured using the basic reproductive rate R_0, which is the average number of individuals that one infected person transmits the virus to. An R_0 value greater than 1 means that the epidemic is growing, whereas a value of less than 1 means it is receding. Naturally, the R_0 depends on the specific viral characteristics but is also influenced to a large extent by the success of policies instituted to promote and maintain social distancing. The R_0 for SARS-CoV-2 is currently estimated to be 2.5 (range 1.8–3.6, depending on the region studied).[6, 44] This is similar to the early phase of SARS (2.0–3.0), which eventually dropped to 1.1 with the implementation of effective control measures.[45] It is higher than that of the 1918 H1N1 influenza (2.0, range 1.2–3.0),[46] the 2009 H1N1 influenza (1.3–1.7),[47] and MERS-CoV (0.69).[48] At the other end of the spectrum, measles, smallpox, rubella, and mumps all have a much higher R_0 than SARS-CoV-2 (Fig. 1.5).[6, 49] SARS-CoV-2 has an incubation period (i.e., time from exposure to symptom onset) similar to that of SARS-CoV and MERS-CoV (mean of 5.1–5.8 days, range 4–12 days),[50] but longer than that of the influenza A viruses (mean of 2 days).[51] Importantly, infectivity starts at 2.3 days before symptom onset and peaks at 0.7 days before symptom onset.[52] This is different from the influenza A pandemics and even SARS where the time from symptom onset to peak infectivity was 2 and 5–7 days, respectively. Both the long incubation period and presymptomatic peak infectivity make contact tracing and effective confinement measures challenging because they both facilitate undetected transmission of the virus (Table 1.1).[44]

- Viral shedding in SARS-CoV-2 infections declines rapidly within the first week after symptom onset. Compared to SARS-CoV, this is one week less in our ability to diagnose acute illness and confine subjects before transmission occurs. Additionally, peak viral shedding in SARS occurred as patients became

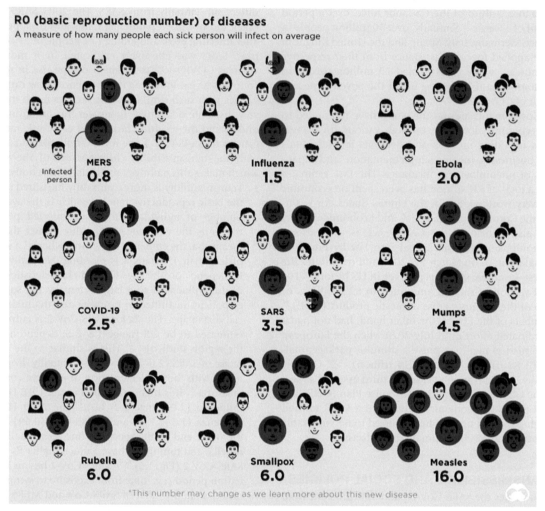

FIG. 1.5 Reproductive numbers (R_0) of several viral diseases. (Modified from LePan N. *Visualizing the History of Pandemics*. Visual Capitalist. https://www.visualcapitalist.com/history-of-pandemics-deadliest/; 2021 Accessed March 5, 2021.)

seriously ill, usually while hospitalized, which helped in their effective isolation, thereby limiting transmission.

- Another important facilitator of transmission is the noted high proportion of asymptomatic or mildly symptomatic cases in COVID-19, which again makes selective confinement and quarantine measures less effective. An important distinction with SARS is the fact that community, and not nosocomial, transmission is the major form of viral spread in COVID-19. Infected individuals are often not aware of their carrier status and therefore, without proper containment measures, can far more easily transmit the virus. To complicate matters, determining the proportion of asymptomatic carriers has been particularly challenging due to ample variability in the definition, reporting, and follow-up of asymptomatic cases in the existing literature. The best estimate seems to hover around 40% of infected cases.[53] However, many of these cases later turn out to have been presymptomatic.

In addition to viral transmissibility, the enforcement of public health measures aimed at confinement and contact tracing of sick and exposed individuals plays a major role in determining the magnitude of spread of airborne-transmitted viruses. This explains why some

TABLE 1.1
Characteristics of SARS-CoV-2, SARS-CoV, and the 1918 and 2009 Pandemic Influenzae.

	SARS-CoV-2	SARS-CoV	Pandemic Influenza 1918	Pandemic Influenza 2009	Interpretation
Transmissibility, R_0	2.5	2.4	2.0	1.7	SARS-CoV-2 has the highest average R_0
Incubation period, days	4–12	2–7	Unknown	2	Longer incubation period; SARS-CoV epidemics form slower
Interval between symptom onset and maximum infectivity, days	0	5–7	2	2	SARS-CoV-2 is harder to contain than SARS-CoV
Proportion with mild illness	High	Low	High	High	Facilitates undetected transmission
Proportion of patients requiring hospitalization	Few (20%)	Most (> 70%)	Few	Few	Concern about capacity in the health sector
Proportion of patients requiring intensive care	1/16,000	Most (40%)	Unknown	1/104,000	Concern about capacity in the health sector
Proportion of deaths in people younger than 65 years out of all deaths	0.6%–2.8%	Unknown	95%	80%	SARS-CoV-2 might cause as many deaths as the 1918 influenza pandemic, but fewer years of life lost and disability-adjusted life-years, as deaths are in the older population with underlying health conditions
Risk factors for severe illness	Age, comorbidity	Age, comorbidity	Age (< 60 years)	Age (< 60 years)	

Modified from Petersen E, Koopmans M, Go U, et al. Comparing SARS-CoV-2 with SARS-CoV and influenza pandemics. *Lancet Infect Dis*. 2020;20(9):e238–e244. doi:10.1016/S1473-3099(20)30484-9.

regions have more successfully curbed the outbreak than others during the COVID-19 pandemic. Several types of containment measures have been put in effect in modern-day epidemics: isolation of ill patients, quarantines of exposed individuals, and community-wide containment measures (social distancing in public spaces, school closures, lockdown of cities/regions, curfews, at-home orders). Historically, in 2003, SARS elicited a rapid and astonishingly effective response from the hardest hit areas, the so-called "hotspots," which at the time were China, Hong Kong, Taiwan, Toronto, and Singapore (in descending order of number of confirmed cases).[54] For instance, China built a one thousand-bed hospital in one week in Beijing and put the capital on lockdown,[55] while Singapore mandated temperature monitoring in all public spaces and hospitals.[56]

In 2020, several societal factors have worked in unison to enable a more rapid transmission of the virus. In the early days of the pandemic, Wuhan, one of the largest metropolizes in China with an increasing connectivity with the world, was home to several superspreading events such as the Spring Festival and a banquet that gathered 40,000 guests before the lockdown, all contributing to the rapid propagation of the virus to other Chinese provinces and countries.[57] It is unclear, however, whether the large-scale protests which took place in the United States in the context of the Black Lives Matter movement had any significant effect on rebounding the number of COVID-19 cases and deaths.

A study published in *Health Affairs* and conducted by the University of Kentucky, University of Louisville, and Georgia State University studied the impact of four public health policies related to social distancing on lowering the COVID-19 case growth rate in the United States.[58] The policies examined were bans on large gatherings, closing restaurants, bars, gyms, entertainment venues, school closures, and stay-at-home orders. The study found that implementing all four policies reduced the daily growth rate by 9.1 percentage points after being in effect for 16–20 days. They concluded that not instituting any of the four policies would lead to a 35-fold faster spread of the virus in the community. A *Cochrane* systematic review of 10 COVID-19 modeling studies from China, the United Kingdom, South Korea, and the cruise ship Diamond Princess arrived at a similar conclusion that the addition to quarantine of control measures, such as travel restrictions, school closures, and social distancing, was more effective than quarantine alone in reducing the number of incident cases and deaths.[59]

TESTING CHALLENGES

Policies on COVID-19 testing have varied widely across countries and regions, and have gone through multiple iterations. These variations in space and time are directly related to availability of testing kits, reagents, laboratory personnel and equipment, and to the understanding of patterns of viral spread in the community informed by epidemiological studies and contact tracing. For instance, the latest US CDC guidelines on testing for SARS-CoV-2 describe five categories of individuals in whom testing is appropriate.[60] These include

- Individuals with symptoms consistent with COVID-19.
- Asymptomatic individuals who were in close contact with persons with known or suspected COVID-19.
- Asymptomatic but vulnerable individuals without known or suspected exposure (i.e., members of ethnic and racial minorities such as African American, Latinos and Hispanics, or Native Americans, and individuals with predisposing medical or social conditions).
- Individuals known to have been infected and being tested to determine resolution of infection.
- Testing for public health purposes and to guide policymaking.

Testing in viral pandemics is paramount in ensuring that infected individuals can be effectively quarantined or isolated, thereby limiting spread to the community, and it also informs policies aimed at removing previously infected individuals from confinement, allowing them to rejoin a workforce that is under unduly strain.

Therefore the availability and accuracy of testing holds a central role in epidemics that cannot be overemphasized. Unfortunately, no test is ever 100% specific and sensitive. In a pandemic, the concept of a test's false positive and negative rates becomes even more relevant as their effect on societies is multiplied. A low sensitivity will lead to fewer infected individuals being appropriately confined, contributing therefore to the propagation of the virus in the community. On the other hand, a low specificity will potentially lead to unnecessary treatment and isolation of healthy individuals, temporarily excluding them from a soaring workforce. Most testing errors are preanalytical, i.e., they occur before the patient sample is analyzed, and account for 46%–68% of all errors that occur during the entire testing process. Most notorious are errors in sample collection, handling, transportation, storage, preparation, exposure to degrading agents, cross contamination, and mismatch.[61–63]

Testing for SARS-CoV-2 comes in three forms: molecular, antigen, and serological (antibody). The molecular and antigen tests are meant to detect viral genome or antigens and therefore, if positive, are diagnostic of an acute infection. Antibody tests, however, detect past exposure to the virus. They are therefore not meant to diagnose an acute illness but can assist in making the diagnosis. Antibody testing becomes important in epidemiological studies and in the determination of disease prevalence in the community. By January 2021, the US Food and Drug Administration (FDA) has not yet approved any COVID-19 test but has granted Emergency Use Authorization (EUA) for over 200 diagnostic tests (molecular and antigen) and 50 serological tests.[64] Many of these tests are laboratory based, and some are point of care (POC) available in clinical settings. Additionally, as of August 2020, the FDA had also authorized the commercialization of eight at-home tests which allows individuals to collect their own nasal swab and saliva specimens and mail them the same day to designated laboratories.[65]

Serological tests are usually done on blood but can also be tested on CSF and other body fluids. Molecular tests are typically carried out on nasopharyngeal (NP), oropharyngeal (OP) and nasal swabs, sputum, tracheal aspirate, bronchoalveolar lavage (BAL), stool, or CSF. Sputum induction is not recommended due to the high risk of aerosolization and exposure to health-care personnel. An individual test's sensitivity and specificity not only depend heavily on the sampling site, but also on whether the test is laboratory or POC based. The determination of sensitivity and specificity for each individual test type is an evolving topic, but we attempt to provide the reader with the most updated data on this matter:

1. **Molecular Tests: Real-Time Reverse Transcription-Polymerase Chain Reaction**

Real-time reverse transcription-polymerase chain reaction (rRT-PCR) remains the gold standard for diagnosing acute infection. Unfortunately, it cannot differentiate between an actively replicating virus and viral remnants. The test's specificity is thought to be very high due to the uniqueness of the SARS-CoV-2 genome primer utilized. Sensitivity, however, varies based on the source of the specimen. In one Chinese study of 205 patients in Wuhan, sensitivity was lowest in the blood (1%), feces (29%), and pharyngeal swab (32%), intermediate in the nasal swab (63%) and sputum (72%), and highest in BAL (93%).[66] Recently, the FDA granted a EUA for a diagnostic method developed by the Yale School of Public Health which detects SARS-CoV-2 in saliva.[67] The test was shown to have similar accuracy when compared to NP swabs (94% positive agreement) and offers the advantages of lower invasiveness,

reduced exposure risk to health-care personnel and costs.[68] rRT-PCR methodology can usually detect the virus in respiratory tract samples from as early as 1 week before symptom onset to 1 week later when tested on an NP specimen. PCR positivity may persist beyond 6 weeks in the stool, sputum, and BAL. While it is unlikely that patients remain infectious for this long, the tests may detect nonviable viral RNA (Fig. 1.6).[69] Laboratory-based rRT-PCR tests only take 4–6 h to complete but the turnaround time from sample collection to results delivery varies greatly and depends on factors such as location, demand, availability of reagents, and batching of samples, and can range from less than 24 h to 5–7 days, even longer occasionally. Commercial POC tests, however, give much faster results (5–30 min). The accuracy of POC tests is believed to be similar to that of laboratory-based tests.

2. **Antigen immune assays**

These are antibody-based tests that detect viral antigens such as SARS-CoV-2's nucleocapsid (N) protein or spike protein, hence imparting a high specificity

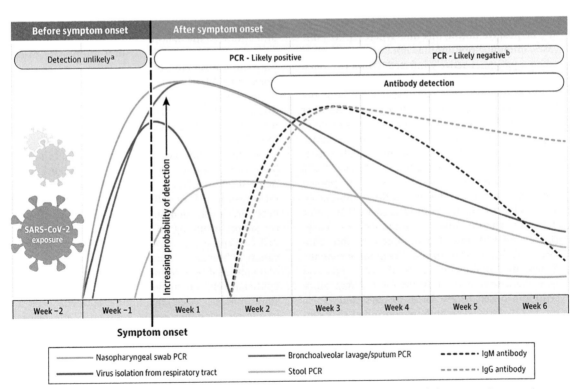

FIG. 1.6 Timeline of diagnostic tests for the detection of SARS-CoV-2 infection relative to symptom onset. (Modified from Sethuraman N, Jeremiah SS, Ryo A. Interpreting diagnostic tests for SARS-CoV-2. *JAMA*. 2020;323(22):2249–2251. doi:10.1001/jama.2020.8259.)

to these tests. Antigen tests can only be processed in high and moderate complexity laboratories. In general, they are less costly, yield faster results (20–60 min) but take longer to develop and are also less sensitive than rRT-PCR.[70]

3. **Antibody tests**

Serological tests detect IgM and IgG antibodies directed at antigenic elements of the virion. They are products of the humoral, B-cell mediated, immune response of the host against the virus. These antibodies last much longer than viral RNA, well beyond a patient's period of maximal infectivity, and therefore can be very useful to determine disease prevalence, even when the patient remains an asymptomatic carrier. IgM immunoglobulins appear as early as 4–7 days from symptom onset, peak at 2–3 weeks, and usually disappear by week 4. IgG takes about 2 weeks to appear and will persist for several weeks to months (Fig. 1.6).[69, 71, 72] While IgM positivity indicates a recent or current infection, IgG positivity indicates recent or previous infection (or vaccinated status). The combination of negative IgM and IgG antibodies does not imply that the patient is not infected as they could still be in the early phase before seroconversion (PCR would usually be positive during this time window). In some cases, immunoglobulins may not even be produced when a patient is actively infected with a pathogen of low virulence because the innate cell-mediated immune response may have cleared the virus before a humoral response could be triggered. Another scenario of lack of antibody production is likely to happen in an immunocompromised or immunosuppressed host. Specificity of the available IgM/IgG tests is high and ranged from 96.6% to 99.7% in one metaanalysis of 40 studies.[73] The pooled sensitivity was lower for lateral-flow immunoassays (LFIA; 66%), the method used in POC tests, than for enzyme-linked immunosorbent assays (ELISA; 84.3%) and chemiluminescent immunoassays (CLIA, 97.8%). In one Cochrane systematic review, the combination of SARS-CoV-2 IgG and IgM had a sensitivity of 30.1% for 1–7 days since symptom onset, 72.2% for 8–14 days, and 91.4% for 15–21 days.[74] The authors concluded that sensitivity was too low for patients presenting within the first week for serological testing to be useful for the diagnosis of COVID-19. Importantly, it is as of yet unclear whether SARS-CoV-2 IgG seropositivity confers any type of immunity to the host preventing reinfection, and how long such immunity would last.[70, 75] Some governments, such as Germany, the United Kingdom, the United States, and Chile, have advocated the use of the so-called "immunity passports" to grant individuals who test positive for SARS-CoV-2 antibodies the carte blanche to return to work or school, travel, and be exempt from social distancing and other types of physical restrictions. However, many experts are voicing their concerns over such initiatives for many reasons.[76, 77] One of them is the fact that the accuracy of antibody tests is suboptimal and that seropositivity does not necessarily equate to immunity. Furthermore, being immune or seropositive does not guarantee that asymptomatic individuals are not able to transmit the virus to others. In addition to the medical concerns, the legal and ethical ramifications of creating such passports are consequential, especially as it is likely to create biased access to employment, health care, and insurance eligibility. They could in fact deepen social discriminations and inequities, rendering underprivileged populations even more vulnerable.

SARS COV-2, A RESPIRATORY PATHOGEN WITH SYSTEMIC COMPLICATIONS

Although COVID-19 infection presents as a mild febrile illness in the majority of patients, around 20% of patients develop severe or critical pulmonary disease warranting hospitalization.[78, 79] Pulmonary complications of COVID-19 infection including acute hypoxic respiratory failure with or without acute respiratory distress syndrome (ARDS) account for the majority of morbidities and fatalities associated with COVID-19 infection.[79–82]

In vitro studies have demonstrated that binding of SARS-CoV-2 surface glycoprotein (S protein) to the ACE2 receptor plays a unique role in facilitating viral invasion of host cells.[83–87] This phenomenon has been previously demonstrated with other coronavirus strains including HCoV-NL63 and SARS-CoV.[88–90] ACE2 receptors are known to be widely expressed in a variety of human cells including type 1 and type 2 alveolar epithelial cells, bronchial epithelial cells, olfactory epithelial cells, enterocytes, endothelial cells, vascular smooth muscle cells, renal tubular epithelial cells, and to a lesser extent glomerular cells, glial cells, neurons, fibroblasts, and macrophages.[91–95] In addition, transmembrane cellular protease/serine subfamily member 2 (TMPRSS2) catalyzes viral S protein priming, promoting viral entry into host cells, thus playing a pivotal role in viral spread to various host cells.[92, 96–98] Tissue and cellular tropisms of SARS-CoV-2 as well as these closely related strains can be explained by the selective expression of ACE2 receptors and TMPRSS2 enzyme among various body cells, distinguishing these strains from other less aggressive common coronavirus strains. Thus the emergence of a variety of extrapulmonary manifestations of COVID-19 infection does not seem surprising. These include gastrointestinal,[99-102] hepatic,[103-106] renal,[107-109] cardiac,[110-113] endocrine,[114, 115] cutaneous,[116-118] hematological,[119, 120] and thromboembolic manifestations,[121-125] which can manifest as the initial presentation of COVID-19 infection in the absence of pulmonary or systemic manifestations of illness. A variety of pathomechanisms have been postulated to play a role in the development of these symptoms. These include direct viral mediated toxic damage,[126-129] dysregulated immune response to infection,[130-134] endothelial cell dysfunction leading to activation of prothrombotic pathways,[135-137] and renin angiotensin aldosterone system (RAAS) dysregulation.[138, 139]

NEUROLOGICAL MANIFESTATIONS OF COVID-19 INFECTION

Multiple neurological manifestations have been reported in association with a group of coronavirus strains prior to the COVID-19 epidemic. These strains include SARS-CoV,[140-142] MERS-CoV,[142-144] HCoV-OC43,[145-148] and HCoV-229E.[148] Detailed descriptions of the various neurological manifestations of the disease will be the object of Chapters 3–11, but we offer here a preamble to the matter.

The reported neurological complications in association with the aforementioned coronaviruses include headache, olfactory dysfunction, ischemic and hemorrhagic strokes, seizures, encephalitis, acute disseminated encephalomyelitis (ADEM), acute inflammatory demyelinating neuropathy (AIDP), acute motor axonal neuropathy (AMAN), and myopathy.[142, 149] These manifestations have all been reported again with COVID-19 infection.[150] The rates of occurrence of neurological manifestations differ widely across the published case series, likely reflecting the variable severity of infection among patients, with reported rates ranging from 4.5% to 67%.[151-156] In addition, there have been numerous reports of a plethora of novel central and peripheral neurological manifestations of COVID-19 infection. The reported central nervous system (CNS) complications include nonspecific encephalopathy,[150-155, 157, 158] acute hemorrhagic necrotizing encephalopathy,[159-161] leukoencephalopathy with or without cerebral microbleeds,[162-165] posterior reversible encephalopathy syndrome (PRES),[166-169] cerebral vasculitis,[170-172]

reversible cerebral vasoconstriction syndrome (RCVS),[173] and mild encephalopathy with reversible splenial lesion (MERS),[174] Wernicke-like syndrome with hypothalamic dysfunction and ophthalmoparesis,[175] and transverse myelitis of varying severity,[176-178] including acute necrotizing myelitis.[179] On the other hand, peripheral nervous system (PNS) complications include the Miller Fisher variant of Guillain-Barré syndrome,[180-183] isolated[184-186] and multiple cranial neuropathies, gustatory dysfunction,[187, 188] polymyositis,[189, 190] rhabdomyolysis,[189, 191, 192] and new onset ocular or generalized myasthenia gravis.[193, 194] Furthermore, there have been few case reports describing the occurrence of a variety of movement disorders in association with COVID-19 infection. These include generalized myoclonus,[195, 196] opsoclonus-myoclonus ataxia syndrome,[197] acute parkinsonian syndrome,[198-200] and tremors associated with gait ataxia.[201] Ellul et al. proposed definitions for the most common neurological syndromes associated with COVID-19 infection in an effort to define the level of certainty of their associations versus their mere coincidence.[202]

It is worth noting that the occurrence of neurological complications is not limited to patients with severe disease and can be seen in patients with mild infection or can even manifest as the initial presentation in otherwise asymptomatic infection.[157, 203, 204] The occurrence of neurological complications in the setting of COVID-19 infection is not limited to the adult population and has also been noted in children, occasionally in association with the multisystem inflammatory syndrome in children (MIS-C).[205-209] More information regarding COVID-19 and neuropediatric disorders will follow in Chapter 8.

The emergence of neurological complications carries significant prognostic implications as the occurrence of few complications including mental status alteration and radiologically proven strokes has been associated with increased in-hospital mortality risk.[210] Preliminary evidence suggests the potential of severe COVID-19 infections to cause long-term cognitive deficits similar to those seen among patients recovering from other critical systemic infections. A preprint study reports the occurrence of executive/attention deficits and sleep disorders in around 30% of COVID-19 survivors at 6-month follow-up.[211] More data is likely to emerge as COVID-19 survivors continue to be followed clinically.

Multiple pathomechanisms are postulated to play a role in the development of neurological complications in patients with COVID-19 infections. As mentioned earlier, ACE2 receptors and TMPRSS2 proteases play a vital role in facilitating viral host cell invasion. ACE2 receptors and TMPRSS2 proteases are highly expressed in olfactory epithelial cells which are commonly infected early in the course of COVID-19 infections, implicating the olfactory pathway as the most likely direct route for invasion of CNS structures in SARS-CoV-2 infections.[212, 213] Recent reports of olfactory bulb atrophy on brain imaging in association with COVID-19 infection further substantiate this hypothesis.[214, 215] Endothelial cells also commonly express ACE2 receptors[91] and TMPRSS2[92, 216] genes, and thus endothelial cell dysfunction has been proposed as a key mechanism in the development of cerebrovascular complications.[135, 136] The detection of viral particles in brain autopsy specimens obtained from deceased COVID-19 patients further corroborates the neuroinvasive potential of the SARS-CoV-2 virus.[217] In addition to promoting viral CNS invasion, blood-brain barrier compromise leads to enhanced CNS permeability to a variety of antigens inciting a local CNS inflammatory response which can potentiate a systemic hyperinflammatory response.[218] Finally, acute cerebral hypoxia likely plays a vital role in the development of acute neuronal injury, as substantiated by the radiological evidence of hypoperfusion in a few patients with COVID-19 infections,[153, 163, 219] and neuropathological evidence of diffuse hypoxic brain injury demonstrated in recent brain autopsy series.[220] These pathomechanisms will be discussed in detail in Chapter 2.

In addition to the recognition of neurological complications, there are additional important considerations for practitioners managing patients with chronic neurological disorders in the COVID pandemic era. Many patients with immune-mediated central and peripheral neurological diseases receive chronic immunosuppressive or immunomodulatory therapies, which may potentially make them more susceptible to COVID-19 infection and its associated complications.[221–223] In addition, many neurological disorders cause swallowing and respiratory difficulties, which can further exacerbate COVID-19-related respiratory complications.[224] Guideline statements are currently available from various neurological subspecialty societies on the care of neurological patients in the COVID-19 epidemic era.[225, 226] These will be discussed in more detail in Chapters 6 and 7.

COVID-19 VACCINES: A NEUROLOGICAL PERSPECTIVE

There has been remarkable unprecedented progress in the development of safe and efficacious vaccines for COVID-19. So far, two of those vaccines have been approved in the United States for emergency use: Pfizer's BNT162b2 and Moderna's mRNA1273. Both vaccines are messenger RNA (mRNA) based and have achieved efficacy rates of around 95% in preventing all COVID-19 infections and 100% in preventing severe infections.[29, 30, 227] Chinese authorities, on the other hand, have recently approved Sinopharm's inactivated vaccine,[228] while British authorities have authorized Oxford-AstraZeneca's adenovirus-vectored vaccine AZD1222 for emergency use.[31, 229] A similarly structured vaccine (Sputnik V) has also been developed and approved in Russia.[27, 230] At least five other vaccines are currently in the advanced stages of development.[231] So far, there has been one report of transverse myelitis possibly linked to AZD1222 vaccine administration and two cases in which neurological complications happened after AZD1222 vaccination but not believed to be related to the vaccine administration, namely one patient with preexisting but unrecognized multiple sclerosis and one patient in whom transverse myelitis developed 68 days post vaccination.[232] Another neurological complication of particular concern—vaccine-induced thrombotic thrombocytopenia—emerged during the rollout of adenovirus-vectored vaccines as several cases of deep vein thromboses, pulmonary embolism and cerebral venous sinus thromboses, were reported in vaccinated young females. Chapter 12 details the development, efficacy, and side effects of the available SARS-CoV-2 vaccines.

HURDLES AND OPPORTUNITIES IN THE CARE OF NEUROLOGICAL PATIENTS

The COVID-19 pandemic impacted the practice of neurology in more than one way. In response to the rapid surge in the number of COVID-19 patients, many neurological and neurosurgical wards and ICUs across the world had to be reassigned to the care of COVID-19 patients. Neurology practitioners and trainees were often deployed to provide care for COVID-19 patients, outside of their usual practice. This reshuffling of clinical responsibilities created challenges for the care of patients with neurological ailments in both hospital and outpatient settings. For instance, in an attempt to social distance and reduce viral transmission, the majority of elective neurological procedures, outpatient therapies, and in-person clinic visits had to be canceled or postponed, limiting the care of patients with chronic neurological diseases. Additionally, the burden imposed on emergency medical services during the COVID-19 surge and patients' own fear of contracting the infection in overwhelmed hospitals and emergency rooms most likely contributed to the delayed presentation of patients with acute neurological symptoms. Ischemic strokes, for instance, were among the most affected diagnoses with health-care systems across the world reporting significant drops in the number of patients seeking medical attention in a timely fashion, thereby limiting their eligibility for acute interventions such as intravenous thrombolysis or endovascular therapies during the pandemic.[233, 234] Novel protocols were established to ensure effective triaging of patients with acute neurological syndromes and provide adequate screening of patients deemed high infectious risk in order to limit transmission within health-care facilities, as was showcased in a paper published by the authors.[235] Details of these protocols are reviewed in the upcoming chapters.

Despite the unprecedented challenges imposed by the COVID-19 pandemic, many opportunities aimed at improving care for patients with neurological diseases emerged in the last year. Telemedicine, for instance, saw a formidable uptake in utilization and proved to be an effective way to provide care while reducing contact and thereby viral transmission. Although not ideal or appropriate in every situation, this oftentimes underused technology helped minimize interruptions in care imposed by social distancing or other confinement measures. The benefits obtained from widespread utilization of telemedicine go well beyond COVID-19 as it provides a valuable alternative for patients with chronic neurologic diseases, limiting unnecessary travel and cost, especially for those with a more clinically stable disease course.[236] The COVID-19 pandemic has also highlighted profound disparities in health-care outcomes across different racial and socioeconomic groups, emphasizing the need to enhance health-care access for the most vulnerable populations.[237-239]

REFERENCES

1. *Timeline of China Releasing Information on COVID-19 and Advancing International Cooperation. National Health Commission of the People's Republic of China;* 2021. http://en.nhc.gov.cn/2020-04/06/c_78861_2.htm. Accessed 1 March 2021.
2. *Severe Acute Respiratory Syndrome Coronavirus 2 Isolate Wuhan-Hu-1, Co—Nucleotide. NCBI;* 2020. https://www.ncbi.nlm.nih.gov/nuccore/1798174254. Accessed 1 March 2021.
3. Joseph A. Woman in Thailand is first case with novel pneumonia virus outside China. *STAT.* 2020. https://www.statnews.com/2020/01/13/woman-with-novel-pneumonia-virus-hospitalized-in-thailand-the-first-case-outside-china/. Accessed 1 March 2021.
4. Holshue ML, DeBolt C, Lindquist S, et al. First case of 2019 novel coronavirus in the United States. *N Engl J Med.* 2020;382(10):929–936. https://doi.org/10.1056/NEJMoa2001191.
5. *Naming the Coronavirus Disease (COVID-19) and the Virus That Causes It.* Who.int.; 2020. https://www.who.int/emergencies/diseases/novel-coronavirus-2019/technical-guidance/naming-the-coronavirus-disease-(covid-2019)-and-the-virus-that-causes-it. Accessed 1 March 2021.
6. LePan N. *Visualizing the History of Pandemics. Visual Capitalist;* 2021. https://www.visualcapitalist.com/history-of-pandemics-deadliest/. Accessed 5 March 2021.
7. Cucinotta D, Vanelli M. WHO declares COVID-19 a pandemic. *Acta Biomed.* 2020;91(1):157–160. 2020 March 19 10.23750/abm.v91i1.9397.
8. Zhou P, Yang XL, Wang XG, et al. A pneumonia outbreak associated with a new coronavirus of probable bat origin. *Nature.* 2020;579(7798):270–273. https://doi.org/10.1038/s41586-020-2012-7.
9. Lau SKP, Luk HKH, Wong ACP, et al. Possible bat origin of severe acute respiratory syndrome coronavirus 2. *Emerg Infect Dis.* 2020;26(7):1542–1547. https://doi.org/10.3201/eid2607.200092.
10. Lu R, Zhao X, Li J, et al. Genomic characterisation and epidemiology of 2019 novel coronavirus: implications for virus origins and receptor binding. *Lancet.* 2020;395(10224):565–574. https://doi.org/10.1016/S0140-6736(20)30251-8.
11. Lam TT, Jia N, Zhang YW, et al. Identifying SARS-CoV-2-related coronaviruses in Malayan pangolins. *Nature.* 2020;583(7815):282–285. https://doi.org/10.1038/s41586-020-2169-0.
12. Andersen KG, Rambaut A, Lipkin WI, Holmes EC, Garry RF. The proximal origin of SARS-CoV-2. *Nat Med.* 2020;26(4):450–452. https://doi.org/10.1038/s41591-020-0820-9.
13. Li Q, Guan X, Wu P, et al. Early transmission dynamics in Wuhan, China, of novel coronavirus-infected pneumonia. *N Engl J Med.* 2020;382(13):1199–1207. https://doi.org/10.1056/NEJMoa2001316.
14. Zhang X, Tan Y, Ling Y, et al. Viral and host factors related to the clinical outcome of COVID-19. *Nature.* 2020;583(7816):437–440. https://doi.org/10.1038/s41586-020-2355-0.
15. *Cases, Data, and Surveillance: SARS-CoV-2 Variants. Centers for Disease Control and Prevention;* 2021. https://www.cdc.gov/coronavirus/2019-ncov/cases-updates/variant-surveillance/variant-info.html#Consequence. Accessed 18 March 2021.
16. *Cases, Data, and Surveillance: Variant Proportions in the U.S. Centers for Disease Control and Prevention;* 2021. https://www.cdc.gov/coronavirus/2019-ncov/cases-updates/variant-proportions.html. Accessed 18 March 2021.
17. Ravelo J, Jerving S. COVID-19—a timeline of the coronavirus outbreak. *Devex.* 2021. https://www.devex.com/news/covid-19-a-timeline-of-the-coronavirus-outbreak-9639. Accessed 1 March 2021.

18. *COVID-19 Map—Johns Hopkins Coronavirus Resource Center. Johns Hopkins Coronavirus Resource Center;* 2021. https://coronavirus.jhu.edu/map.html. Accessed 1 March 2021.

19. A timeline of the coronavirus pandemic. *NY Times.* 2020. https://www.nytimes.com/article/coronavirus-timeline.html. Accessed 1 March 2021.

20. *WHO Director-General's Opening Remarks at the Media Briefing on COVID-19—11 March 2020.* WHO; 2020. https://www.who.int/dg/speeches/detail/who-director-general-s-opening-remarks-at-the-media-briefing-on-covid-19- - -11-march-2020. Accessed 1 March 2021.

21. IHME. *COVID-19 Projections. Institute for Health Metrics and Evaluation;* 2021. http://covid19.healthdata.org/united-states-of-america?view=resource-use&tab=trend&resource=all_resources. Accessed 1 March 2021.

22. Irish J. After retesting samples, French hospital discovers COVID-19 case from December. *Reuters.* 2020. 4 May https://www.reuters.com/article/us-health-coronavirus-france/after-retesting-samples-french-hospital-discovers-covid-19-case-from-december-idUSKBN22G20L.

23. mRNA-1273 Study Group. An mRNA vaccine against SARS-CoV-2—preliminary report. *N Engl J Med.* 2020. https://doi.org/10.1056/NEJMoa2022483. Jul 14, NEJMoa2022483.

24. *Coronavirus (COVID-19) Update: FDA Revokes Emergency Use Authorization for Chloroquine and Hydroxychloroquine. U.S. Food and Drug Administration;* 2021. https://www.fda.gov/news-events/press-announcements/coronavirus-covid-19-update-fda-revokes-emergency-use-authorization-chloroquine-and. Accessed 1 March 2021.

25. RECOVERY Collaborative Group, Horby P, Lim WS, et al. Dexamethasone in hospitalized patients with covid-19. *N Engl J Med.* 2021;384(8):693–704. https://doi.org/10.1056/NEJMoa2021436.

26. Folegatti PM, Ewer KJ, Aley PK, et al. Safety and immunogenicity of the ChAdOx1 nCoV-19 vaccine against SARS-CoV-2: a preliminary report of a phase 1/2, single-blind, randomised controlled trial. *Lancet.* 2020;396(10249):467–478. https://doi.org/10.1016/S0140-6736(20)31604-4. [published correction appears in Lancet. 2020 Aug 15;396(10249):466] [published correction appears in Lancet. 2020 Dec 12;396(10266):1884].

27. Logunov DY, Dolzhikova IV, Shcheblyakov DV, et al. Safety and efficacy of an rAd26 and rAd5 vector-based heterologous prime-boost COVID-19 vaccine: an interim analysis of a randomised controlled phase 3 trial in Russia. *Lancet.* 2021;397(10275):671–681. https://doi.org/10.1016/S0140-6736(21)00234-8. [published correction appears in Lancet. 2021 Feb 20;397(10275):670].

28. RECOVERY Collaborative Group. Lopinavir-ritonavir in patients admitted to hospital with COVID-19 (RECOVERY): a randomised, controlled, open-label, platform trial. *Lancet.* 2020;396(10259):1345–1352. https://doi.org/10.1016/S0140-6736(20)32013-4 [published online ahead of print, 2020 Oct 5].

29. Polack FP, Thomas SJ, Kitchin N, et al. Safety and efficacy of the BNT162b2 mRNA covid-19 vaccine. *N Engl J Med.* 2020;383(27):2603–2615. https://doi.org/10.1056/NEJMoa2034577.

30. *Moderna's COVID-19 Vaccine Candidate Meets Its Primary Efficacy Endpoint in the First Interim Analysis of the Phase 3 COVE Study.* Moderna; 2020. https://investors.modernatx.com/news-releases/news-release-details/modernas-covid-19-vaccine-candidate-meets-its-primary-efficacy. Accessed 2 March 2021.

31. Voysey M, Clemens SAC, Madhi SA, et al. Safety and efficacy of the ChAdOx1 nCoV-19 vaccine (AZD1222) against SARS-CoV-2: an interim analysis of four randomised controlled trials in Brazil, South Africa, and the UK. *Lancet.* 2021;397(10269):99–111. https://doi.org/10.1016/S0140-6736(20)32661-1 [published correction appears in Lancet. 2021 Jan 9;397(10269):98].

32. Winck B. IMF says 'Great Lockdown' global recession will be worst economic meltdown since Great Depression. *Bus Insid.* 2020. https://www.businessinsider.com/imf-economic-outlook-great-lockdown-worst-recession-century-coronavirus-pandemic-2020-4. Accessed 2 March 2021.

33. Jackson J, Weiss M, Schwarzenberg A, Nelson R, Sutter K, Sutherland M. *Global Economic Effects of COVID-19. Congressional Research Service;* 2021. https://fas.org/sgp/crs/row/R46270.pdf. Accessed 2 March 2021.

34. Economic data, commodities and markets. *De Economist.* 2020. https://www.economist.com/economic-and-financial-indicators/2020/05/14/economic-data-commodities-and-markets. Accessed 2 March 2021.

35. *Civilian Unemployment Rate.* U.S. Bureau of Labor Statistics; 2020. https://www.bls.gov/charts/employment-situation/civilian-unemployment-rate.htm. Accessed 2 March 2021.

36. Romm T, Stein J, Werner E. 2.4 million Americans filed jobless claims last week, bringing nine-week total to 38.6 million. *Wash Post.* 2020. https://www.washingtonpost.com/business/2020/05/21/unemployment-claims-coronavirus/. Accessed 2 March 2021.

37. Hall B. Coronavirus shutdown poses threat to 59m jobs in Europe, report warns. *Financial Times.* 2021. https://www.ft.com/content/36239c82-84ae-4cc9-89bc-8e71e53d6649. Accessed 2 March 2021.

38. Stott M. Coronavirus set to push 29m Latin Americans into poverty. *Financial Times.* 2020. https://www.ft.com/content/3bf48b80-8fba-410c-9bb8-31e33fffc3b8. Accessed 2 March 2021.

39. *World Economic Outlook. International Monetary Fund;* 2020. https://www.imf.org/en/Publications/WEO/Issues/2020/06/24/WEOUpdateJune2020. Accessed 2 March 2021.

40. *CARES Act.* Congress.gov; 2020. https://www.congress.gov/116/bills/s3548/BILLS-116s3548is.pdf. Accessed 2 March 2021.

41. Cochrane E, Stolberg S. $2 Trillion coronavirus stimulus bill is signed into law. *NY Times.* 2020. https://www.nytimes.com/2020/03/27/us/politics/coronavirus-house-voting.html. Accessed 2 March 2021.

42. *Coronavirus Response. European Commission;* 2021. https://ec.europa.eu/info/live-work-travel-eu/coronavirus-response_en. Accessed 2 March 2021.

43. *UN Issues $10.3B Coronavirus Appeal and Warns of the Price of Inaction. OCHA;* 2020. https://www.unocha.org/story/un-issues-103b-coronavirus-appeal-and-warns-price-inaction. Accessed 2 March 2021.

44. Petersen E, Koopmans M, Go U, et al. Comparing SARS-CoV-2 with SARS-CoV and influenza pandemics. *Lancet Infect Dis.* 2020;20(9):e238–e244. https://doi.org/10.1016/S1473-3099(20)30484-9.

45. *Consensus Document on the Epidemiology of Severe Acute Respiratory Syndrome (SARS). WHO;* 2021. https://www.who.int/csr/sars/WHOconsensus.pdf?ua=1. Accessed 2 March 2021.

46. Vynnycky E, Trindall A, Mangtani P. Estimates of the reproduction numbers of Spanish influenza using morbidity data. *Int J Epidemiol.* 2007;36(4):881–889. https://doi.org/10.1093/ije/dym071.

47. Yang Y, Sugimoto JD, Halloran ME, et al. The transmissibility and control of pandemic influenza A (H1N1) virus. *Science.* 2009;326(5953):729–733. https://doi.org/10.1126/science.1177373.

48. Breban R, Riou J, Fontanet A. Interhuman transmissibility of Middle East respiratory syndrome coronavirus: estimation of pandemic risk. *Lancet.* 2013;382(9893):694–699. https://doi.org/10.1016/S0140-6736(13)61492-0.

49. Callaway E, Cyranoski D, Mallapaty S, Stoye E, Tollefson J. The coronavirus pandemic in five powerful charts. *Nature.* 2020. https://www.nature.com/articles/d41586-020-00758-2. Accessed 2 March 2021.

50. Jiang X, Rayner S, Luo MH. Does SARS-CoV-2 have a longer incubation period than SARS and MERS? *J Med Virol.* 2020;92(5):476–478. https://doi.org/10.1002/jmv.25708.

51. Lessler J, Reich NG, Brookmeyer R, Perl TM, Nelson KE, Cummings DA. Incubation periods of acute respiratory viral infections: a systematic review. *Lancet Infect Dis.* 2009;9(5):291–300. https://doi.org/10.1016/S1473-3099(09)70069-6.

52. He X, Lau EHY, Wu P, et al. Temporal dynamics in viral shedding and transmissibility of COVID-19. *Nat Med.* 2020;26(5):672–675. https://doi.org/10.1038/s41591-020-0869-5 [published correction appears in Nat Med. 2020 Sep;26(9):1491-1493].

53. *Healthcare Workers. Centers for Disease Control and Prevention;* 2020. https://www.cdc.gov/coronavirus/2019-ncov/hcp/planning-scenarios.html. Accessed 2 March 2021.

54. Wendorf M, Lang F, Papadopoulos L, Wendorf M, McFadden C. *The 2003 SARS Outbreak: A Timeline.* Interesting Engineering; 2020. https://interestingengineering.com/the-2003-sars-outbreak-a-timeline. Accessed 2 March 2021.

55. Kahn J. The SARS epidemic: treatment; beijing hurries to build hospital complex for increasing number of SARS patients. *NY Times.* 2003. https://www.nytimes.com/2003/04/27/world/sars-epidemic-treatment-beijing-hurries-build-hospital-complex-for-increasing.html. Accessed 2 March 2021.

56. Gopalakrishna G, Choo P, Leo YS, et al. SARS transmission and hospital containment. *Emerg Infect Dis.* 2004;10(3):395–400. https://doi.org/10.3201/eid1003.030650.

57. Deng L. China's coronavirus response is questioned: 'everyone was blindly optimistic'. *WSJ.* 2020. https://www.wsj.com/articles/china-contends-with-questions-over-response-to-viral-outbreak-11579825832. Accessed 2 March 2021.

58. Courtemanche C, Garuccio J, Le A, Pinkston J, Yelowitz A. Strong social distancing measures in the United States reduced the COVID-19 growth rate. *Health Aff (Millwood).* 2020;39(7):1237–1246. https://doi.org/10.1377/hlthaff.2020.00608.

59. Nussbaumer-Streit B, Mayr V, Dobrescu AI, et al. Quarantine alone or in combination with other public health measures to control COVID-19: a rapid review. *Cochrane Database Syst Rev.* 2020;4(4):CD013574. https://doi.org/10.1002/14651858.CD013574.

60. *Evaluating and Testing Persons for Coronavirus Disease 2019 (COVID-19). Centers for Disease Control and Prevention;* March 9, 2020. www.cdc.gov/coronavirus/2019-nCoV/hcp/clinical-criteria.html.

61. Lippi G, von Meyer A, Cadamuro J, Simundic AM, European Federation of Clinical Chemistry and Laboratory Medicine (EFLM) Working Group for Preanalytical Phase (WG-PRE). PREDICT: a checklist for preventing preanalytical diagnostic errors in clinical trials. *Clin Chem Lab Med.* 2020;58(4):518–526. https://doi.org/10.1515/cclm-2019-1089.

62. Plebani M. Errors in clinical laboratories or errors in laboratory medicine? *Clin Chem Lab Med.* 2006;44(6):750–759. https://doi.org/10.1515/CCLM.2006.123.

63. van Zyl G, Maritz J, Newman H, Preiser W. Lessons in diagnostic virology: expected and unexpected sources of error. *Rev Med Virol.* 2019;29(4):e2052. https://doi.org/10.1002/rmv.2052.

64. Billingsley A. *The Latest in Coronavirus (COVID-19) Testing Methods and Availability. GoodRx;* 2021. https://www.goodrx.com/blog/coronavirus-covid-19-testing-updates-methods-cost-availability/. Accessed 2 March 2021.

65. Li D, Can I. *Test for Coronavirus At Home? The State of At-Home COVID-19 Tests. GoodRx;* 2020. https://www.goodrx.com/blog/coronavirus-at-home-tests/. Accessed 2 March 2021.

66. Wang W, Xu Y, Gao R, et al. Detection of SARS-CoV-2 in different types of clinical specimens. *JAMA.* 2020;323(18):1843–1844. https://doi.org/10.1001/jama.2020.3786.

67. *Coronavirus (COVID-19) Update: FDA Issues Emergency Use Authorization to Yale School of Public Health for SalivaDirect, Which Uses a New Method of Saliva Sample Processing. U.S. Food and Drug Administration;* 2020. https://www.fda.gov/news-events/press-announcements/coronavirus-covid-19-update-fda-issues-emergency-use-authorization-yale-school-public-health. Accessed 2 March 2021.

68. Vogels CBF, Watkins AE, Harden CA, et al. SalivaDirect: a simplified and flexible platform to enhance SARS-CoV-2 testing capacity. *Med (N Y)*. 2020. https://doi.org/10.1016/j.medj.2020.12.010 [published online ahead of print, 2020 Dec 26].

69. Sethuraman N, Jeremiah SS, Ryo A. Interpreting diagnostic tests for SARS-CoV-2. *JAMA*. 2020;323(22):2249–2251. https://doi.org/10.1001/jama.2020.8259.

70. *Testing Guide. AAFP*; 2021. https://www.aafp.org/patient-care/emergency/2019-coronavirus/covid-19_resources/covid-19--testing.html. Accessed 2 March 2021.

71. Xiao AT, Gao C, Zhang S. Profile of specific antibodies to SARS-CoV-2: the first report. *J Infect*. 2020;81(1):147–178. https://doi.org/10.1016/j.jinf.2020.03.012.

72. *Coronavirus Testing Explained*. Confirmbiosciences.com; 2020. https://www.confirmbiosciences.com/wp-content/uploads/2020/04/coronavirus-testing-explained-infographic.pdf. Accessed 2 March 2021.

73. Lisboa Bastos M, Tavaziva G, Abidi SK, et al. Diagnostic accuracy of serological tests for covid-19: systematic review and meta-analysis. *BMJ*. 2020;370:m2516. https://doi.org/10.1136/bmj.m2516.

74. Deeks JJ, Dinnes J, Takwoingi Y, et al. Antibody tests for identification of current and past infection with SARS-CoV-2. *Cochrane Database Syst Rev*. 2020;6(6):CD013652. https://doi.org/10.1002/14651858.CD013652.

75. *"Immunity Passports" in the Context of COVID-19*. WHO; 2020. https://www.who.int/news-room/commentaries/detail/immunity-passports-in-the-context-of-covid-19. Accessed 2 March 2021.

76. Phelan AL. COVID-19 immunity passports and vaccination certificates: scientific, equitable, and legal challenges. *Lancet*. 2020;395(10237):1595–1598. https://doi.org/10.1016/S0140-6736(20)31034-5.

77. Buchanan PM. Why 'immunity passports' won't be the golden tickets to travel after all. *CNBC*. 2020. https://www.cnbc.com/2020/06/04/covid-19-update-will-immunity-passports-let-people-travel-again.html. Accessed 2 March 2021.

78. Clark A, Jit M, Warren-Gash C, et al. Global, regional, and national estimates of the population at increased risk of severe COVID-19 due to underlying health conditions in 2020: a modelling study. *Lancet Glob Health*. 2020;8(8):e1003–e1017. https://doi.org/10.1016/S2214-109X(20)30264-3.

79. Guan WJ, Ni ZY, Hu Y, et al. Clinical characteristics of coronavirus disease 2019 in China. *N Engl J Med*. 2020;382(18):1708–1720. https://doi.org/10.1056/NEJMoa2002032.

80. Richardson S, Hirsch JS, Narasimhan M, et al. Presenting characteristics, comorbidities, and outcomes among 5700 patients hospitalized with COVID-19 in the New York City Area. *JAMA*. 2020;323(20):2052–2059. https://doi.org/10.1001/jama.2020.6775 [published correction appears in JAMA. 2020 May 26;323(20):2098].

81. Myers LC, Parodi SM, Escobar GJ, Liu VX. Characteristics of hospitalized adults with covid-19 in an integrated health care system in California. *JAMA*. 2020;323(21):2195–2198. https://doi.org/10.1001/jama.2020.7202.

82. Grasselli G, Zangrillo A, Zanella A, et al. Baseline characteristics and outcomes of 1591 patients infected with SARS-CoV-2 admitted to ICUs of the Lombardy Region, Italy. *JAMA*. 2020;323(16):1574–1581. https://doi.org/10.1001/jama.2020.5394.

83. Yang J, Petitjean SJL, Koehler M, et al. Molecular interaction and inhibition of SARS-CoV-2 binding to the ACE2 receptor. *Nat Commun*. 2020;11(1):4541. https://doi.org/10.1038/s41467-020-18319-6.

84. Verdecchia P, Cavallini C, Spanevello A, Angeli F. The pivotal link between ACE2 deficiency and SARS-CoV-2 infection. *Eur J Intern Med*. 2020;76:14–20.

85. Sharifkashani S, Bafrani MA, Khaboushan AS, et al. Angiotensin-converting enzyme 2 (ACE2) receptor and SARS-CoV-2: potential therapeutic targeting. *Eur J Pharmacol*. 2020;884:173455. https://doi.org/10.1016/j.ejphar.2020.173455.

86. Rivellese F, Prediletto E. ACE2 at the centre of COVID-19 from paucisymptomatic infections to severe pneumonia. *Autoimmun Rev*. 2020;19(6):102536. https://doi.org/10.1016/j.autrev.2020.102536.

87. Chung MK, Karnik S, Saef J, et al. SARS-CoV-2 and ACE2: the biology and clinical data settling the ARB and ACEI controversy. *EBioMedicine*. 2020;58:102907. https://doi.org/10.1016/j.ebiom.2020.102907.

88. Hofmann H, Pyrc K, van der Hoek L, Geier M, Berkhout B, Pöhlmann S. Human coronavirus NL63 employs the severe acute respiratory syndrome coronavirus receptor for cellular entry. *Proc Natl Acad Sci USA*. 2005;102(22):7988–7993. https://doi.org/10.1073/pnas.0409465102.

89. Li F, Li W, Farzan M, Harrison SC. Structure of SARS coronavirus spike receptor-binding domain complexed with receptor. *Science*. 2005;309(5742):1864–1868. https://doi.org/10.1126/science.1116480.

90. Jia HP, Look DC, Shi L, et al. ACE2 receptor expression and severe acute respiratory syndrome coronavirus infection depend on differentiation of human airway epithelia. *J Virol*. 2005;79(23):14614–14621. https://doi.org/10.1128/JVI.79.23.14614-14621.2005.

91. Hamming I, Timens W, Bulthuis ML, Lely AT, Navis G, van Goor H. Tissue distribution of ACE2 protein, the functional receptor for SARS coronavirus. A first step in understanding SARS pathogenesis. *J Pathol*. 2004;203(2):631–637. https://doi.org/10.1002/path.1570.

92. Dong M, Zhang J, Ma X, et al. ACE2, TMPRSS2 distribution and extrapulmonary organ injury in patients with COVID-19. *Biomed Pharmacother*. 2020;131:110678. https://doi.org/10.1016/j.biopha.2020.110678.

93. Gupta A, Madhavan MV, Sehgal K, et al. Extrapulmonary manifestations of COVID-19. *Nat Med*. 2020;26(7):1017–1032. https://doi.org/10.1038/s41591-020-0968-3.

94. Ziegler CGK, Allon SJ, Nyquist SK, et al. SARS-CoV-2 receptor ACE2 is an interferon-stimulated gene in human airway epithelial cells and is detected in specific cell subsets across tissues. *Cell*. 2020;181(5):1016–1035.e19. https://doi.org/10.1016/j.cell.2020.04.035.

95. Xu J, Lazartigues E. Expression of ACE2 in human neurons supports the neuro-invasive potential of COVID-19

virus [published online ahead of print 2020 Jul 4]. *Cell Mol Neurobiol.* 2020;1–5. https://doi.org/10.1007/s10571-020-00915-1.

96. Zang R, Gomez Castro MF, McCune BT, et al. TMPRSS2 and TMPRSS4 promote SARS-CoV-2 infection of human small intestinal enterocytes. *Sci Immunol.* 2020;5(47):eabc3582. https://doi.org/10.1126/sciimmunol.abc3582.

97. Hoffmann M, Kleine-Weber H, Schroeder S, et al. SARS-CoV-2 cell entry depends on ACE2 and TMPRSS2 and is blocked by a clinically proven protease inhibitor. *Cell.* 2020;181(2):271–280.e8. https://doi.org/10.1016/j.cell.2020.02.052.

98. Baughn LB, Sharma N, Elhaik E, Sekulic A, Bryce AH, Fonseca R. Targeting TMPRSS2 in SARS-CoV-2 infection. *Mayo Clin Proc.* 2020;95(9):1989–1999. https://doi.org/10.1016/j.mayocp.2020.06.018.

99. Zhang H, Liao YS, Gong J, Liu J, Xia X, Zhang H. Clinical characteristics of coronavirus disease (COVID-19) patients with gastrointestinal symptoms: a report of 164 cases. *Dig Liver Dis.* 2020;52(10):1076–1079. https://doi.org/10.1016/j.dld.2020.04.034.

100. Henry BM, de Oliveira MHS, Benoit J, Lippi G. Gastrointestinal symptoms associated with severity of coronavirus disease 2019 (COVID-19): a pooled analysis. *Intern Emerg Med.* 2020;15(5):857–859. https://doi.org/10.1007/s11739-020-02329-9.

101. Parasa S, Desai M, Thoguluva Chandrasekar V, et al. Prevalence of gastrointestinal symptoms and fecal viral shedding in patients with coronavirus disease 2019: a systematic review and meta-analysis. *JAMA Netw Open.* 2020;3(6):e2011335. https://doi.org/10.1001/jamanetworkopen.2020.11335.

102. Galanopoulos M, Gkeros F, Doukatas A, et al. COVID-19 pandemic: pathophysiology and manifestations from the gastrointestinal tract. *World J Gastroenterol.* 2020;26(31):4579–4588. https://doi.org/10.3748/wjg.v26.i31.4579.

103. Tian D, Ye Q. Hepatic complications of COVID-19 and its treatment. *J Med Virol.* 2020;92(10):1818–1824. https://doi.org/10.1002/jmv.26036.

104. Li Y, Xiao SY. Hepatic involvement in COVID-19 patients: pathology, pathogenesis, and clinical implications. *J Med Virol.* 2020;92(9):1491–1494. https://doi.org/10.1002/jmv.25973.

105. Kullar R, Patel AP, Saab S. Hepatic injury in patients with COVID-19. *J Clin Gastroenterol.* 2020;54(10):841–849. https://doi.org/10.1097/MCG.0000000000001432.

106. Velarde-Ruiz Velasco JA, García-Jiménez ES, Remes-Troche JM. Hepatic manifestations and impact of COVID-19 on the cirrhotic patient. Manifestaciones hepáticas y repercusión en el paciente cirrótico de COVID-19. *Rev Gastroenterol Mex.* 2020;85(3):303–311. https://doi.org/10.1016/j.rgmx.2020.05.002.

107. Yang X, Jin Y, Li R, Zhang Z, Sun R, Chen D. Prevalence and impact of acute renal impairment on COVID-19: a systematic review and meta-analysis. *Crit Care.* 2020;24(1):356. https://doi.org/10.1186/s13054-020-03065-4.

108. Pei G, Zhang Z, Peng J, et al. Renal involvement and early prognosis in patients with COVID-19 pneumonia. *J Am Soc Nephrol.* 2020;31(6):1157–1165. https://doi.org/10.1681/ASN.2020030276.

109. Duarte PMA, Bastos Filho FAG, Duarte JVA, et al. Renal changes in COVID-19 infection. *Rev Assoc Med Bras.* 2020;66(10):1335–1337. https://doi.org/10.1590/1806-9282.66.10.1335.

110. Wei JF, Huang FY, Xiong TY, et al. Acute myocardial injury is common in patients with COVID-19 and impairs their prognosis. *Heart.* 2020;106(15):1154–1159. https://doi.org/10.1136/heartjnl-2020-317007.

111. Guo T, Fan Y, Chen M, et al. Cardiovascular implications of fatal outcomes of patients with coronavirus disease 2019 (COVID-19). *JAMA Cardiol.* 2020;5(7):811–818. https://doi.org/10.1001/jamacardio.2020.1017 [published correction appears in JAMA Cardiol. 2020 Jul 1;5(7):848].

112. Lavie CJ, Sanchis-Gomar F, Lippi G. Cardiac injury in COVID-19-echoing prognostication. *J Am Coll Cardiol.* 2020;76(18):2056–2059. https://doi.org/10.1016/j.jacc.2020.08.068.

113. Lala A, Johnson KW, Januzzi JL, et al. Prevalence and impact of myocardial injury in patients hospitalized with COVID-19 infection. *J Am Coll Cardiol.* 2020;76(5):533–546. https://doi.org/10.1016/j.jacc.2020.06.007.

114. Bellastella G, Maiorino MI, Esposito K. Endocrine complications of COVID-19: what happens to the thyroid and adrenal glands? *J Endocrinol Investig.* 2020;43(8):1169–1170. https://doi.org/10.1007/s40618-020-01311-8.

115. Bansal R, Gubbi S, Muniyappa R. Metabolic syndrome and COVID 19: endocrine-immune-vascular interactions shapes clinical course. *Endocrinology.* 2020;161(10):bqaa112. https://doi.org/10.1210/endocr/bqaa11.

116. Sanghvi AR. COVID-19: an overview for dermatologists. *Int J Dermatol.* 2020;59(12):1437–1449. https://doi.org/10.1111/ijd.15257.

117. Tang K, Wang Y, Zhang H, Zheng Q, Fang R, Sun Q. Cutaneous manifestations of the coronavirus disease 2019 (COVID-19): a brief review. *Dermatol Ther.* 2020;33(4):e13528. https://doi.org/10.1111/dth.13528.

118. Rahimi H, Tehranchinia Z. A comprehensive review of cutaneous manifestations associated with COVID-19. *Biomed Res Int.* 2020;2020:1236520. https://doi.org/10.1155/2020/1236520.

119. Mina A, van Besien K, Platanias LC. Hematological manifestations of COVID-19. *Leuk Lymphoma.* 2020;61(12):2790–2798. https://doi.org/10.1080/10428194.2020.1788017.

120. Yuan X, Huang W, Ye B, et al. Changes of hematological and immunological parameters in COVID-19 patients. *Int J Hematol.* 2020;112(4):553–559. https://doi.org/10.1007/s12185-020-02930-w.

121. Tal S, Spectre G, Kornowski R, Perl L. Venous thromboembolism complicated with COVID-19: what do we know so far? *Acta Haematol.* 2020;143(5):417–424. https://doi.org/10.1159/000508233.

122. Sridharan GK, Vegunta R, Rokkam VRP, et al. Venous thromboembolism in hospitalized COVID-19 Patients. *Am J Ther.* 2020;27(6):e599–e610. https://doi.org/10.1097/MJT.0000000000001295.

123. Rieder M, Goller I, Jeserich M, et al. Rate of venous thromboembolism in a prospective all-comers cohort with COVID-19. *J Thromb Thrombolysis.* 2020;50(3):558–566. https://doi.org/10.1007/s11239-020-02202-8.

124. Llitjos JF, Leclerc M, Chochois C, et al. High incidence of venous thromboembolic events in anticoagulated severe COVID-19 patients. *J Thromb Haemost.* 2020;18(7):1743–1746. https://doi.org/10.1111/jth.14869.

125. Hasan SS, Radford S, Kow CS, Zaidi STR. Venous thromboembolism in critically ill COVID-19 patients receiving prophylactic or therapeutic anticoagulation: a systematic review and meta-analysis. *J Thromb Thrombolysis.* 2020;50(4):814–821. https://doi.org/10.1007/s11239-020-02235-z.

126. Yuki K, Fujiogi M, Koutsogiannaki S. COVID-19 pathophysiology: a review. *Clin Immunol.* 2020;215:108427. https://doi.org/10.1016/j.clim.2020.108427.

127. Bohn MK, Hall A, Sepiashvili L, Jung B, Steele S, Adeli K. Pathophysiology of COVID-19: mechanisms underlying disease severity and progression. *Physiology (Bethesda).* 2020;35(5):288–301. https://doi.org/10.1152/physiol.00019.2020.

128. Borczuk AC, Salvatore SP, Seshan SV, et al. COVID-19 pulmonary pathology: a multi-institutional autopsy cohort from Italy and New York City. *Mod Pathol.* 2020;33(11):2156–2168. https://doi.org/10.1038/s41379-020-00661-1.

129. Alharthy A, Faqihi F, Memish ZA, Karakitsos D. Lung injury in COVID-19—an emerging hypothesis. *ACS Chem Neurosci.* 2020;11(15):2156–2158. https://doi.org/10.1021/acschemneuro.0c00422.

130. Mortaz E, Tabarsi P, Varahram M, Folkerts G, Adcock IM. The immune response and immunopathology of COVID-19. *Front Immunol.* 2020;11:2037. https://doi.org/10.3389/fimmu.2020.02037.

131. Chowdhury MA, Hossain N, Kashem MA, Shahid MA, Alam A. Immune response in COVID-19: a review. *J Infect Public Health.* 2020;13(11):1619–1629. https://doi.org/10.1016/j.jiph.2020.07.001.

132. Azkur AK, Akdis M, Azkur D, et al. Immune response to SARS-CoV-2 and mechanisms of immunopathological changes in COVID-19. *Allergy.* 2020;75(7):1564–1581. https://doi.org/10.1111/all.14364.

133. McGonagle D, O'Donnell JS, Sharif K, Emery P, Bridgewood C. Immune mechanisms of pulmonary intravascular coagulopathy in COVID-19 pneumonia. *Lancet Rheumatol.* 2020;2(7):e437–e445. https://doi.org/10.1016/S2665-9913(20)30121-1.

134. Fajgenbaum DC, June CH. Cytokine storm. *N Engl J Med.* 2020;383(23):2255–2273. https://doi.org/10.1056/NEJMra2026131.

135. Varga Z, Flammer AJ, Steiger P, et al. Endothelial cell infection and endotheliitis in COVID-19. *Lancet.* 2020;395(10234):1417–1418. https://doi.org/10.1016/S0140-6736(20)30937-5.

136. Jin Y, Ji W, Yang H, Chen S, Zhang W, Duan G. Endothelial activation and dysfunction in COVID-19: from basic mechanisms to potential therapeutic approaches. *Signal Transduct Target Ther.* 2020;5(1):293. https://doi.org/10.1038/s41392-020-00454-7.

137. Del Turco S, Vianello A, Ragusa R, Caselli C, Basta G. COVID-19 and cardiovascular consequences: is the endothelial dysfunction the hardest challenge? *Thromb Res.* 2020;196:143–151. https://doi.org/10.1016/j.thromres.2020.08.039.

138. Brojakowska A, Narula J, Shimony R, Bander J. Clinical implications of SARS-CoV-2 interaction with renin angiotensin system: JACC review topic of the week. *J Am Coll Cardiol.* 2020;75(24):3085–3095. https://doi.org/10.1016/j.jacc.2020.04.028.

139. Augoustides JGT. The renin-angiotensin-aldosterone system in coronavirus infection-current considerations during the pandemic. *J Cardiothorac Vasc Anesth.* 2020;34(7):1717–1719. https://doi.org/10.1053/j.jvca.2020.04.010.

140. Tsai LK, Hsieh ST, Chang YC. Neurological manifestations in severe acute respiratory syndrome. *Acta Neurol Taiwanica.* 2005;14(3):113–119.

141. Tsai LK, Hsieh ST, Chao CC, et al. Neuromuscular disorders in severe acute respiratory syndrome. *Arch Neurol.* 2004;61(11):1669–1673. https://doi.org/10.1001/archneur.61.11.1669.

142. Alshebri MS, Alshouimi RA, Alhumidi HA, Alshaya AI. Neurological complications of SARS-CoV, MERS-CoV, and COVID-19. *SN Compr Clin Med.* 2020;1–11. https://doi.org/10.1007/s42399-020-00589-2 [published online ahead of print, 2020 Oct 16].

143. Algahtani H, Subahi A, Shirah B. Neurological complications of Middle East Respiratory Syndrome coronavirus: a report of two cases and review of the literature. *Case Rep Neurol Med.* 2016;2016:3502683. https://doi.org/10.1155/2016/3502683.

144. Arabi YM, Harthi A, Hussein J, et al. Severe neurologic syndrome associated with Middle East respiratory syndrome coronavirus (MERS-CoV). *Infection.* 2015;43(4):495–501. https://doi.org/10.1007/s15010-015-0720-y.

145. Morfopoulou S, Brown JR, Davies EG, et al. Human coronavirus OC43 associated with fatal encephalitis. *N Engl J Med.* 2016;375(5):497–498. https://doi.org/10.1056/NEJMc1509458.

146. Nilsson A, Edner N, Albert J, Ternhag A. Fatal encephalitis associated with coronavirus OC43 in an immunocompromised child. *Infect Dis (Lond).* 2020;52(6):419–422. https://doi.org/10.1080/23744235.2020.1729403.

147. Arbour N, Day R, Newcombe J, Talbot PJ. Neuroinvasion by human respiratory coronaviruses. *J Virol.* 2000;74(19):8913–8921. https://doi.org/10.1128/jvi.74.19.8913-8921.2000.

148. Bonavia A, Arbour N, Yong VW, Talbot PJ. Infection of primary cultures of human neural cells by human

coronaviruses 229E and OC43. *J Virol.* 1997;71(1):800–806. https://doi.org/10.1128/JVI.71.1.800-806.1997.

149. Morgello S. Coronaviruses and the central nervous system. *J Neurovirol.* 2020;26(4):459–473. https://doi.org/10.1007/s13365-020-00868-7.

150. Verstrepen K, Baisier L, De Cauwer H. Neurological manifestations of COVID-19, SARS and MERS. *Acta Neurol Belg.* 2020;120(5):1051–1060. https://doi.org/10.1007/s13760-020-01412-4 [published correction appears in Acta Neurol Belg. 2020 Jul 21].

151. Mao L, Jin H, Wang M, et al. Neurologic manifestations of hospitalized patients with coronavirus disease 2019 in Wuhan, China. *JAMA Neurol.* 2020;77(6):683–690. https://doi.org/10.1001/jamaneurol.2020.1127.

152. Xiong W, Mu J, Guo J, et al. New onset neurologic events in people with COVID-19 in 3 regions in China. *Neurology.* 2020;95(11):e1479–e1487. https://doi.org/10.1212/WNL.0000000000010034.

153. Helms J, Kremer S, Merdji H, et al. Neurologic features in severe SARS-CoV-2 infection. *N Engl J Med.* 2020;382(23):2268–2270. https://doi.org/10.1056/NEJMc2008597.

154. Romero-Sánchez CM, Díaz-Maroto I, Fernández-Díaz E, et al. Neurologic manifestations in hospitalized patients with COVID-19: the ALBACOVID registry. *Neurology.* 2020;95(8):e1060–e1070. https://doi.org/10.1212/WNL.0000000000009937.

155. Liotta EM, Batra A, Clark JR, et al. Frequent neurologic manifestations and encephalopathy-associated morbidity in Covid-19 patients. *Ann Clin Transl Neurol.* 2020;7(11):2221–2230. https://doi.org/10.1002/acn3.51210.

156. Karadaş Ö, Öztürk B, Sonkaya AR. A prospective clinical study of detailed neurological manifestations in patients with COVID-19. *Neurol Sci.* 2020;41(8):1991–1995. https://doi.org/10.1007/s10072-020-04547-7.

157. Varatharaj A, Thomas N, Ellul MA, et al. Neurological and neuropsychiatric complications of COVID-19 in 153 patients: a UK-wide surveillance study. *Lancet Psychiatry.* 2020;7(10):875–882. https://doi.org/10.1016/S2215-0366(20)30287-X [published correction appears in Lancet Psychiatry. 2020 Jul 14].

158. Garg RK, Paliwal VK, Gupta A. Encephalopathy in patients with COVID-19: a review. *J Med Virol.* 2021;93(1):206–222. https://doi.org/10.1002/jmv.26207.

159. Poyiadji N, Shahin G, Noujaim D, Stone M, Patel S, Griffith B. COVID-19-associated acute hemorrhagic necrotizing encephalopathy: imaging features. *Radiology.* 2020;296(2):E119–E120. https://doi.org/10.1148/radiol.2020201187.

160. Dixon L, Varley J, Gontsarova A, et al. COVID-19-related acute necrotizing encephalopathy with brain stem involvement in a patient with aplastic anemia. *Neurol Neuroimmunol Neuroinflamm.* 2020;7(5):e789. https://doi.org/10.1212/NXI.0000000000000789.

161. Krett JD, Jewett GAE, Elton-Lacasse C, et al. Hemorrhagic encephalopathy associated with COVID-19. *J Neuroimmunol.* 2020;346:577326. https://doi.org/10.1016/j.jneuroim.2020.577326 [published online ahead of print, 2020 Jul 14].

162. Sachs JR, Gibbs KW, Swor DE, et al. COVID-19-associated Leukoencephalopathy. *Radiology.* 2020;296(3):E184–E185. https://doi.org/10.1148/radiol.2020201753.

163. Lang M, Buch K, Li MD, et al. Leukoencephalopathy associated with severe COVID-19 infection: sequela of hypoxemia? *AJNR Am J Neuroradiol.* 2020;41(9):1641–1645. https://doi.org/10.3174/ajnr.A6671.

164. Radmanesh A, Derman A, Lui YW, et al. COVID-19-associated diffuse leukoencephalopathy and microhemorrhages. *Radiology.* 2020;297(1):E223–E227. https://doi.org/10.1148/radiol.2020202040.

165. Agarwal S, Jain R, Dogra S, et al. Cerebral microbleeds and leukoencephalopathy in critically Ill patients with COVID-19. *Stroke.* 2020;51(9):2649–2655. https://doi.org/10.1161/STROKEAHA.120.030940.

166. Princiotta Cariddi L, Tabaee Damavandi P, Carimati F, et al. Reversible encephalopathy syndrome (PRES) in a COVID-19 patient. *J Neurol.* 2020;267(11):3157–3160. https://doi.org/10.1007/s00415-020-10001-7.

167. Franceschi AM, Ahmed O, Giliberto L, Castillo M. Hemorrhagic posterior reversible encephalopathy syndrome as a manifestation of COVID-19 infection. *AJNR Am J Neuroradiol.* 2020;41(7):1173–1176. https://doi.org/10.3174/ajnr.A6595.

168. D'Amore F, Vinacci G, Agosti E, et al. Pressing issues in COVID-19: probable cause to seize SARS-CoV-2 for its preferential involvement of posterior circulation manifesting as severe posterior reversible encephalopathy syndrome and posterior strokes. *AJNR Am J Neuroradiol.* 2020;41(10):1800–1803. https://doi.org/10.3174/ajnr.A6679.

169. Anand P, Lau KHV, Chung DY, et al. Posterior reversible encephalopathy syndrome in patients with coronavirus disease 2019: two cases and a review of the literature. *J Stroke Cerebrovasc Dis.* 2020;29(11):105212. https://doi.org/10.1016/j.jstrokecerebrovasdis.2020.105212.

170. Lersy F, Anheim M, Willaume T, et al. Cerebral vasculitis of medium-sized vessels as a possible mechanism of brain damage in COVID-19 patients [published online ahead of print, 2020 Dec 16]. *J Neuroradiol.* 2020. https://doi.org/10.1016/j.neurad.2020.11.004. S0150-9861(20)30287-X.

171. Hanafi R, Roger PA, Perin B, et al. COVID-19 neurologic complication with CNS vasculitis-like pattern. *AJNR Am J Neuroradiol.* 2020;41(8):1384–1387. https://doi.org/10.3174/ajnr.A6651.

172. Yagita Y. COVID-19-related cerebrovascular disease and vasculitis. *Brain Nerve.* 2020;72(10):1039–1043. https://doi.org/10.11477/mf.1416201645.

173. Dakay K, Kaur G, Gulko E, et al. Reversible cerebral vasoconstriction syndrome and dissection in the setting of COVID-19 infection. *J Stroke Cerebrovasc Dis.* 2020;29(9):105011. https://doi.org/10.1016/j.jstrokecerebrovasdis.2020.105011.

174. Kakadia B, Ahmed J, Siegal T, Jovin TG, Thon JM. Mild encephalopathy with reversible splenium lesion (MERS) in a patient with COVID-19. *J Clin Neurosci.* 2020;79:272–274. https://doi.org/10.1016/j.jocn.2020.07.009.

175. Pascual-Goñi E, Fortea J, Martínez-Domeño A, et al. COVID-19-associated ophthalmoparesis and hypothalamic involvement. *Neurol Neuroimmunol Neuroinflamm.* 2020;7(5):e823. https://doi.org/10.1212/NXI.0000000000000823.

176. Valiuddin H, Skwirsk B, Paz-Arabo P. Acute transverse myelitis associated with SARS-CoV-2: a case-report. *Brain Behav Immun Health.* 2020;5:100091. https://doi.org/10.1016/j.bbih.2020.100091.

177. Chakraborty U, Chandra A, Ray AK, Biswas P. COVID-19-associated acute transverse myelitis: a rare entity. *BMJ Case Rep.* 2020;13(8):e238668. https://doi.org/10.1136/bcr-2020-238668.

178. AlKetbi R, AlNuaimi D, AlMulla M, et al. Acute myelitis as a neurological complication of Covid-19: a case report and MRI findings. *Radiol Case Rep.* 2020;15(9):1591–1595. https://doi.org/10.1016/j.radcr.2020.06.001.

179. Sotoca J, Rodríguez-Álvarez Y. COVID-19-associated acute necrotizing myelitis. *Neurol Neuroimmunol Neuroinflamm.* 2020;7(5):e803. https://doi.org/10.1212/NXI.0000000000000803.

180. Ray A. Miller Fisher syndrome and COVID-19: is there a link? *BMJ Case Rep.* 2020;13(8):e236419. https://doi.org/10.1136/bcr-2020-236419.

181. Fernández-Domínguez J, Ameijide-Sanluis E, García-Cabo C, García-Rodríguez R, Mateos V. Miller-Fisher-like syndrome related to SARS-CoV-2 infection (COVID 19). *J Neurol.* 2020;267(9):2495–2496. https://doi.org/10.1007/s00415-020-09912-2.

182. Gutiérrez-Ortiz C, Méndez-Guerrero A, Rodrigo-Rey S, et al. Miller Fisher syndrome and polyneuritis cranialis in COVID-19. *Neurology.* 2020;95(5):e601–e605. https://doi.org/10.1212/WNL.0000000000009619.

183. Lantos JE, Strauss SB, Lin E. COVID-19-associated Miller Fisher syndrome: MRI findings. *AJNR Am J Neuroradiol.* 2020;41(7):1184–1186. https://doi.org/10.3174/ajnr.A6609.

184. Fitzpatrick JC, Comstock JM, Longmuir RA, Donahue SP, Fitzpatrick JM, Bond 3rd JB. Cranial nerve III palsy in the setting of COVID 19 infection [published online ahead of print, 2020 Oct 13]. *J Neuroophthalmol.* 2020. https://doi.org/10.1097/WNO.0000000000001160.

185. Dinkin M, Gao V, Kahan J, et al. COVID-19 presenting with ophthalmoparesis from cranial nerve palsy. *Neurology.* 2020;95(5):221–223. https://doi.org/10.1212/WNL.0000000000009700.

186. Greer CE, Bhatt JM, Oliveira CA, Dinkin MJ. Isolated cranial nerve 6 palsy in 6 patients with COVID-19 infection. *J Neuroophthalmol.* 2020;40(4):520–522. https://doi.org/10.1097/WNO.0000000000001146.

187. Mehraeen E, Behnezhad F, Salehi MA, Noori T, Harandi H, SeyedAlinaghi S. Olfactory and gustatory dysfunctions due to the coronavirus disease (COVID-19): a review of current evidence. *Eur Arch Otorhinolaryngol.* 2021;278(2):307–312. https://doi.org/10.1007/s00405-020-06120-6.

188. Lechien JR, Chiesa-Estomba CM, De Siati DR, et al. Olfactory and gustatory dysfunctions as a clinical presentation of mild-to-moderate forms of the coronavirus disease (COVID-19): a multicenter European study. *Eur Arch Otorhinolaryngol.* 2020;277(8):2251–2261. https://doi.org/10.1007/s00405-020-05965-1.

189. Zhang Q, Shan KS, Minalyan A, O'Sullivan C, Nace T. A rare presentation of coronavirus disease 2019 (COVID-19) induced viral myositis with subsequent rhabdomyolysis. *Cureus.* 2020;12(5):e8074. https://doi.org/10.7759/cureus.8074.

190. Beydon M, Chevalier K, Al Tabaa O, et al. Myositis as a manifestation of SARS-CoV-2. *Ann Rheum Dis.* 2020. annrheumdis-2020-217573.

191. Valente-Acosta B, Moreno-Sanchez F, Fueyo-Rodriguez O, Palomar-Lever A. Rhabdomyolysis as an initial presentation in a patient diagnosed with COVID-19. *BMJ Case Rep.* 2020;13(6). https://doi.org/10.1136/bcr-2020-236719.

192. Jin M, Tong Q. Rhabdomyolysis as potential late complication associated with COVID-19. *Emerg Infect Dis.* 2020;26(7):1618–1620. https://doi.org/10.3201/eid2607.200445.

193. Sriwastava S, Tandon M, Kataria S, Daimee M, Sultan S. New onset of ocular myasthenia gravis in a patient with COVID-19: a novel case report and literature review. *J Neurol Oct.* 2020;12:1–7. https://doi.org/10.1007/s00415-020-10263-1.

194. Huber M, Rogozinski S, Puppe W, et al. Postinfectious onset of myasthenia gravis in a COVID-19 patient. *Front Neurol.* 2020;11:576153. https://doi.org/10.3389/fneur.2020.576153.

195. Rábano-Suárez P, Bermejo-Guerrero L, Méndez-Guerrero A, et al. Generalized myoclonus in COVID-19. *Neurology.* 2020;95(6):e767–e772. https://doi.org/10.1212/wnl.0000000000009829.

196. Anand P, Zakaria A, Benameur K, et al. Myoclonus in patients with coronavirus disease 2019: a multicenter case series. *Crit Care Med.* 2020;48(11):1664–1669. https://doi.org/10.1097/CCM.0000000000004570.

197. Shah PB, Desai SD. Opsoclonus myoclonus ataxia syndrome in the setting of COVID-19 infection. *Neurology.* 2021;96(1):33. https://doi.org/10.1212/wnl.0000000000010978.

198. Faber I, Brandão PRP, Menegatti F, de Carvalho Bispo DD, Maluf FB, Cardoso F. Coronavirus disease 2019 and parkinsonism: a non-post-encephalitic case. *Mov Disord.* 2020;35(10):1721–1722. https://doi.org/10.1002/mds.28277.

199. Cohen ME, Eichel R, Steiner-Birmanns B, et al. A case of probable Parkinson's disease after SARS-CoV-2 infection. *Lancet Neurol.* 2020;19(10):804–805. https://doi.org/10.1016/S1474-4422(20)30305-7.

200. Méndez-Guerrero A, Laespada-García MI, Gómez-Grande A, et al. Acute hypokinetic-rigid syndrome following

SARS-CoV-2 infection. *Neurology.* 2020;95(15):e2109–e2118. https://doi.org/10.1212/wnl.0000000000010282.

201. Diezma-Martín AM, Morales-Casado MI, García Alvarado N, Vadillo Bermejo A, López-Ariztegui N, Sepúlveda Berrocal MA. Tremor and ataxia in COVID-19. *Neurologia.* 2020;35(6):409–410. https://doi.org/10.1016/j.nrleng.2020.06.004 [English Edition].

202. Ellul MA, Benjamin L, Singh B, et al. Neurological associations of COVID-19. *Lancet Neurol.* 2020;19(9):767–783. https://doi.org/10.1016/S1474-4422(20)30221-0.

203. Anand P, Zhou L, Bhadelia N, Hamer DH, Greer DM, Cervantes-Arslanian AM. Neurologic findings among inpatients with COVID-19 at a safety-net US hospital. *Neurol Clin Pract.* 2020. https://doi.org/10.1212/cpj.0000000000001031.

204. Gaughan M, Connolly S, Direkze S, Kinsella JA. Acute new-onset symptomatic seizures in the context of mild COVID-19 infection. *J Neurol.* 2020;1–3. https://doi.org/10.1007/s00415-020-10214-w.

205. Abel D, Shen MY, Abid Z, et al. Encephalopathy and bilateral thalamic lesions in a child with MIS-C associated with COVID-19. *Neurology.* 2020;95(16):745–748. https://doi.org/10.1212/wnl.0000000000010652.

206. Ahmed M, Advani S, Moreira A, et al. Multisystem inflammatory syndrome in children: a systematic review. *EClinicalMedicine.* 2020;26:100527. https://doi.org/10.1016/j.eclinm.2020.100527.

207. Panda PK, Sharawat IK, Panda P, Natarajan V, Bhakat R, Dawman L. Neurological complications of SARS-CoV-2 infection in children: a systematic review and meta-analysis. *J Trop Pediatr.* 2020;fmaa070. https://doi.org/10.1093/tropej/fmaa070.

208. Chen T-H. Neurological involvement associated with COVID-19 infection in children. *J Neurol Sci.* 2020;418:117096. https://doi.org/10.1016/j.jns.2020.117096.

209. Abdel-Mannan O, Eyre M, Löbel U, et al. Neurologic and radiographic findings associated with COVID-19 infection in children. *JAMA Neurol.* 2020;77(11):1440–1445. https://doi.org/10.1001/jamaneurol.2020.2687.

210. Eskandar EN, Altschul DJ, de La Garza RR, et al. Neurologic syndromes predict higher in-hospital mortality in COVID-19. *Neurology.* 2020. https://doi.org/10.1212/wnl.0000000000011356.

211. Pilotto A, Cristillo V, Piccinelli SC, et al. COVID-19 severity impacts on long-term neurological manifestation after hospitalisation. *medRxiv.* 2021. https://doi.org/10.1101/2020.12.27.20248903.

212. Chen M, Shen W, Rowan NR, et al. Elevated ACE-2 expression in the olfactory neuroepithelium: implications for anosmia and upper respiratory SARS-CoV-2 entry and replication. *Eur Respir J.* 2020;56(3):2001948. https://doi.org/10.1183/13993003.01948-2020.

213. Bilinska K, Jakubowska P, Von Bartheld CS, Butowt R. Expression of the SARS-CoV-2 entry proteins, ACE2 and TMPRSS2, in cells of the olfactory epithelium: identification of cell types and trends with age. *ACS Chem Neurosci.* 2020;11(11):1555–1562. https://doi.org/10.1021/acschemneuro.0c00210.

214. Kandemirli SG, Altundag A, Yildirim D, Tekcan Sanli DE, Saatci O. Olfactory bulb MRI and paranasal sinus CT findings in persistent COVID-19 anosmia. *Acad Radiol.* 2021;28(1):28–35. https://doi.org/10.1016/j.acra.2020.10.006.

215. Chiu A, Fischbein N, Wintermark M, Zaharchuk G, Yun PT, Zeineh M. COVID-19-induced anosmia associated with olfactory bulb atrophy. *Neuroradiology.* 2020;1–2. https://doi.org/10.1007/s00234-020-02554-1.

216. Strope JD, Chau CH, Figg WD. TMPRSS2: potential biomarker for COVID-19 outcomes. *J Clin Pharmacol.* 2020;60(7):801–807. https://doi.org/10.1002/jcph.1641.

217. Matschke J, Lütgehetmann M, Hagel C, et al. Neuropathology of patients with COVID-19 in Germany: a post-mortem case series. *Lancet Neurol.* 2020;19(11):919–929. https://doi.org/10.1016/S1474-4422(20)30308-2.

218. Alquisiras-Burgos I, Peralta-Arrieta I, Alonso-Palomares LA, Zacapala-Gómez AE, Salmerón-Bárcenas EG, Aguilera P. Neurological complications associated with the blood-brain barrier damage induced by the inflammatory response during SARS-CoV-2 infection. *Mol Neurobiol.* 2020;1–16. https://doi.org/10.1007/s12035-020-02134-.

219. Soldatelli MD, Amaral LFD, Veiga VC, Rojas SSO, Omar S, Marussi VHR. Neurovascular and perfusion imaging findings in coronavirus disease 2019: case report and literature review. *Neuroradiol J.* 2020;33(5):368–373. https://doi.org/10.1177/1971400920941652.

220. Solomon IH, Normandin E, Bhattacharyya S, et al. Neuropathological features of covid-19. *N Engl J Med.* 2020;383(10):989–992. https://doi.org/10.1056/NEJMc2019373.

221. Cajamarca-Baron J, Guavita-Navarro D, Buitrago-Bohorquez J, et al. SARS-CoV-2 (COVID-19) in patients with some degree of immunosuppression [SARS-CoV-2 (COVID-19) en pacientes con algún grado de inmunosupresión]. *Reumatol Clin.* 2020. https://doi.org/10.1016/j.reumae.2020.08.001.

222. Barzegar M, Mirmosayyeb O, Ghajarzadeh M, et al. Characteristics of COVID-19 disease in multiple sclerosis patients. *Mult Scler Relat Disord.* 2020;45:102276. https://doi.org/10.1016/j.msard.2020.102276.

223. Anand P, Slama MCC, Kaku M, et al. COVID-19 in patients with myasthenia gravis. *Muscle Nerve.* 2020. https://doi.org/10.1002/mus.26918. May 11.

224. Costamagna G, Abati E, Bresolin N, Comi GP, Corti S. Management of patients with neuromuscular disorders at the time of the SARS-CoV-2 pandemic. *J Neurol.* 2021;268(5):1580–1591. https://doi.org/10.1007/s00415-020-10149-2.

225. *MS Treatment Guidelines During Coronavirus. National Multiple Sclerosis Society;* 2020. https://www.nationalmssociety.org/coronavirus-covid-19-information/multiple-sclerosis-and-coronavirus/ms-treatment-guidelines-during-coronavirus. Accessed 18 March 2021.

226. Jacob S, Muppidi S, Guidon A, et al. Guidance for the management of myasthenia gravis (MG) and Lambert-Eaton myasthenic syndrome (LEMS) during the COVID-19 pandemic. *J Neurol Sci.* 2020;412. https://doi.org/10.1016/j.jns.2020.116803.

227. Widge AT, Rouphael NG, Jackson LA, et al. Durability of responses after SARS-CoV-2 mRNA-1273 vaccination. *N Engl J Med.* 2020;384(1):80–82. https://doi.org/10.1056/NEJMc2032195.

228. Wee S, Qin A. China approves covid-19 vaccine as it moves to inoculate millions. *NY Times.* 2021. https://www.nytimes.com/2020/12/30/business/china-vaccine.html#:~:text=The%20Chinese%20government%20said%20on,vaccines%20but%20lacked%20crucial%20details. Accessed 18 March 2021.

229. UK A. *AstraZeneca's COVID-19 Vaccine Authorised for Emergency Supply in the UK.* AstraZeneca; 2020. https://www.astrazeneca.com/media-centre/press-releases/2020/astrazenecas-covid-19-vaccine-authorised-in-uk.html. Accessed 18 March 2021.

230. Burki TK. The Russian vaccine for COVID-19. *Lancet Respir Med.* 2020;8(11):e85–e86. https://doi.org/10.1016/S2213-2600(20)30402-1.

231. Krammer F. SARS-CoV-2 vaccines in development. *Nature.* 2020;586(7830):516–527. https://doi.org/10.1038/s41586-020-2798-3.

232. Zhao J, Li H, Kung D, Fisher M, Shen Y, Liu R. Impact of the COVID-19 epidemic on stroke care and potential solutions. *Stroke.* 2020;51(7):1996–2001. https://doi.org/10.1161/STROKEAHA.120.030225.

233. Baracchini C, Pieroni A, Viaro F, et al. Acute stroke management pathway during Coronavirus-19 pandemic. *Neurol Sci.* 2020;1–3. https://doi.org/10.1007/s10072-020-04375-9.

234. Kerleroux B, Fabacher T, Bricout N, et al. Mechanical thrombectomy for acute ischemic stroke amid the COVID-19 outbreak. *Stroke.* 2020;51(7):2012–2017. https://doi.org/10.1161/STROKEAHA.120.030373.

235. Ramadan AR, Alsrouji OK, Cerghet M, et al. Tales of a department: how the COVID-19 pandemic transformed Detroit's Henry Ford Hospital, Department of Neurology-part I: the surge. *BMJ Neurol Open.* 2020;2(1):e000070. https://doi.org/10.1136/bmjno-2020-000070.

236. Bloem BR, Dorsey ER, Okun MS. The coronavirus disease 2019 crisis as catalyst for telemedicine for chronic neurological disorders. *JAMA Neurol.* 2020;77(8):927–928. https://doi.org/10.1001/jamaneurol.2020.1452.

237. Cummings C, Almallouhi E, Kasab SA, Spiotta AM, Holmstedt CA. Blacks are less likely to present with strokes during the COVID-19 pandemic. *Stroke.* 2020;51(10):3107–3111. https://doi.org/10.1161/STROKEAHA.120.031121.

238. Dmytriw AA, Phan K, Schirmer C, et al. Ischaemic stroke associated with COVID-19 and racial outcome disparity in North America. *J Neurol Neurosurg Psychiatry.* 2020;91(12):1362–1364. https://doi.org/10.1136/jnnp-2020-324653.

239. Aboul Nour H, Affan M, Mohamed G, et al. Impact of the COVID-19 pandemic on acute stroke care, time metrics, outcomes, and racial disparities in a Southeast Michigan Health System. *J Stroke Cerebrovasc Dis.* 2021;30(6):105746. https://doi.org/10.1016/j.jstrokecerebrovasdis.2021.105746.

CHAPTER 2

Neuropathogenesis of SARS-CoV-2 Infection

INSHA ZAHOOR • MIRELA CERGHET • SHAILENDRA GIRI
Department of Neurology, Henry Ford Hospital, Detroit, MI, United States

INTRODUCTION

The severe acute respiratory syndrome coronavirus 2 (SARS-CoV-2) is responsible for causing the novel coronavirus disease 2019 (COVID-19) that became a global concern after it emerged from Wuhan, China in December 2019.[1] Its high community transmission propelled its spread across several countries, gripping the world in a major health crisis that was eventually declared a pandemic by the World Health Organization (WHO). The ongoing pandemic of COVID-19 has presented new challenges to scientists. Currently, there is a lack of information about the different aspects of SARS-CoV-2 to enable researchers worldwide to understand the virus as they race to find an effective vaccine. With each passing day, new features are being unraveled about its behavior, and new information gathered as the virus evolves across different populations. While there is no specific treatment available, those employed are based on prior experience from other viral infections and depend on the severity of the case being presented.[2] Clinical and epidemiological findings have revealed that some patients are asymptomatic, and others have mild symptoms such as fever, fatigue, sore throat, and dry cough, and recover on minimal medical intervention. In contrast, many others show rapid deterioration and develop complications that include gastrointestinal, cardiovascular, dermatologic, and neurological disturbances, along with respiratory, renal, and liver dysfunction, which can lead to sepsis, encephalitis, and death.[3-7]

There is a soaring mortality rate associated with SARS-CoV-2 infection, and the number of infected cases is still rising across different parts of the world. Based on the hospital admission data, epidemiologists have reported that elderly patients and people of any age with underlying comorbidities are highly susceptible to the complications associated with COVID-19.[8-10]

These comorbid conditions include hypertension, cardiovascular disease, diabetes, chronic respiratory disease, liver disease, hemoglobin disorders, cancer, renal disease, neurological diseases, and obesity and may affect disease outcomes.[3, 11-15] Indeed there is concern that patients on immunosuppressive therapies for inflammatory conditions such as multiple sclerosis (MS), neuromyelitis optica spectrum disorder (NMOSD), myasthenia gravis, and chronic inflammatory demyelinating polyneuropathy (CIDP) may have a higher risk of infection or develop a severe COVID-19.[16, 17] However, data is lacking and so far there is no supporting evidence. Overall, these comorbid conditions lead to a weakened immune state, which decreases the ability to fight the viral infection. Given the robust immune response incurred by the virus, it is currently unclear if treatment with specific immunomodulators that are used to treat chronic autoimmune disorders predisposes patients to severe SARS-CoV-2 infection, or protects the host by dampening immune cell activation.

A peculiar feature of COVID-19 is the heterogeneous spectrum of clinical manifestations that affect different organ systems.[18] It appears that SARS-CoV-2 primarily starts as an infection in the upper respiratory tract, which then moves to the lower respiratory tract from where it can also invade the nervous system.[19] Hospitalization data strongly suggests that the neurological symptoms of the SARS-CoV-2 cannot be overlooked, yet there is a huge debate regarding the neurological impact of the virus. In this chapter, we provide an overview of studies that assessed the neuroinvasive potential of COVID-19 and discuss possible neuropathogenic mechanisms used by SARS-CoV-2 to invade the nervous system. As we grapple with the effects of this novel virus and the unique challenges of diagnosing and managing COVID-19, it is critical that all of the effects of this novel virus on the nervous system are considered so that these can be better managed and the outcomes of individuals infected with the virus can be improved.

THE NEUROINVASIVE POTENTIAL OF CORONAVIRUSES (COV)

To understand the neuroinvasiveness of coronaviruses (CoV), it is essential to consider their structural features. The electron microscopic structure of CoV appears as an enveloped particle having a spherical, oval, or pleomorphic crown-like shape with a diameter ranging between 80 and 120 nm.[20] These structural features are encoded by the genome of CoV, which is comprised of a single-stranded nonsegmented positive-sense RNA of about 27–32 kb. The entire genome is bound by the nucleocapsid (N) protein to form a helical symmetric nucleocapsid.[20, 21] The surface is coated with large projections of membrane glycoproteins, termed spike (S) proteins, and some CoV even have shorter projections of the hemagglutinin-esterase (HE) protein.[21] The S protein is the primary facilitator for entry into the host cell by mediating binding to target receptors present on the cellular surface.[22] The outer viral envelope contains the membrane (M) and envelope (E) proteins. The M protein is a type III transmembrane glycoprotein that helps maintain the CoV conformation and antigenicity, whereas the E protein acts as an ion-channeling viroporin that is involved in envelope formation, budding, and pathogenesis, and interacts with other CoV proteins and host proteins.[23] The N protein interacts with the M protein to stabilize the assembly of envelope complexes during the formation of new viral particles.[24] Together, each of these four key structural proteins (N, S, E, M) confer unique properties to CoV for invading the host and spreading the infection to different tissues.[21-24]

SARS-CoV-2 is the newest addition to the beta-CoV genus as the seventh member of the family of human CoV (HCoV), which consists of respiratory viruses including HCoV-229E (named after a student specimen coded 229E), HCoV-OC43 (organ culture 43), HCoV-NL63 (NetherLand 63), HCoV-HKU1 (Hong Kong University 1), SARS-CoV (severe acute respiratory syndrome), and MERS-CoV (Middle East respiratory syndrome).[25-27] The genomic data of SARS-CoV-2 shows sequence similarity of 79%–80% to SARS-CoV, 50% to MERS-CoV, and the highest similarity of 96% to a bat family of CoV.[28, 29] SARS-CoV, MERS-CoV, and SARS-CoV-2 cause a severe respiratory illness that hints toward their lethal nature, making them highly pathogenic. At the same time, other members of the family

have been associated with a mild or moderate form of respiratory disease. To understand the neuropathogenesis of novel SARS-CoV-2 infection, it is important to familiarize ourselves with the impact of other members of the CoV family on the nervous system and what is known from past experience with SARS and MERS, the relevant aspects of which are included here.

Several reports have shown neurovirulence of CoV in pediatric and adult cases with no evidence for a direct link.[30, 31] In a study by Li et al. cytokine profiles were determined in the central nervous system (CNS) and respiratory tract of hospitalized pediatric cases with CNS illness and CoV infection.[32] Cytokine profiling in the serum showed significantly higher granulocyte colony-stimulating factor (G-CSF) in individuals infected with CoV that had complications in the CNS or respiratory tract, compared to healthy subjects, although levels were markedly higher in those with CNS complications. Further, the levels of cytokines such as interleukins (IL-6, IL-8), monocyte chemoattractant protein-1 (MCP-1), and granulocyte-macrophage colony-stimulating factor (GM-CSF) were significantly higher in the cerebrospinal fluid (CSF) of patients with CNS infection relative to levels in the serum. It is noteworthy that this report was the first to have found a high incidence of CoV infection in pediatric cases with CNS illness, showing characteristic cytokine profiles in the CSF, which suggests the host immune response, plays a role in the progression of the infection and its associated complications.

Similarly, multiple reports suggest an association of CoV infection with chronic CNS diseases, including MS, encephalitis, acute flaccid paralysis, Guillain-Barré syndrome (GBS), acute disseminated encephalomyelitis (ADEM), hemorrhage, seizures, and stroke.[30, 33–41] The initial reports on SARS patients have shown evidence of SARS-CoV infection in neurons in the brain, as detected by the presence of viral particles and genetic material using electron microscopy, immunohistochemistry, and polymerase chain reaction (PCR).[42-46] Interestingly, autopsy reports of SARS patients have also shown cerebral edema and meningeal vasodilation, as well as virus-infiltrated monocytes and lymphocytes in the vessel wall, viral particles in the brain, and changes in neurons with demyelinating nerve fibers.[43, 47] Clinical findings have found that SARS-CoV can even cause neurological complications such as encephalitis, axonopathic polyneuropathy, myopathy or rhabdomyolysis, aortic ischemic stroke, and olfactory neuropathy.[48, 49] The neuroinvasive potential of MERS-CoV was shown in a retrospective study in which 25.7% of infected patients developed confusion, and

8.6% had seizures.[50] Another study found a delayed appearance of neurological features after the presentation of respiratory symptoms in 20% of patients with MERS, including disturbances in consciousness, neuropathy, ischemic stroke, paralysis, and GBS.[51] Inoculation of SARS-CoV and MERS-CoV in transgenic mice through the intranasal route has revealed the ability of these viruses to infect brain areas such as the thalamus and brainstem through olfactory nerves.[32, 44, 45] The mice induced with low doses of MERS-CoV showed that the viral particles were confined to the brain region only, not lungs, strongly hinting that neuroinvasion-induced mortality in the infected mice.[32]

Despite the neurological impact, the exact route of infection used by SARS-CoV and MERS-CoV for neuroinvasion in humans is unknown. Studies suggest that the hematogenous or lymphatic route of infection does not play a significant role in driving initial CNS infection due to the absence of virus in nonneuronal cells in the infected areas of the brain.[42, 43, 46] Some studies suggest that CoV may invade the CNS through a synaptic route by infecting the peripheral nerve terminals.[52, 53] Although the exact mechanisms by which CoV affects the nervous system remain unclear, the above findings demonstrate that infection with SARS-CoV and MERS-CoV is associated with neurological manifestations and complications, which support recent findings of brain invasion in patients infected with SARS-CoV-2.

THE NEUROINVASIVE POTENTIAL OF SARS-COV-2

There is limited knowledge about the emergence of SARS-CoV-2; however, it is believed that it evolved from other CoV such as SARS-CoV and/or MERS-CoV through a series of mutagenic events. As such, it behaves similarly to these viruses in terms of its pathogenicity, structure, and route of infection.[28, 54, 55] Given the evidence that SARS-CoV and MERS-CoV are neurotropic viruses, this suggests the same may be true of SARS-CoV-2. Epidemiological findings show that the median duration of disease progression from the onset of illness was 5 days to dyspnea, 7 days to hospital admission, and 8 days to the intensive care unit.[56] Notably, this latency period is likely long enough for viral particles to invade the nervous system and damage the neurons.[6, 57, 58]

The effect of SARS-CoV-2 on the nervous system can be gauged at three levels: symptoms arising due to viral infection, collateral effect on the nervous system from the immune response to the virus, and complications in patients with neurological comorbidities. It has now become clear that in addition to having a major impact on the respiratory and cardiovascular systems, it also affects the nervous system. Altogether, the clinical and experimental studies report commonly observed manifestations and postinfection complications that clearly reflect neurovirulence in COVID-19, including headache, stroke, nausea, dizziness, vomiting, disturbed olfaction, seizures, disturbed sensorium, altered consciousness, ataxia, encephalopathy/encephalitis, hypogeusia, hypoplasia, neuralgia, myelitis, and skeletal muscle symptoms.[5, 6, 11, 56, 59–64] Findings from some of the major studies highlighting the neurological impact of SARS-CoV-2 infection are summarized in Table 2.1 and will be further detailed throughout this volume.

Additional neurologic complications have been reported in studies of infected patients with SARS-CoV-2 that have used neuroimaging with computerized tomography (CT) and magnetic resonance imaging (MRI) along with electroencephalogram (EEG) data. These have reported hemorrhagic necrotizing encephalopathy, epileptogenicity, and encephalomalacia, which could be the outcome of the severe cytokine storm observed in some COVID-19 cases.[71, 72] There have also been reports of a temporary loss of speech, confusion, lethargy, and signs of disorientation, with brain scans showing injury to the thalamus accompanied by hemorrhage and necrotizing encephalopathy.[86, 87] Even though there are only a few reports confirming that the neurovirulence in COVID-19 is primarily linked to encephalitis and meningitis, its lethal impact cannot be underlooked.

As will be discussed in more detail in Chapter 10, there is also mounting evidence of changes in olfaction and taste in SARS-CoV-2-infected patients, and in some cases, patients have experienced a bitter taste while fighting off the infection. This sets the basis for anosmia and dysgeusia observed in some infected patients, possibly due to reduced sensitivity of neurosensory reflexes by SARS-CoV-2.[70, 88, 89] This is partially supported by data from experimental animals infected with SARS-CoV or MERS-CoV, where olfactory nerves were shown as a route of brain invasion.[44, 45, 90]

Several reports indicate the presence of virus particles in various parts of the nervous system, such as the brain and CSF, which could incur damage. To this end, a putative route of infection of the brain by SARS-CoV-2 has been proposed, and it is suggested that isolating viral particles from the endothelium of cerebral microcirculation, CSF, glial cells, and neuronal tissue would serve as confirmatory evidence for the neurotrophic potential of SARS-CoV-2.[19] Pathological findings from postmortem analysis of COVID-19 patients

TABLE 2.1
Major Studies[a] Reporting Neurological Manifestations of SARS-CoV-2.

Study	Neurological Findings	Sample Size
Mao et al.[59]	Dizziness, headache, hypogeusia, hyposmia, impaired consciousness, ischemic stroke, cerebral hemorrhage, and skeletal muscle injury	214
Li et al.[60]	Acute ischemic stroke and intracerebral hemorrhage	219
Chen et al.[65]	Disturbed consciousness	113
Helms et al.[61]	Encephalopathy, ischemic stroke, dysexecutive syndrome, corticospinal tract signs, agitation, and confusion	58
Varatharaj et al.[66]	Ischemic stroke, intracerebral hemorrhage, CNS vasculitis, unspecified encephalopathy, encephalitis, and altered mental status	125
Xiang et al.[67]	Encephalitis	1
Ye et al.[68]	Encephalitis	1
Coolen et al.[69]	Hemorrhagic lesions, posterior reversible encephalopathy syndrome-related brain lesions, and asymmetric olfactory bulbs	19
Giacomelli et al.[70]	Dysgeusia, hyposmia, anosmia, and ageusia	59
Filatov et al.[71]	Encephalopathy	1
Poyiadji et al.[72]	Acute hemorrhagic necrotizing encephalopathy	1
Alkeridy[73]	Delirium	1
Benameur et al.[74]	Encephalopathy and encephalitis	3
Moriguchi et al.[75]	Meningitis/encephalitis	1
Oxley et al.[76]	Large-vessel stroke	5
Tun et al.[77]	Acute ischemic stroke	4
Avula et al.[78]	Acute stroke	4
Gutierrez-Ortiz et al.[79]	Miller-Fisher syndrome and polyneuritis cranialis	2
Virani et al.[80]	Guillain-Barre syndrome	1
Padroni et al.[81]	Guillain-Barre syndrome	1
Zhao et al.[82]	Guillain-Barre syndrome	1
Farhadian et al.[83]	Encephalopathy and seizures	1
Parsons et al.[84]	Acute disseminated encephalomyelitis	1
Zhang et al.[85]	Acute disseminated encephalomyelitis	1

[a]This table covers some main studies on neuroinvasion by SARS-CoV-2, which were published till July 2020.

have shown neurodegeneration and edema in the brain tissue.[91] The first report of viral encephalitis that appeared to be the result of direct SARS-CoV-2 invasion of the brain was reported from China's Beijing Ditan Hospital, where the presence of the virus was revealed in the CSF of a patient by PCR-based genome sequencing.[67] Similarly, imaging data on brain autopsies of 19 cases have shown brain lesions in eight patients, which were related to hemorrhagic and posterior reversible encephalopathy syndrome.[69] Taken together, these observations point to a viral-mediated blood-brain barrier (BBB) disruption, enhancing its permeability and thus contributing to the localized edema and inflammatory response seen within the parenchyma. Further, it has not yet been fully discerned if respiratory failure in COVID-19 is linked to the neurovirulence potential of SARS-CoV-2.[92] Thus, continued investigation to determine the causes of these neurological symptoms is required in order to fully understand the overall effects of SARS-CoV-2.

Intriguingly, dysregulated metabolism at a neuropeptide and neurotransmitter level has also been linked to disease severity in COVID-19 patients.[93, 94] Proteomic and metabolic alterations have been reported in the sera of severe cases of COVID-19 that were linked to serotonin, kynurenine, tryptophan, and polyamine pathways.[93] These findings have also highlighted the role of platelets in SARS-CoV-2 infection, which was in consensus with clinical studies showing complications in coagulopathy and delirium, with a possible link to altered neurotransmitters like serotonin.[73, 95] Similarly, aberrations in the biosynthesis of the neurotransmitter dopamine have also been linked with certain pathophysiological processes of SARS-CoV-2.[96] Considering the neurovirulence of SARS-CoV-2 infection, it is unclear if metabolic alterations occur in the peripheral blood circulation, and if altered metabolites cross the BBB and impact the nervous system. A recent study has performed metabolite profiling in the CSF and in blood samples from severe SARS-CoV-2 infection cases and delirium-prone patients,[97] which provides clues into the altered brain metabolism observed in these patients. This demonstrated a significant difference in the concentrations of metabolites such as acylcarnitines and polyamines, particularly phenethylamine (PEA) between the CSF and blood in delirium-prone patients compared to healthy controls. The observed difference was linked to altered activity of the enzyme monoamine oxidase B (MAOB) that is involved in platelet regulation and coagulation and in the metabolism of neurotransmitters, with known association with delirium, anosmia, neuropsychiatric disorders, and neurodegenerative diseases.[98–105] Notably, the computational structural analysis showed significant similarity between the angiotensin-converting enzyme 2 (ACE2), which mediates the entry of SARS-CoV-2 into host cells, and MAOB, with 95% similarity observed in the SARS-CoV-2 spike protein binding region of ACE2. This suggests that SARS-CoV-2 interacts with MAOB through its spike protein and alters its activity at the molecular level, setting up the ground for neurological complications in COVID-19.

To find promising drug targets for treating SARS-CoV-2, it is crucial to understand the mechanisms of neuroinvasion by the virus and the impact it has on the nervous system. It will also be interesting to explore the interactions between the BBB and SARS-CoV-2 proteins in gaining access to the nervous system. Thus far, there has been no evidence of direct meningeal invasion of SARS-CoV-2, making it unclear if reported neurological features, such as headache or encephalopathy, are a consequence of the systemic inflammatory response

or are secondary to CNS investment by the virus.[106] It is also possible that respiratory muscle injury and/or reduced sensorium may be responsible for the observed respiratory failure in COVID-19 patients.[107] In light of the possible involvement of the neuromuscular system in COVID-19 patients, neurophysiological assessment should be included in patients that present with the disease.[107] Ultimately, understanding the neuroinvasive propensity of SARS-CoV-2 may provide clues for the treatment and prevention of COVID-19 transmissions.

MECHANISMS OF NEUROINVASION AND NEUROPATHOLOGY BY SARS-COV-2

Despite the neurotropic behavior of CoV,[16] the precise route of neuroinvasion has not yet been elucidated. There is not much known about the specific mechanism of nervous system invasion by SARS-CoV-2, which compels for a comprehensive investigation into viral-host interactions. However, based on the structural similarity and sequence homology of SARS-CoV-2 to SARS-CoV and MERS-CoV, it is expected to show similar neurotropism and adopt similar pathogenic mechanisms for invading the nervous system.[28, 54, 106, 108–110] Uncovering the specific signatures of SARS-CoV-2 infection and the precise mechanisms responsible for its neurovirulence in COVID-19 will help guide the rapid development of target-based antibodies and drugs. Thus far, anecdotal observations have put forth postulated mechanisms responsible for neuroinvasion by SARS-Co-V-2 and the consequent neuropathological damage to the nervous system. Accordingly, mechanisms of SARS-CoV-2 neuropathogenesis seem multifactorial, for which we have provided a comprehensive summary from the literature published so far in this regard.

Involvement of the Angiotensin-Converting Enzyme 2 (ACE2) Receptor

It is already established that receptor-mediated endocytosis is one of the most common mechanisms used by viruses such as SARS-CoV to enter into the host system.[45, 111, 112] The primary mechanism used by SARS-CoV-2 for entry into human host cells is potentially through binding of the S1 protein to the entry receptor, ACE2, which is present on the surface of target cells. Subsequently, using host enzyme transmembrane serine protease 2 (TMPRSS2) or furin, the cleavage sites on the S protein are broken for priming and fusion of host and viral membranes.[109, 113, 114] The binding of the virus to the ACE2 receptor is followed by its internalization into the host cell, where it releases its RNA into the cytoplasm, which is followed by the multiplication of new viral particles that are subsequently released in the bloodstream.[19] Goblet and ciliated ACE2-expressing nasal epithelial cells act as portals for SARS-CoV-2.[115] The binding affinity of the SARS-CoV-2 S protein with ACE2 was found to be significantly higher (10- to 20-fold) than the S protein of the SARS-CoV.[114] Also, pair-wise sequence alignments have shown high similarity between the sequences of S proteins of SARS-CoV-2 and sequences from other CoV which could explain the high binding affinity of the SARS-CoV-2 S protein to the ACE2 receptor present on human cells.

ACE2 is broadly expressed on the cellular epithelia of airways, oral mucosa, nasal mucosa, nasopharynx, lungs, kidneys, spleen, liver, stomach, small intestine, colon, cardiac tissues, nervous system (glial cells and spinal neurons), vascular endothelium, lymph nodes, monocytes, macrophages, thymus, and skeletal system.[116–119] It acts as a cardio-cerebral vascular protection factor by regulating hypertension and antiatherosclerotic mechanisms through negative regulation of the renin-angiotensin system (RAS). Specifically, ACE2 cleaves the active forms of angiotensin (Ang I and Ang II) to generate inactive nonapeptide Ang1-9 and heptapeptide Ang1-7, respectively.[120] Ang II plays a key role in driving vasoconstriction, the pathogenesis of cardiovascular diseases, and oxidative stress by binding to the angiotensin II receptor type 1 (AT1R); however, its cleavage changes it into an inactive form that counteracts the negative effects of the ACE/AngII/AT1R axis.[121, 122] When ACE2 acts as an entry receptor for SARS-CoV-2, its internalization downregulates its function, making it unavailable to confer protection afforded by Ang II cleavage. Accordingly, loss of ACE2 can be detrimental to the normal function of the cardiocerebral system, leading to the dysregulation of RAS, making SARS-CoV-2-infected patients more susceptible to complications such as headaches.[123]

Viral attachment to ACE2 can damage neuronal tissue, which can have far-reaching consequences on the nervous system. The viral attack may also destroy ACE2 receptors and the endothelial lining of capillaries, leading to vasodilation, increasing the luminal pressure of cerebral vessels, and thus, the risk of a cerebral hemorrhage.[110] It can also invade the CNS by targeting the vascular system and damaging the BBB, causing viral encephalitis.[19] The damage to cerebral capillaries by the direct viral attack can also result in bleeding that can be fatal for infected SARS-CoV-2 patients.[19] It may even activate the trigeminovascular pathway, which can cause headaches.[123] Similarly, the binding of SARS-CoV-2 to spinal cord membranes through ACE2 can lead to myelitis. The dysfunction of ACE2/Ang1-7/Mas receptor

axis has been reported in various conditions such as stroke, cognitive decline, pain, Alzheimer's disease, and Parkinson's disease.[124, 125] The enhanced expression of AT1R in the autopsied brain tissue of Alzheimer's and aged Parkinson's patients has been linked with neuroinflammation due to the impact of AT1R signaling on dopaminergic neurons. Also, reports have linked a decline in cognitive impairment and improved synaptic transmission with inhibition of the AT1R signaling axis. Based on these findings, the interaction of viral particles with the ACE2 receptor may partly explain some of the neurological manifestations of SARS-CoV-2 infection.

ACE2 is also a primary receptor for cell attachment and invasion by CoV and influenza viruses.[111, 112, 114] However, MERS-CoV attaches to target cells through dipeptidyl peptidase 4 (DPP4, also known as CD26), which is expressed on the epithelia of the lower respiratory tract, small intestine, liver, kidney, and immune cells.[126, 127] It is noteworthy that neither the ACE2 nor DPP4 receptor alone is sufficient for attachment and host infectivity, as some reports have found no infection by SARS-CoV or MERS-CoV in ACE2 expressing cell lines (endothelial and intestinal cells). Conversely, infection was reported in hepatocytes or cells of the CNS expressing ACE2 or DPP4 in insignificant levels.[128–131] Thus, the gaps in our understanding of the ACE2 receptor and its function in the neuropathological consequences of SARS-CoV-2 infection call for in-depth analysis of this interaction.

Direct Injury Upon SARS-CoV-2 Infection Through CNS Invasion

The detection of viral genetic material and proteins in CSF and brain samples strongly indicate the neurotropic potential of such viruses to directly invade the nervous system.[132] The first case of viral encephalitis by SARS-CoV-2, reported from China's Beijing Ditan Hospital, suggests it directly invaded the brain. The virus was detected in the CSF of a patient by PCR-based genome sequencing,[67] and was further supported by another report from Japan.[75] In this study, the authors detected the virus in the CSF of a patient with meningitis, but without isolation of the virus in a nasopharyngeal swab, raising the possibility that infection occurred as a result of direct invasion of the nervous system.[75] These reports raise the possibility that the virus can spread from the respiratory tract to the nervous system, which has made the neuroinvasive potential of SARS-CoV-2 the focus of many discussions worldwide.

There can be several routes by which SARS-CoV-2 can invade the CNS, the diagrammatic representation

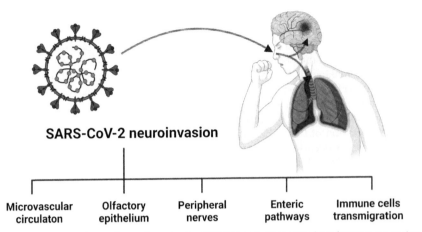

SARS-CoV-2 neuroinvasion

| Microvascular circulaton | Olfactory epithelium | Peripheral nerves | Enteric pathways | Immune cells transmigration |

FIG. 2.1 Possible mechanisms of neuroinvasion by SARS-CoV-2. Viral entry into the nervous system is mediated by different routes of transmission: Microvascular transmission involves the interaction of the virus with the entry receptor, ACE2, present on the endothelial cells of BBB, allowing it to gain entry into the CNS; the intranasal route of neuroinvasion occurs through olfactory receptor neurons present in the olfactory epithelium of the nasal cavity; transsynaptic mode of transmission through peripheral nerves; the gut-brain axis can serve as an alternate route for viral infection of the nervous system through enterocytes; and immune cells such as monocytes/macrophages and activated T lymphocytes infected by the virus can cross the BBB and infect nerve cells (Created with BioRender.com (2020); https://app.biorender.com).

of which is given in Fig. 2.1. Neuronal pathways hold significance for spreading the viral infection from the periphery to the nervous system, particularly for viruses with neuroinvasive potential. These can include hematogenous and retrograde or anterograde transport via motor proteins, dynein, and kinesins that may involve sensory or motor nerve endings.[133, 134] The hematogenous route involves direct infection of endothelial cells of the BBB, or epithelial cells of the blood-CSF barrier in the choroid plexus, as well as manipulation of the innate immune system by inflammatory cells that manage to gain access into the CNS in a process called myeloid cell trafficking. This involves transcytosis via endocytic vesicles across the brain microvascular endothelial cells and pericytes.[30, 134]

1) Microvascular Route: Ultrastructural analysis of autopsied brains using transmission electron microscopy has identified viral particles in neural and capillary endothelial cells in frontal lobe sections of the brain (not CSF) by RT-PCR. This supports the theory that SARS-CoV-2 harbors neurovirulence and indicates the possibility that it uses a hematogenous route to invade the brain.[135] Indeed, several reports have suggested that the neurotropism of SARS-CoV-2 is due to its ability to cross the BBB by a hematogenous route that involves the microvascular circulation.[19, 32, 46, 136–140] The slow flow of blood in capillaries aids in receptor-virus interaction followed by viral budding from the endothelium

and its entry in the brain where it interacts with ACE2 receptor on neurons. The resulting damage to the capillary endothelium and neurons leads to its dissemination across the nervous system. Currently, there is not enough evidence to support the ability of SARS-CoV-2 to invade the CNS through a vascular route involving microvascular endothelial cells of BBB as these have minimal or no expression of ACE2 or DPP4. Despite that, some reports have still observed infectivity by other viruses such as SARS-CoV and MERS-CoV.[128–131] Also, ACE2 and CD209L receptors have been found to facilitate the entry of SARS-CoV into the CNS.[30, 132, 141] Given these observations, the vascular route remains a possible mechanism for neuroinvasion by SARS-CoV-2.

2) Olfactory Nerve Route: Alternative to a vascular route of infection, other reports have suggested SARS-CoV-2 mediates neuroinvasion through retrograde axonal transport. In this context, the virus is likely to travel from axon terminals down the axon to the neuron cell bodies located in the CNS and would typically involve olfactory or respiratory neurons, or those of the enteric nervous system. In particular, afferent nerve endings of the vagus nerve from the lungs may be targeted.[30, 35, 36, 43, 54, 107, 134, 142, 143] Similar to the mechanism used by the influenza A virus, SARS-CoV-2 may pass the olfactory network via receptor neurons across the cribriform plate of the ethmoid bone to either the olfactory bulb situated in the forebrain, the trigeminal nerves which

reside in the nasal cavity, or sensory fibers of the vagus nerve in the brain stem.[30, 35, 36, 43, 134, 143] The anatomical features of the nasal cavity and the forebrain connect the nasal epithelium with the CNS through the olfactory bulb and nerves, making viral entry into the brain possible through the olfactory tract.[30, 132, 143] This route of transport via olfactory neurons appears to be more efficient for invasion due to its close proximity to the brain and the expression of the ACE2 receptor on olfactory cilia cells, as has been found in patients with MERS-CoV infection and which is somewhat supported by signs of anosmia and hyposmia in COVID-19 patients.[59, 90] Animal experiments on CoV have demonstrated that they can reach the brain and CSF within 7 days through the olfactory bulb and nerves (olfactory epithelium or cribriform bone), resulting in CNS inflammation and demyelination.[44, 45, 90] Notably, the removal of the olfactory bulb in mice limited the entry of the virus into the CNS.[35] In C57BL/6J mice, the host receptors for SARS-CoV-2, ACE2, and TMPRSS2, are expressed in sustentacular cells of the olfactory epithelium, but only minimal or no expression of these is observed in olfactory receptor neurons.[144] This provides additional evidence that SARS-CoV-2 can utilize the olfactory route for infection, which could explain the disturbing olfaction in infected patients. Of note, expression of these receptors was increased in older animals, which is consistent with an increased vulnerability to SARS-CoV-2 infection in elderly patients. Higher expression of ACE2 in murine olfactory epithelium compared to the respiratory epithelium was also shown in this study. However, the mechanism behind the spread of SARS-CoV-2 from the olfactory epithelium to olfactory receptor neurons requires continued investigation. If this finding holds true in humans, the olfactory epithelium may be a potential source of tissue in which to detect SARS-CoV-2 in the early stages of infection, and in individuals who are asymptomatic, potentially reducing the rate of false negatives.[144]

3) Peripheral Nerve Route: Another possible route by which SARS-CoV-2 may gain access to the CNS is through a transsynaptic mode of transmission involving retrograde neuronal transport across axons into the medulla oblongata, through synapses connected to peripheral nerve terminals of the respiratory network, as found in rats injected with hemagglutinating encephalomyelitis virus (HEV).[52, 53] Through this route, SARS-CoV-2 can spread to the medullary cardiorespiratory center from the mechanoreceptors and chemoreceptors in the lung and lower respiratory airways.[54] 4) Enteric Pathway: Additionally, the gut-brain axis has been postulated as an alternate door for neuroinvasion

by SARS-CoV-2, as enterocytes send signals through the enteric nervous system, including sympathetic afferent fibers based on observations such as the relatively higher expression of the ACE2 receptor on enterocytes lining the gastrointestinal tract compared to the cells of the lungs, worse outcomes in infected patients with digestive symptoms and acute respiratory distress, and the ability of viral infection and replication in intestinal cells.[142, 145] Based on prior observations for other viruses, the exosomal transport pathway is also considered as a presumed route for systemic dissemination and CNS invasion by SARS-CoV-2, to which there is no confirmatory evidence so far.[146] 5) Immune Cell Transmigration Route: Finally, SARS-CoV-2 may invade the CNS through the cellular route of peripheral immune cell transmigration, as is known for MERS-CoV infection. In this case, once peripheral myeloid immune cells (monocytes and macrophages) are infected by the virus, they act as a viral reservoir, spreading the viruses to distant tissues by crossing the BBB.[30, 147–149]

The lack of major histocompatibility complex antigens, the dense parenchymal structure of the brain, and the unique homeostatic features of nerve cells, together with the presence of nonpermeable blood vessels in the CNS enable these cells to avoid death while maintaining the survival of viral particles.[150, 151] Viral entry into the CNS involves modulating the BBB by cytokines to increase its permeability, augmenting its direct entry into the brain.[152] Overall, there are multiple potential mechanisms by which SARS-CoV-2 invades the nervous system. Despite the route used for invasion, once the virus finds access to CNS, it can infect brain cells, such as astrocytes and microglia, leading to activation of immune cells that produce inflammatory mediators, cytokines, chemokines, and free radicals, thus triggering a cascade of neuroinflammation and neurodegeneration.

Molecular Mimicry

Once SARS-CoV-2 infection occurs, there are chances of a virus-induced autoreactive process that may cause autoimmunity, as has been reported for other CoV infections, including SARS-CoV and MERS-CoV.[49, 51] The most widely debated mechanism for this autoreactive process is that of molecular mimicry, similar to that observed in SARS, where T-cell receptors (TCR) specific for viral epitopes cross-react to normal host epitopes (self-antigens) with similar molecular patterns and elicit an unwanted autoimmune response.[153, 154] The antibodies produced in response to an immune reaction against viral proteins might show cross-reactivity against self-proteins, generating an acute autoimmune reaction. The rapid and robust activation of the innate and acquired immune systems leading to a hyper-inflammatory response upon SARS-CoV-2 infection supports this response and could be a reason for the neurological complications observed in COVID-19 patients.[155–157] Epidemiological and clinical reports have suggested the course of the disease worsens in the presence of comorbid conditions. This could be due to heightened stress on endothelial cells, somehow favoring molecular mimicry as seen during the infective process.[158–162]

The absence of detectable virus in the CSF samples from patients infected with SARS-CoV-2 who present with neurological symptoms supports an indirect role of virus-induced autoimmunity that contributes to neurological manifestations.[83] A recent study has shown the presence of autoantibodies against CNS antigens in the serum and CSF of 11 patients with severe COVID-19 accompanied with neurological symptoms.[163] They also observed increased levels of neurofilament light chain, which reflects signs of inflammation in the CSF, providing evidence for virus-induced autoimmunity. A current hypothesis in the field is that molecular mimicry, together with hypoxia and systemic inflammatory response, leads to a raging cytokine storm syndrome in patients, which could be responsible for increased disease severity and additional complications such as acute pulmonary embolism, microvascular thrombosis, disseminated intravascular coagulation (DIC), and multiple organ dysfunction.[158, 164] In support of this, one of the neurological complications of SARS-CoV-2 is GBS, the pathogenesis of which involves molecular mimicry to elicit an autoimmune response.[165, 166] In addition, other mechanisms of neuropathology due to virus-induced CNS autoimmunity may involve bystander activation of immune cells and epitope spreading.[167] Further work, therefore, is needed to explore the role of human epitopes of self-proteins in an autoimmune response, as these could be targeted for vaccine development and drug design to treat COVID-19.[158]

Immune-Mediated Injury by Cytokine Storm

In addition to the virus-induced inflammatory rampage that causes immunopathological changes in the lungs, the exaggerated immune response in the body that is caused by viral infections can severely damage the nervous system.[168] Several viral infections, including CoV that cause severe pneumonia, have been linked to the development of an overly robust immune response in the form of systemic inflammatory response syndrome (SIRS). The viral-induced cytokine storm observed in SARS-CoV and SARS-CoV-2 infections has resulted in higher mortality due

to multiple organ dysfunction.[65, 169] In this context, early intervention using antiinflammatory drugs may reduce damage to the nervous system.[170, 171] This is in part because SARS-CoV-2 infection is believed to indirectly damage the nervous system by causing a massive inflammatory response in the host that results in a surge in the production of proinflammatory cytokines, recruitment of proinflammatory macrophages and granulocytes to CNS, aberrant activation of macrophages, and induction of chemokine/cytokine response, termed as the "cytokine storm" syndrome.[155, 172] These events are suggestive of macrophage activation syndrome (MAS) or of secondary hemophagocytic lymphohistiocytosis (sHLH), as is observed in histological profiles from autopsies of COVID-19 patients, potentially due to an imbalance in immune responses leading to tissue damage.[171, 173] Notably, the infected monocytes, macrophages, microglia, astrocytes, endothelial cells, and weakened BBB play a crucial role in inducing a proinflammatory state inside the brain, thereby causing chronic inflammation and damage to the nervous system in the form of acute necrotizing encephalopathy.[72, 174]

Immunological profiling of SARS-CoV-2-infected patients has shown a positive correlation between the production of a cytokine storm with the severity and progression of ARDS, and fatality. Severely ill COVID-19 patients and those requiring intensive care have shown elevated levels of alanine aminotransferase (ALT), lactate dehydrogenase (LDH), C-reactive protein (CRP), ferritin, D-dimer, TNF-α, IL-1, IL-2, IL-6, IL-7, IL-8, IL-4, IL-10, IL-2R, IL-1B, interferon-gamma (IFN-γ)-induced protein 10 (IP-10), G-CSF, MCP-1, MCP-3, macrophage inflammatory protein 1-alpha (MIP-1-A), and MIP-1B.[4, 6, 155, 172, 175–178] There are also reports of immune dysregulation by SARS-CoV-2 that primarily affects T lymphocytes, such as a significant reduction in the numbers of CD4 + and CD8 + T cells (lymphopenia) and a decrease in IFN-γ production by CD4 + T cells, particularly in severe cases where intensive care is required as opposed to more moderate cases. Similarly, a decrease in type-1 IFN response in severely ill patients has also been observed for SARS-CoV.[4, 179–181] These events may reduce the control of viral replication and further enhance the production of proinflammatory cytokines, particularly TNF-α, IL-6, and IL-10, potentiating virus-induced injury.[157] These reports demonstrate that TNF-α- and IL-6-driven inflammatory responses, along with an impaired type-1 IFN response are hallmarks of severe cases of COVID-19.

In addition to driving inflammation, the elevated levels of these inflammatory cytokines can have other detrimental consequences. TNF-α may also cause apoptosis in T cells by interacting with TNF-receptor 1 (TNFR1) present on their surface.[182, 183] It has been suggested that IL-10, an inhibitory cytokine, can cause T-cell depletion, which may be the reason for the high levels of the T-cell exhaustion markers, programmed cell death protein 1 (PD-1), and T-cell immunoglobulin and mucin-domain containing-3 (Tim-3) in SARS-CoV-2-infected patients.[179] The incessant synthesis of IL-6 may have pathological implications as is observed in chronic inflammation and infection.[184, 185] The overall compounded effect of this hypercytokinemia may, in turn, cause lymphocytopenia, as is being observed in SARS-CoV-2 patients, which can lead to a substantial weakening of the host immune response.[16]

In vitro findings have shown that upon CoV infection, activated glial cells produce elevated levels of proinflammatory cytokines, such as IL-6, IL-2, IL-15, and TNF-α, which, at high enough levels, can cause brain damage.[35] Cytokine dysregulation, particularly IL-6 and TNF-α, has been linked to cytokine storm-mediated encephalitis.[6] Neuroinvasion by SARS-CoV-2 can activate CD4 + T cells, which can stimulate macrophages to produce IL-6, one of the key mediators of cytokine storm, via activation of GM-CSF, thus contributing to MAS. To this end, elevated levels of IL-6 are consistently observed during the course of COVID-19 in nonsurvivors compared to survivors and are positively correlated with disease severity.[4, 10, 13, 65, 110, 155, 176, 186] The increased levels of IL-6 can have pathological implications that can lead to vascular leakage, activation of the complement and coagulation pathways, DIC, and multiple organ failure.[171, 187] The contributions of IL-6 are further made evident by the improved outcomes observed in patients with severe cases of COVID-19 that have also been treated with the IL-6 receptor antagonist, tocilizumab.[188]

The immunological findings of a female patient presenting with seizure and acute encephalopathy have related neurological features to increased neuroinflammation due to a host-mediated immune response, and not neuroinvasion by SARS-CoV-2. Immunological analysis of this patient showed elevated levels of the proinflammatory chemokine MCP-1 in the CSF, but not in the plasma when compared to three control samples; however, there was no evidence of SARS-CoV-2 in the CSF of the patient.[83] Simultaneously, this patient exhibited elevated levels of IL-6, IL-8, and IP-10 in both the CSF and plasma compared to controls. While at present this is an isolated case, it certainly suggests that targeting host inflammatory responses may be a beneficial practice to alleviate many of the complications that arise in tissues other than the respiratory tract.

Additional analysis of serological and inflammatory proteins in CSF samples from SARS-CoV-2-infected patients with neurologic complications such as encephalopathy and encephalitis shows elevated levels of anti-S1 IgM, IL-6, IL-8, IL-10, IP-10, and TNF-α, providing evidence for peri-infectious and/or postinfectious inflammatory changes in the CSF during the course of the disease.[74] Altogether, it seems that the severe complications from SARS-CoV-2 infection are the outcome of a virus-induced cytokine storm that causes immune dysregulation, an altered T-cell response, an aberrant chemokine/cytokine response, proinflammatory monocyte-macrophage accumulation, disturbed homeostasis, and epithelial and endothelial cell apoptosis that results in vascular leakage and alveolar edema causing hypoxia. Ultimately, all of this can result in ARDS and even extrapulmonary multiple organ failure, which contributes to the severe disease course, worse clinical outcomes, a poor prognosis, disease exacerbation, and even mortality.[16, 155, 177, 179, 189] The immune dysregulation observed in some COVID-19 patients could have a role in the neurovirulence of SARS-CoV-2 that may cause neuropathological changes resulting in confusion and disturbed consciousness due to a weakened T-cell response that is unable to eliminate the virus from the brain, leading to neurologic dysfunction.[16] As a result, the present treatment strategies are exclusively aimed at containing the inflammatory rampage induced by SARS-CoV-2, which would also prevent neural damage and its manifestations. To better understand the neuropathology of SARS-CoV-2 infection, a comprehensive immunological profiling in the peripheral circulation and nervous system of COVID-19 patients is required, supported by postmortem studies.

Hypoxia-Mediated Injury

Despite some reports suggesting direct CNS damage by SARS-CoV-2, there is still no clear evidence in support of that theory, requiring consideration of indirect mechanisms by which nervous system damage occurs.[110] Hypoxia is evidently a direct consequence of the wide spectrum of pulmonary system involvement, ranging from mild dysfunction in gas exchange to the diffuse alveolar, interstitial inflammation, and membrane formation seen in severe ARDS 192, but it may also occur as a result of direct infection of medullary cardiorespiratory centers by SARS-CoV-2, resulting in dysregulation of respiratory control, hypoventilation, and cardiopulmonary failure.[54, 107] The precipitating factors for hypoxia-mediated brain injury due to defunct gas exchange and lactic acid accumulation include vasodilation, hypercarbia, interstitial edema, neuronal swelling, brain edema, ischemia, and congestion, raised intracranial pressure, and heightened anaerobic metabolism in the mitochondria of brain cells, all of which eventually damages the CNS and leads to neuropsychiatric manifestations in patients with COVID-19.[190, 191] The persistent hypoxic condition worsens cerebral edema, and together with intracranial hypertension, causes a decline in brain function inducing a comatose state. Due to the severe hypoxia observed in SARS-CoV-2-infected patients, hypoxia-mediated brain injury is one potential neuropathological mechanism causing nerve damage and other neurological morbidities in COVID-19.[110, 192]

Indirect Viral Injury due to Systemic Sickness

The systemic immune response can have several detrimental effects on the nervous system, exhibiting different neurological manifestations in patients, including acute ischemic stroke, intracerebral hemorrhage, and cerebral venous sinus thrombosis.[59, 76, 77] Coagulation abnormalities in the form of hypercoagulability have been observed in severe cases of SARS-CoV-2 infection with different pathogenic mechanisms which will be further detailed in Chapter 3.[18, 193] The prolonged virus-induced inflammation can activate the coagulation system due to the presence of elevated levels of cytokines, particularly IL-6, which can also suppress the fibrinolytic system. While entering the host cells via interaction with ACE2 receptors, the virus causes pulmonary and peripheral endothelial injury, which can activate the coagulation system by exposing tissue factors involved in coagulation and other related pathways. This induces hypercoagulability, particularly in severe cases, causing elevated levels of D-dimer, fibrinogen, anticardiolipin, and anti-β2-glycoprotein 1 (β2GP1) antibodies, eventually resulting in DIC.[194, 195] The dysfunctional coagulation that occurs during SARS-CoV-2 infection potentiates the risk of ischemic stroke even in young patients who are otherwise less susceptible to vascular risk factors and injury.[78, 194] In addition, the binding of SARS-CoV-2 to the ACE2 receptor causes its downregulation, leading to overactivation of the RAS and underactivation of alternative RAS signaling in the brain. The resulting imbalance in vasodilation, oxidative stress, and thrombogenesis may be responsible for the occurrence of strokes that are observed in some patients with COVID-19.[196]

Unintended Host Immune Response After an Acute Infection

Owing to the neurotrophic potential of CoV, these viruses can damage tissue in the nervous system due to unintended host immune responses that occur after the remission of an acute infection, causing severe neurological manifestations such as postinfectious ADEM, brainstem encephalitis, and GBS.[34, 38, 41, 51, 197] Along similar lines, SARS-CoV-2 can also cause these manifestations; although considering the hypothetical nature of the neuropathological implications of infection, it is premature to make any conclusive statement in that regard.[108] Nevertheless, it is important to consider the complications that arise in COVID-19 patients upon such neurological manifestations. GBS is an autoimmune disease primarily affecting the PNS and has a severe impact on respiratory muscles due to its neuromuscular effects. This causes respiratory insufficiency and further contributes to breathing issues experienced by SARS-CoV-2-infected patients, thereby worsening the disease course.[198] A recent review has reported that upper respiratory infection or enteritis occurs prior to GBS development in about 2/3 of patients.[199] And there are umpteen reports stating that the presence of GBS and its variants, including Miller-Fisher syndrome, in SARS-CoV-2-infected patients are the result of indirect viral nerve injury. The first of these was a report from China, where a patient showed COVID-19 symptoms 7 days after admission to the hospital, suggestive of a para-infectious profile where both conditions occurred within a close time frame reflecting their concomitant presence.[79, 80, 82, 166, 200] Another report from Italy describes a neurological manifestation in the form of GBS in an aged female patient that appeared to occur after the patient had made a complete recovery from COVID-19.[81] Further, case reports have also suggested an association of COVID-19 with ADEM.[84, 85] There is the possibility that the neuromuscular and autonomic dysfunction could worsen disease outcomes and even cause cardio-respiratory failure in COVID-19 patients. Thus, the aforementioned studies clearly highlight the derailed immune response in SARS-CoV-2 patients that form the basis for the severe neurological complications and manifestations that are being increasingly reported worldwide. An outline of the various postulated mechanisms involved in the neuropathogenesis of SARS-CoV-2 is shown in Fig. 2.2.

CONCLUSIONS

Typically, infection with SARS-CoV-2 is associated with respiratory symptoms; however, there are many reports of extrapulmonary manifestations which may impact the nervous system and cause neurologic disorders. As the above-discussed studies convey, the neurological manifestations and complications of COVID-19 are

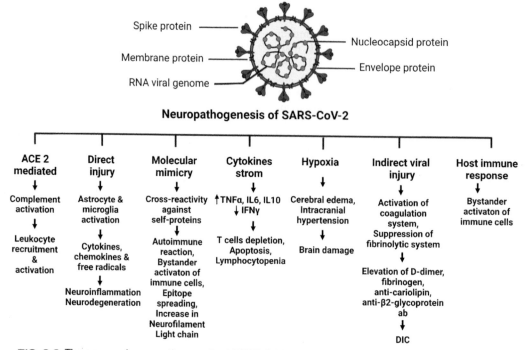

FIG. 2.2 The proposed neuropathogenesis of SARS-CoV-2. The damaging effect of SARS-CoV-2 infection on the nervous system happens through different mechanisms, as described in detail in the text: ACE2 attachment of the virus through its spike (S) protein leads to its entry into the host system; direct viral infection of the nervous system; molecular mimicry; excess immune response in the form of cytokine storm; hypoxic brain injury; indirect viral injury due to systemic sickness; and unintended postinfection host immune response (Created with BioRender.com (2020); https://app.biorender.com).

nonspecific as reflected by the clinical heterogeneity of the disease. Based on the hospitalization reports available so far, the neurologic presentations of COVID-19 are numerous and include disturbed consciousness, headache, acute cerebrovascular diseases, cranial nerve dysfunction, and meningoencephalitis. In addition, impaired taste and smell may be present in both mild and moderate cases without the presence of nasal symptoms. Due to the highly dysregulated immune response in severe cases of SARS-CoV-2 infection, neurological manifestations are quite prevalent. However, as of yet, there is no evidence of direct neural injury by the virus, suggesting that the neurological effects of SARS-CoV-2 are, at minimum, secondary injuries caused by disturbed cellular homeostasis due to a potent systemic immune response. Thus, the host-virus interactions need to be thoroughly investigated by developing disease models to explore the mechanisms of neuroinvasion and to determine if neuropathology observed in the patients is the outcome of direct injury or immune-mediated implication.

Around the world, people are adopting social distancing measures to stop the spread of this highly contagious disease. In light of the information described above, it seems pertinent that we begin to take into account the presenting neurological features of COVID-19 patients, as these may be evident before the typical respiratory symptoms and could help prevent or dilute inadvertent exposure of the virus among the population. At the very least, exercising precaution when prescribing medications for such cases is warranted. In addition, knowledge about possible mechanisms of neuroinvasion is equally important in understanding potential targets for drug design. As there is minimal understanding of the mechanisms involved in the neuropathogenesis of SARS-CoV-2 and the respiratory failure that occurs, further studies in patients and animal models of the disease are needed to aid in appropriate, immediate, and individualized treatment strategies that are based on the stage of the disease, nervous tissue involvement, and severity of the symptoms. Neurologic testing, CSF analysis, and postmortem examination of nerve tissue from areas of the brain and spinal cord in infected patients will help in determining if a central mechanism is responsible for neuroinvasion-based acute respiratory failure. This would also help prioritize hospitalizations and requirements for intensive care, which might alleviate some of the burdens on the health-care system.

Currently, the greatest challenge in understanding the fatal neuropathological implications that arise in COVID-19 patients lies in the lack of information regarding SARS-CoV-2 infection and the disease it causes. Despite the proposed mechanisms, the precise pathway of neuroinvasion adopted by SARS-CoV-2 is still not known. Given the minimal information available about SARS-CoV-2, knowledge regarding its neurological impact is crucial for planning treatment and rehabilitation strategies for underlying comorbidities and postinfection complications.

DEDICATION

While putting forth information on different aspects of COVID-19, it was gut-wrenching to read about countless lives that succumbed to this invisible enemy that has shackled humanity. This health crisis has negatively impacted millions of lives worldwide, yet its consideration has become the new normal of our lives. It is important to remember that the number of infections, and more importantly, deaths that are being reported are not mere figures; they represent human lives. While it is straightforward to sum up the numbers and descriptions in written form, courage must be mustered to let the scientific community explore this hidden enemy using a priceless human life. Behind every research paper, case report, series, and press briefing, there is the loss of a precious life, someone who is a family member, a friend, a colleague, and more essentially, a human being. At the heart of it all, this pandemic enforces the message of being humane, living each day as if it is the last day of our lives, and being thankful for what we have while being hopeful about the future. Not everyone is privileged to fulfill their desires and live life the way they wanted. As a token of appreciation, we would like to dedicate this piece of writing to the essence of being human.

Roy T. Bennett has rightly said:

Be the reason someone smiles. Be the reason someone feels loved and believes in the goodness in people.

DISCLOSURE OF INTERESTS

All authors declare they have no conflict of interest.

ETHICAL APPROVAL FOR STUDIES

This article does not contain any studies with human and animal participants performed by any of the authors.

REFERENCES

1. Thompson R. Pandemic potential of 2019-nCoV. *Lancet Infect Dis.* 2020;20(3):280.
2. COVID-19 Treatment Guidelines Panel. *Coronavirus Disease 2019 (COVID-19) Treatment Guidelines.* National Institutes of Health; 2020. Available at https://www.covid19treatmentguidelines.nih.gov/. Accessed June 2020.
3. Cai Q, Chen F, Wang T, et al. Obesity and COVID-19 severity in a designated hospital in Shenzhen, China. *Diabetes Care.* 2020;43(7):1392–1398.
4. Chen G, Wu D, Guo W, et al. Clinical and immunological features of severe and moderate coronavirus disease 2019. *J Clin Invest.* 2020;130(5):2620–2629.
5. Chen N, Zhou M, Dong X, et al. Epidemiological and clinical characteristics of 99 cases of 2019 novel coronavirus pneumonia in Wuhan, China: a descriptive study. *Lancet.* 2020;395(10223):507–513.
6. Huang C, Wang Y, Li X, et al. Clinical features of patients infected with 2019 novel coronavirus in Wuhan, China. *Lancet.* 2020;395(10223):497–506.
7. Wei YY, Wang RR, Zhang DW, et al. Risk factors for severe COVID-19: Evidence from 167 hospitalized patients in Anhui, China. *J Infect.* 2020;81(1):e89–e92.
8. Du RH, Liang LR, Yang CQ, et al. Predictors of mortality for patients with COVID-19 pneumonia caused by SARS-CoV-2: a prospective cohort study. *Eur Respir J.* 2020;55(5).
9. Liu Y, Mao B, Liang S, et al. Association between age and clinical characteristics and outcomes of COVID-19. *Eur Respir J.* 2020;55(5).
10. Zhou F, Yu T, Du R, et al. Clinical course and risk factors for mortality of adult inpatients with COVID-19 in Wuhan, China: a retrospective cohort study. *Lancet.* 2020;395(10229):1054–1062.
11. Guan WJ, Ni ZY, Hu Y, et al. Clinical characteristics of coronavirus disease 2019 in China. *N Engl J Med.* 2020;382(18):1708–1720.
12. Centers for Disease Control and Prevention. *Coronavirus disease 2019 (COVID-19): People who are at higher risk for severe illness;* 2020. Available at https://www.cdc.gov/coronavirus/2019-ncov/need-extra-precautions/people-at-higher-risk.html. Accessed June 2020.
13. Wu C, Chen X, Cai Y, et al. Risk factors associated with acute respiratory distress syndrome and death in patients with coronavirus disease 2019 pneumonia in Wuhan, China. *JAMA Intern Med.* 2020;180(7):934–943.
14. Yang X, Yu Y, Xu J, et al. Clinical course and outcomes of critically ill patients with SARS-CoV-2 pneumonia in Wuhan, China: a single-centered, retrospective, observational study. *Lancet Respir Med.* 2020;8(5):475–481.

15. Zhang JJ, Dong X, Cao YY, et al. Clinical characteristics of 140 patients infected with SARS-CoV-2 in Wuhan, China. *Allergy.* 2020;75(7):1730–1741.

16. Koralnik IJ, Tyler KL. COVID-19: A Global Threat to the Nervous System. *Ann Neurol.* 2020;88(1):1–11.

17. Korsukewitz C, Reddel SW, Bar-Or A, Wiendl H. Neurological immunotherapy in the era of COVID-19 - looking for consensus in the literature. *Nat Rev Neurol.* 2020;16(9):493–505.

18. Cao W, Li T. COVID-19: towards understanding of pathogenesis. *Cell Res.* 2020;30(5):367–369.

19. Baig AM, Khaleeq A, Ali U, Syeda H. Evidence of the COVID-19 virus targeting the CNS: tissue distribution, host-virus interaction, and proposed neurotropic mechanisms. *ACS Chem Neurosci.* 2020;11(7):995–998.

20. Liu DX, Liang JQ, Fung TS. Human coronavirus-229E, -OC43, -NL63, and -HKU1 (*Coronaviridae*). *Encyclopedia Virol.* 2021;428–440.

21. Schoeman D, Fielding BC. Coronavirus envelope protein: current knowledge. *Virol J.* 2019;16(1):69.

22. de Haan CA, Smeets M, Vernooij F, Vennema H, Rottier PJ. Mapping of the coronavirus membrane protein domains involved in interaction with the spike protein. *J Virol.* 1999;73(9):7441–7452.

23. Alsaadi EAJ, Jones IM. Membrane binding proteins of coronaviruses. *Futur Virol.* 2019;14(4):275–286.

24. Arndt AL, Larson BJ, Hogue BG. A conserved domain in the coronavirus membrane protein tail is important for virus assembly. *J Virol.* 2010;84(21):11418–11428.

25. Corman VM, Lienau J, Witzenrath M. Coronaviruses as the cause of respiratory infections. *Internist (Berl).* 2019;60(11):1136–1145.

26. Matoba Y, Abiko C, Ikeda T, et al. Detection of the human coronavirus 229E, HKU1, NL63, and OC43 between 2010 and 2013 in Yamagata, Japan. *Jpn J Infect Dis.* 2015;68(2):138–141.

27. Myint SH. *Human coronavirus infections The Coronaviridae.* Springer; 1995:389–401.

28. Wu A, Peng Y, Huang B, et al. Genome composition and divergence of the novel coronavirus (2019-nCoV) originating in China. *Cell Host Microbe.* 2020;27(3):325–328.

29. Zhou P, Yang XL, Wang XG, et al. A pneumonia outbreak associated with a new coronavirus of probable bat origin. *Nature.* 2020;579(7798):270–273.

30. Desforges M, Le Coupanec A, Dubeau P, et al. Human coronaviruses and other respiratory viruses: underestimated opportunistic pathogens of the central nervous system? *Viruses.* 2019;12(1).

31. Principi N, Bosis S, Esposito S. Effects of coronavirus infections in children. Emerg Infect Dis. 16(2):183-188.

32. Li Y, Li H, Fan R, et al. Coronavirus infections in the central nervous system and respiratory tract show distinct features in hospitalized children. *Intervirology.* 2016;59(3):163–169.

33. Algahtani H, Subahi A, Shirah B. Neurological complications of middle east respiratory syndrome coronavirus: a report of two cases and review of the literature. *Case Rep Neurol Med.* 2016;2016:3502683.

34. Arabi YM, Harthi A, Hussein J, et al. Severe neurologic syndrome associated with Middle East respiratory syndrome corona virus (MERS-CoV). *Infection.* 2015;43(4):495–501.

35. Bohmwald K, Galvez NMS, Rios M, Kalergis AM. Neurologic alterations due to respiratory virus infections. *Front Cell Neurosci.* 2018;12:386.

36. Desforges M, Le Coupanec A, Stodola JK, Meessen-Pinard M, Talbot PJ. Human coronaviruses: viral and cellular factors involved in neuroinvasiveness and neuropathogenesis. *Virus Res.* 2014;194:145–158.

37. Lau KK, Yu WC, Chu CM, Lau ST, Sheng B, Yuen KY. Possible central nervous system infection by SARS coronavirus. *Emerg Infect Dis.* 2004;10(2):342–344.

38. Morfopoulou S, Brown JR, Davies EG, et al. Human coronavirus OC43 associated with fatal encephalitis. *N Engl J Med.* 2016;375(5):497–498.

39. Sharma K, Tengsupakul S, Sanchez O, Phaltas R, Maertens P. Guillain-Barre syndrome with unilateral peripheral facial and bulbar palsy in a child: a case report. *SAGE Open Med Case Rep.* 2019;7. 2050313X19838750.

40. Turgay C, Emine T, Ozlem K, Muhammet SP, Haydar AT. A rare cause of acute flaccid paralysis: human coronaviruses. *J Pediatr Neurosci.* 2015;10(3):280–281.

41. Yeh EA, Collins A, Cohen ME, Duffner PK, Faden H. Detection of coronavirus in the central nervous system of a child with acute disseminated encephalomyelitis. *Pediatrics.* 2004;113(1 Pt 1):e73–e76.

42. Ding Y, He L, Zhang Q, et al. Organ distribution of severe acute respiratory syndrome (SARS) associated coronavirus (SARS-CoV) in SARS patients: implications for pathogenesis and virus transmission pathways. *J Pathol.* 2004;203(2):622–630.

43. Gu J, Gong E, Zhang B, et al. Multiple organ infection and the pathogenesis of SARS. *J Exp Med.* 2005;202(3):415–424.

44. McCray Jr PB, Pewe L, Wohlford-Lenane C, et al. Lethal infection of K18-hACE2 mice infected with severe acute respiratory syndrome coronavirus. *J Virol.* 2007;81(2):813–821.

45. Netland J, Meyerholz DK, Moore S, Cassell M, Perlman S. Severe acute respiratory syndrome coronavirus infection causes neuronal death in the absence of encephalitis in mice transgenic for human ACE2. *J Virol.* 2008;82(15):7264–7275.

46. Xu J, Zhong S, Liu J, et al. Detection of severe acute respiratory syndrome coronavirus in the brain: potential role of the chemokine mig in pathogenesis. *Clin Infect Dis.* 2005;41(8):1089–1096.

47. Zhang QL, Ding YQ, Hou JL, et al. Detection of severe acute respiratory syndrome (SARS)-associated coronavirus RNA in autopsy tissues with in situ hybridization. *Di Yi Jun Yi Da Xue Xue Bao.* 2003;23(11):1125–1127.

48. Hwang CS. Olfactory neuropathy in severe acute respiratory syndrome: report of A case. *Acta Neurol Taiwanica.* 2006;15(1):26–28.

49. Tsai LK, Hsieh ST, Chang YC. Neurological manifestations in severe acute respiratory syndrome. *Acta Neurol Taiwanica.* 2005;14(3):113–119.

50. Saad M, Omrani AS, Baig K, et al. Clinical aspects and outcomes of 70 patients with Middle East respiratory syndrome coronavirus infection: a single-center experience in Saudi Arabia. *Int J Infect Dis.* 2014;29:301–306.

51. Kim JE, Heo JH, Kim HO, et al. Neurological complications during treatment of middle east respiratory syndrome. *J Clin Neurol.* 2017;13(3):227–233.

52. Li YC, Bai WZ, Hirano N, et al. Neurotropic virus tracing suggests a membranous-coating-mediated mechanism for transsynaptic communication. *J Comp Neurol.* 2013;521(1):203–212.

53. Matsuda K, Park CH, Sunden Y, et al. The vagus nerve is one route of transneural invasion for intranasally inoculated influenza a virus in mice. *Vet Pathol.* 2004;41(2):101–107.

54. Li YC, Bai WZ, Hashikawa T. The neuroinvasive potential of SARS-CoV2 may play a role in the respiratory failure of COVID-19 patients. *J Med Virol.* 2020;92(6):552–555.

55. Yuan Y, Cao D, Zhang Y, et al. Cryo-EM structures of MERS-CoV and SARS-CoV spike glycoproteins reveal the dynamic receptor binding domains. *Nat Commun.* 2017;8:15092.

56. Wang D, Hu B, Hu C, et al. Clinical characteristics of 138 hospitalized patients with 2019 novel coronavirus-infected pneumonia in Wuhan, China. *JAMA.* 2020;323(11):1061–1069.

57. Dube M, Le Coupanec A, Wong AHM, Rini JM, Desforges M, Talbot PJ. Axonal transport enables neuron-to-neuron propagation of human coronavirus OC43. *J Virol.* 2018;92(17).

58. Talbot PJ, Ekande S, Cashman NR, Mounir S, Stewart JN. Neurotropism of human coronavirus 229E. *Adv Exp Med Biol.* 1993;342:339–346.

59. Mao L, Jin H, Wang M, et al. Neurologic manifestations of hospitalized patients with coronavirus disease 2019 in Wuhan, China. *JAMA Neurol.* 2020;77(6):683–690.

60. Li Y, Li M, Wang M, et al. Acute cerebrovascular disease following COVID-19: a single center, retrospective, observational study. *Stroke Vasc Neurol.* 2020;5(3):279–284.

61. Helms J, Kremer S, Merdji H, et al. Neurologic features in severe SARS-CoV-2 infection. *N Engl J Med.* 2020;382(23):2268–2270.

62. Woelfel R, Corman VM, Wea G. Clinical presentation and virological assessment of hospitalized cases of coronavirus disease 2019 in a travel-associated transmission cluster. *Nature.* 2020;581(7809):465–469.

63. Xu XW, Wu XX, Jiang XG, et al. Clinical findings in a group of patients infected with the 2019 novel coronavirus (SARS-Cov-2) outside of Wuhan, China: retrospective case series. *BMJ.* 2020;368:m606.

64. Yang W, Cao Q, Qin L, et al. Clinical characteristics and imaging manifestations of the 2019 novel coronavirus disease (COVID-19):A multi-center study in Wenzhou city, Zhejiang, China. *J Infect.* 2020;80(4):388–393.

65. Chen T, Wu D, Chen H, et al. Clinical characteristics of 113 deceased patients with coronavirus disease 2019: retrospective study. *BMJ.* 2020;368:m1091.

66. Varatharaj A, Thomas N, Ellul MA, et al. Neurological and neuropsychiatric complications of COVID-19 in 153 patients: a UK-wide surveillance study. *Lancet Psychiatry.* 2020;7(10):875–882.

67. Xiang P, Xu XM, Gao LL, Wang HZ, Xiong HF, RHea L. First case of 2019 novel coronavirus disease with encephalitis. *ChinaXiv T20200300015.* 2020.

68. Ye M, Ren Y, Lv T. Encephalitis as a clinical manifestation of COVID-19. *Brain Behav Immun.* 2020;88:945–946.

69. Coolen T, Lolli V, Sadeghi N, et al. Early postmortem brain MRI findings in COVID-19 non-survivors. *Neurology.* 2020;95(14):e2016–e2027.

70. Giacomelli A, Pezzati L, Conti F, et al. Self-reported olfactory and taste disorders in SARS-CoV-2 patients: a cross-sectional study. *Clin Infect Dis.* 2020;71(15):889–890.

71. Filatov A, Sharma P, Hindi F, Espinosa PS. Neurological complications of coronavirus disease (COVID-19): encephalopathy. *Cureus.* 2020;12(3), e7352.

72. Poyiadji N, Shahin G, Noujaim D, Stone M, Patel S, Griffith B. COVID-19-associated acute hemorrhagic necrotizing encephalopathy: CT and MRI features. *Radiology.* 2020;201187.

73. Alkeridy WA, Almaghlouth I, Alrashed R, et al. A unique presentation of delirium in a patient with otherwise asymptomatic COVID-19. *J Am Geriatr Soc.* 2020;68(7):1382–1384.

74. Benameur K, Agarwal A, Auld SC, et al. Encephalopathy and encephalitis associated with cerebrospinal fluid cytokine alterations and coronavirus disease, Atlanta, Georgia, USA, 2020. *Emerg Infect Dis.* 2020;26(9).

75. Moriguchi T, Harii N, Goto J, et al. A first case of meningitis/encephalitis associated with SARS-Coronavirus-2. *Int J Infect Dis.* 2020;94:55–58.

76. Oxley TJ, Mocco J, Majidi S, et al. Large-vessel stroke as a presenting feature of Covid-19 in the young. *N Engl J Med.* 2020;382(20), e60.

77. Tun CA, UnlUba SY, Alemdar M, AkyUz E. Coexistence of COVID-19 and acute ischemic stroke report of four cases. *J Clin Neurosci.* 2020;77:227–229.

78. Avula A, Nalleballe K, Narula K, et al. COVID-19 presenting as stroke. *Brain Behav Immun.* 2020;87:115–119.

79. Gutierrez-Ortiz C, Mendez A, Rodrigo-Rey S, et al. Miller Fisher Syndrome and polyneuritis cranialis in COVID-19. *Neurology.* 2020;95(5):e601–e605.

80. Virani A, Rabold E, Hanson T, et al. Guillain-Barre Syndrome associated with SARS-CoV-2 infection. *IDCases.* 2020;e00771.

81. Padroni M, Mastrangelo V, Asioli GM, et al. Guillain-Barre syndrome following COVID-19: new infection, old complication? *J Neurol.* 2020;267(7):1877–1879.

82. Zhao H, Shen D, Zhou H, Liu J, Chen S. Guillain-Barre syndrome associated with SARS-CoV-2 infection: causality or coincidence? *Lancet Neurol.* 2020;19(5):383–384.

83. Farhadian S, Glick LR, Vogels CBF, et al. Acute encephalopathy with elevated CSF inflammatory markers as the initial presentation of COVID-19. *BMC Neurol.* 2020;20(1):248.

84. Parsons T, Banks S, Bae C, Gelber J, Alahmadi H, Tichauer M. COVID-19-associated acute disseminated encephalomyelitis (ADEM). *J Neurol.* 2020;267(10):2799–2802.

85. Zhang T, Hirsh E, Zandieh S, Rodricks BM. COVID-19-associated acute multi-infarct encephalopathy in an asymptomatic CADASIL patient. *Neurocrit Care.* 2021; 34(3):1099–1102.

86. Lanese N. *Woman with COVID-19 developed a rare brain condition. Doctors suspect a link.* Available via DIALOG https://www.livescience.com/woman-with-covid19-coronavirus-had-rare-braindisease.html. Accessed June 2020.

87. Rahhal N. *Coronavirus may cause brain damage by triggering dangerous inflammation that can cause bleeds and cell death.* Available via DIALOG https://www.dailymail.co.uk/health/article-8181257/Coronavirus-damage-brains-patients-reportssuggests.html. Accessed June 2020.

88. Hopkins C, Kumar N. *Loss of sense of smell as marker of COVID-19 infection.* Available at https://www.entuk.org/sites/default/files/files/Loss%20of%20sense%20of%20smell%20as%20marker%20of%20COVID.pdf. Accessed June 2020.

89. Ryan WM. *There's a new symptom of coronavirus, doctors say: Sudden loss of smell or taste.* Available at https://www.usatoday.com/story/news/health/2020/03/24/coronavirus-symptoms-loss-smell-taste/2897385001/. Accessed June 2020.

90. Li K, Wohlford-Lenane C, Perlman S, et al. Middle east respiratory syndrome coronavirus causes multiple organ damage and lethal disease in mice transgenic for human dipeptidyl peptidase 4. *J Infect Dis.* 2016;213(5):712–722.

91. Xu Z, Shi L, Wang Y, et al. Pathological findings of COVID-19 associated with acute respiratory distress syndrome. *Lancet Respir Med.* 2020;8(4):420–422.

92. Turtle L. Respiratory failure alone does not suggest central nervous system invasion by SARS-CoV-2. *J Med Virol.* 2020;92(7):705–706.

93. Shen B, Yi X, Sun Y, et al. Proteomic and metabolomic characterization of COVID-19 patient sera. *Cell.* 2020;182(1):59–72.e15.

94. Wu D, Shu T, Yang X, et al. Plasma metabolomic and lipidomic alterations associated with COVID-19. *Natl Sci Rev.* 2020;nwaa086.

95. Becker RC. COVID-19 update: Covid-19-associated coagulopathy. *J Thromb Thrombolysis.* 2020;50(1):54–67.

96. Nataf S. An alteration of the dopamine synthetic pathway is possibly involved in the pathophysiology of COVID-19. *J Med Virol.* 2020;92(10):1743–1744.

97. Cuperlovic-Culf M, Cunningham EL, Teimoorinia H, et al. Metabolomics and computational analysis of the role of monoamine oxidase activity in delirium and SARS-COV-2 infection. *Sci Rep.* 2021;11(1):10629.

98. Brunner HG, Nelen M, Breakefield XO, Ropers HH, van Oost BA. Abnormal behavior associated with a point mutation in the structural gene for monoamine oxidase A. *Science.* 1993;262(5133):578–580.

99. Deshwal S, Forkink M, Hu CH, et al. Monoamine oxidase-dependent endoplasmic reticulum-mitochondria dysfunction and mast cell degranulation lead to adverse cardiac remodeling in diabetes. *Cell Death Differ.* 2018;25(9):1671–1685.

100. Ketzef M, Spigolon G, Johansson Y, Bonito-Oliva A, Fisone G, Silberberg G. Dopamine depletion impairs bilateral sensory processing in the striatum in a pathway-dependent manner. *Neuron.* 2017;94(4):855–865. e855.

101. Leiter O, Walker TL. Platelets in neurodegenerative conditions-friend or foe? *Front Immunol.* 2020;11:747.

102. Naoi M, Maruyama W, Inaba-Hasegawa K, Akao Y. Type A monoamine oxidase regulates life and death of neurons in neurodegeneration and neuroprotection. *Int Rev Neurobiol.* 2011;100:85–106.

103. Schedin-Weiss S, Inoue M, Hromadkova L, et al. Monoamine oxidase B is elevated in Alzheimer disease neurons, is associated with gamma-secretase and regulates neuronal amyloid beta-peptide levels. *Alzheimers Res Ther.* 2017;9(1):57.

104. Shih JC, Chen K, Ridd MJ. Monoamine oxidase: from genes to behavior. *Annu Rev Neurosci.* 1999;22:197–217.

105. Yeung AWK, Georgieva MG, Atanasov AG, Tzvetkov NT. Monoamine oxidases (MAOs) as privileged molecular targets in neuroscience: research literature analysis. *Front Mol Neurosci.* 2019;12:143.

106. Sun T, Guan J, You C. The neuroinvasive potential of severe acute respiratory syndrome coronavirus 2. *Brain Behav Immun.* 2020;88:59.

107. Li YC, Bai WZ, Hashikawa T. Response to Commentary on "The neuroinvasive potential of SARS-CoV-2 may play a role in the respiratory failure of COVID-19 patients". *J Med Virol.* 2020;92(7):707–709.

108. Ahmed MU, Hanif M, Ali MJ, et al. Neurological manifestations of COVID-19 (SARS-CoV-2): a review. *Front Neurol.* 2020;11:518.

109. Wan Y, Shang J, Graham R, Baric RS, Li F. Receptor recognition by the novel coronavirus from Wuhan: an analysis based on decade-long structural studies of SARS coronavirus. *J Virol.* 2020;94(7).

110. Wu Y, Xu X, Chen Z, et al. Nervous system involvement after infection with COVID-19 and other coronaviruses. *Brain Behav Immun.* 2020;87:18–22.

111. Turner AJ, Hiscox JA, Hooper NM. ACE2: from vasopeptidase to SARS virus receptor. *Trends Pharmacol Sci.* 2004;25(6):291–294.

112. Yang P, Gu H, Zhao Z, et al. Angiotensin-converting enzyme 2 (ACE2) mediates influenza H7N9 virus-induced acute lung injury. *Sci Rep.* 2014;4:7027.

113. Hoffmann M, Kleine-Weber H, Schroeder S, et al. SARS-CoV-2 cell entry depends on ACE2 and TMPRSS2 and is blocked by a clinically proven protease inhibitor. *Cell.* 2020;181(2):271–280. e278.

114. Wrapp D, Wang N, Corbett KS, et al. Cryo-EM structure of the 2019-nCoV spike in the prefusion conformation. *Science.* 2020;367(6483):1260–1263.

115. Sungnak W, Huang N, Becavin C, et al. SARS-CoV-2 entry factors are highly expressed in nasal epithelial cells together with innate immune genes. *Nat Med.* 2020;26(5):681–687.

116. Donoghue M, Hsieh F, Baronas E, et al. A novel angiotensin-converting enzyme-related carboxypeptidase (ACE2) converts angiotensin I to angiotensin 1-9. *Circ Res.* 2000;87(5):E1–E9.

117. Hamming I, Timens W, Bulthuis ML, Lely AT, Navis G, van Goor H. Tissue distribution of ACE2 protein, the functional receptor for SARS coronavirus. A first step in understanding SARS pathogenesis. *J Pathol.* 2004;203(2):631–637.

118. Harmer D, Gilbert M, Borman R, Clark KL. Quantitative mRNA expression profiling of ACE 2, a novel homologue of angiotensin converting enzyme. *FEBS Lett.* 2002;532(1-2):107–110.

119. Miller AJ, Arnold AC. The renin-angiotensin system in cardiovascular autonomic control: recent developments and clinical implications. *Clin Auton Res.* 2019; 29(2):231–243.

120. Vaduganathan M, Vardeny O, Michel T, McMurray JJV, Pfeffer MA, Solomon SD. Renin-angiotensin-aldosterone system inhibitors in patients with Covid-19. *N Engl J Med.* 2020;382(17):1653–1659.

121. Xu P, Sriramula S, Lazartigues E. ACE2/ANG-(1-7)/Mas pathway in the brain: the axis of good. *Am J Phys Regul Integr Comp Phys.* 2011;300(4):R804–R817.

122. Zhang H, Penninger JM, Li Y, Zhong N, Slutsky AS. Angiotensin-converting enzyme 2 (ACE2) as a SARS-CoV-2 receptor: molecular mechanisms and potential therapeutic target. *Intensive Care Med.* 2020;46(4):586–590.

123. Bolay H, Gül A, Baykan B. COVID-19 is a real headache! *Headache.* 2020;60(7):1415–1421.

124. Bali A, Singh N, Jaggi AS. Renin-angiotensin system in pain: existing in a double life? *J Renin-Angiotensin-Aldosterone Syst.* 2014;15(4):329–340.

125. Jackson L, Eldahshan W, Fagan SC, Ergul A. Within the brain: the renin angiotensin system. *Int J Mol Sci.* 2018;19(3).

126. Boonacker E, Van Noorden CJ. The multifunctional or moonlighting protein CD26/DPPIV. *Eur J Cell Biol.* 2003;82(2):53–73.

127. Mattern T, Scholz W, Feller AC, Flad HD, Ulmer AJ. Expression of CD26 (dipeptidyl peptidase IV) on resting and activated human T-lymphocytes. *Scand J Immunol.* 1991;33(6):737–748.

128. Bernstein HG, Dobrowolny H, Keilhoff G, Steiner J. Dipeptidyl peptidase IV, which probably plays important roles in Alzheimer disease (AD) pathology, is upregulated in AD brain neurons and associates with amyloid plaques. *Neurochem Int.* 2018;114:55–57.

129. Chan PK, To KF, Lo AW, et al. Persistent infection of SARS coronavirus in colonic cells in vitro. *J Med Virol.* 2004;74(1):1–7.

130. Ding Y, Wang H, Shen H, et al. The clinical pathology of severe acute respiratory syndrome (SARS): a report from China. *J Pathol.* 2003;200(3):282–289.

131. To KF, Lo AW. Exploring the pathogenesis of severe acute respiratory syndrome (SARS): the tissue distribution of the coronavirus (SARS-CoV) and its putative receptor, angiotensin-converting enzyme 2 (ACE2). *J Pathol.* 2004;203(3):740–743.

132. Koyuncu OO, Hogue IB, Enquist LW. Virus infections in the nervous system. *Cell Host Microbe.* 2013;13(4): 379–393.

133. Morris M, Zohrabian VM. Neuroradiologists, be mindful of the neuroinvasive potential of COVID-19. *AJNR Am J Neuroradiol.* 2020;41(6):E37–E39.

134. Swanson 2nd PA, McGavern DB. Viral diseases of the central nervous system. *Curr Opin Virol.* 2015;11:44–54.

135. Paniz-Mondolfi A, Bryce C, Grimes Z, et al. Central nervous system involvement by severe acute respiratory syndrome coronavirus-2 (SARS-CoV-2). *J Med Virol.* 2020;92(7):699–702.

136. Cabirac GF, Soike KF, Zhang JY, et al. Entry of coronavirus into primate CNS following peripheral infection. *Microb Pathog.* 1994;16(5):349–357.

137. Cavanagh D. Coronaviruses in poultry and other birds. *Avian Pathol.* 2005;34(6):439–448.

138. Desforges M, Favreau DJ, Brison É, et al. *Human coronaviruses: respiratory pathogens revisited as infectious neuroinvasive, neurotropic, and neurovirulent agents neuroviral infections.* CRC Press; 2013:112–141.

139. Niu J, Shen L, Huang B, et al. Non-invasive bioluminescence imaging of HCoV-OC43 infection and therapy in the central nervous system of live mice. *Antivir Res.* 2020;173:104646.

140. Talbot PJ, Desforges M, Brison E, Jacomy H, Tkachev S. Coronaviruses as encephalitis-inducing infectious agents. *Nonflavirus Encephalitis In-Tech.* 2011;185–202.

141. Li J, Gao J, Xu YP, Zhou TL, Jin YY, Lou JN. Expression of severe acute respiratory syndrome coronavirus receptors, ACE2 and CD209L in different organ derived microvascular endothelial cells. *Zhonghua Yi Xue Za Zhi.* 2007;87(12):833–837.

142. Esposito G, Pesce M, Seguella L, Sanseverino W, Lu J, Sarnelli G. Can the enteric nervous system be an alternative entrance door in SARS-CoV2 neuroinvasion? *Brain Behav Immun.* 2020;87:93–94.

143. Mori I. Transolfactory neuroinvasion by viruses threatens the human brain. *Acta Virol.* 2015;59(4):338–349.

144. Bilinska K, Jakubowska P, Von Bartheld CS, Butowt R. Expression of the SARS-CoV-2 entry proteins, ACE2 and TMPRSS2, in cells of the olfactory epithelium: identification of cell types and trends with age. *ACS Chem Neurosci.* 2020;11(11):1555–1562.

145. Jin X, Lian JS, Hu JH, et al. Epidemiological, clinical and virological characteristics of 74 cases of coronavirus-infected disease 2019 (COVID-19) with gastrointestinal symptoms. *Gut.* 2020;69(6):1002–1009.

146. Alenquer M, Amorim MJ. Exosome Biogenesis, Regulation, and Function in Viral Infection. *Viruses.* 2015;7(9):5066–5083.

147. Chan JF, Chan KH, Choi GK, et al. Differential cell line susceptibility to the emerging novel human betacoronavirus 2c EMC/2012: implications for disease pathogenesis and clinical manifestation. *J Infect Dis.* 2013;207(11):1743–1752.

148. Collins AR. In vitro detection of apoptosis in monocytes/macrophages infected with human coronavirus. *Clin Diagn Lab Immunol.* 2002;9(6):1392–1395.

149. Desforges M, Miletti TC, Gagnon M, Talbot PJ. Activation of human monocytes after infection by human coronavirus 229E. *Virus Res.* 2007;130(1-2):228–240.

150. Reinhold AK, Rittner HL. Barrier function in the peripheral and central nervous system-a review. *Pflugers Arch.* 2017;469(1):123–134.

151. Wuthrich C, Batson S, Koralnik IJ. Lack of major histocompatibility complex class I upregulation and restrictive infection by JC virus hamper detection of neurons by T lymphocytes in the central nervous system. *J Neuropathol Exp Neurol.* 2015;74(8):791–803.

152. Unni SK, Ruzek D, Chhatbar C, Mishra R, Johri MK, Singh SK. Japanese encephalitis virus: from genome to infectome. *Microbes Infect.* 2011;13(4):312–321.

153. Chew FT, Ong SY, Hew CL. Severe acute respiratory syndrome coronavirus and viral mimicry. *Lancet.* 2003; 361(9374):2081.

154. Cappello F. Is COVID-19 a proteiform disease inducing also molecular mimicry phenomena? *Cell Stress Chaperones.* 2020;25(3):381–382.

155. Chen C, Zhang XR, Ju ZY, He WF. Advances in the research of mechanism and related immunotherapy on the cytokine storm induced by coronavirus disease 2019. *Zhonghua Shao Shang Za Zhi.* 2020;36(6):471–475.

156. Kadkhoda K. COVID-19: an immunopathological view. *mSphere.* 2020;5(2).

157. Pedersen SF, Ho YC. SARS-CoV-2: a storm is raging. *J Clin Invest.* 2020;130(5):2202–2205.

158. Cappello F. COVID-19 and molecular mimicry: the Columbus' egg? *J Clin Neurosci.* 2020;77:246.

159. Delunardo F, Scalzi V, Capozzi A, et al. Streptococcal-vimentin cross-reactive antibodies induce microvascular cardiac endothelial proinflammatory phenotype in rheumatic heart disease. *Clin Exp Immunol.* 2013; 173(3):419–429.

160. Kotlarz A, Tukaj S, Krzewski K, Brycka E, Lipinska B. Human Hsp40 proteins, DNAJA1 and DNAJA2, as potential targets of the immune response triggered by bacterial DnaJ in rheumatoid arthritis. *Cell Stress Chaperones.* 2013;18(5):653–659.

161. Mayr M, Metzler B, Kiechl S, et al. Endothelial cytotoxicity mediated by serum antibodies to heat shock proteins of Escherichia coli and Chlamydia pneumoniae: immune reactions to heat shock proteins as a possible link between infection and atherosclerosis. *Circulation.* 1999;99(12):1560–1566.

162. Sun X, Welsh MJ, Benndorf R. Conformational changes resulting from pseudophosphorylation of mammalian small heat shock proteins- a two-hybrid study. *Cell Stress Chaperones.* 2006;11(1):61–70.

163. Franke C, Ferse C, Kreye C, et al. High frequency of cerebrospinal fluid autoantibodies in COVID-19 patients with neurological symptoms. *Brain Behav Immun.* 2021;93:415–419.

164. Pomara C, Li Volti G, Cappello F. COVID-19 deaths: are we sure it is pneumonia? Please, autopsy, autopsy, autopsy! *J Clin Med.* 2020;9(5).

165. Hahn AF. Guillain-Barre syndrome. *Lancet.* 1998;352(9128): 635–641.

166. Sedaghat Z, Karimi N. Guillain Barre syndrome associated with COVID-19 infection: a case report. *J Clin Neurosci.* 2020;76:233–235.

167. Getts DR, Chastain EM, Terry RL, Miller SD. Virus infection, antiviral immunity, and autoimmunity. *Immunol Rev.* 2013;255(1):197–209.

168. Klein RS, Garber C, Howard N. Infectious immunity in the central nervous system and brain function. *Nat Immunol.* 2017;18(2):132–141.

169. Yin CH, Wang C, Tang Z, Wen Y, Zhang SW, Wang BE. Clinical analysis of multiple organ dysfunction syndrome in patients suffering from SARS. *Zhongguo Wei Zhong Bing Ji Jiu Yi Xue.* 2004;16(11):646–650.

170. Fu Y, Cheng Y, Wu Y. Understanding SARS-CoV-2-mediated inflammatory responses: from mechanisms to potential therapeutic tools. *Virol Sin.* 2020;35(3):266–271.

171. Mehta P, McAuley DF, Brown M, et al. COVID-19: consider cytokine storm syndromes and immunosuppression. *Lancet.* 2020;395(10229):1033–1034.

172. Ye Q, Wang B, Mao J. The pathogenesis and treatment of the `Cytokine Storm' in COVID-19. *J Infect.* 2020;80(6):607–613.

173. Bryce C, Grimes Z, Eea P. Pathophysiology of SARS-CoV-2:targeting of endothelial cells renders a complex disease with thrombotic microangiopathy and aberrant immune response. The Mount Sinai COVID-19 autopsy experience. *medRxiv.* 2020.

174. Li Y, Fu L, Gonzales DM, Lavi E. Coronavirus neurovirulence correlates with the ability of the virus to induce proinflammatory cytokine signals from astrocytes and microglia. *J Virol.* 2004;78(7):3398–3406.

175. Coperchini F, Chiovato L, Croce L, Magri F, Rotondi M. The cytokine storm in COVID-19: an overview of the involvement of the chemokine/chemokine-receptor system. *Cytokine Growth Factor Rev.* 2020;53:25–32.

176. Ruan Q, Yang K, Wang W, Jiang L, Song J. Clinical predictors of mortality due to COVID-19 based on an analysis of data of 150 patients from Wuhan, China. *Intensive Care Med.* 2020;46(5):846–848.

177. Trouillet-Assant S, Viel S, Gaymard A, et al. Type I IFN immunoprofiling in COVID-19 patients. *J Allergy Clin Immunol.* 2020;146(1):206–208.e2.

178. Yang Y, Shen C, Li J, et al. Plasma IP-10 and MCP-3 levels are highly associated with disease severity and predict the progression of COVID-19. *J Allergy Clin Immunol.* 2020;146(1):119–127.e4.

179. Diao B, Wang C, Tan Y, et al. Reduction and functional exhaustion of T cells in patients with coronavirus disease 2019 (COVID-19). *Front Immunol.* 2020;11:827.

180. Channappanavar R, Fehr AR, Vijay R, et al. Dysregulated type I interferon and inflammatory monocyte-macrophage responses cause lethal pneumonia in SARS-CoV-infected mice. *Cell Host Microbe.* 2016;19(2):181–193.

181. Liu Z, Long W, Tu M, et al. Lymphocyte subset (CD4 +, CD8 +) counts reflect the severity of infection and predict the clinical outcomes in patients with COVID-19. *J Infect.* 2020;81(2):318–356.
182. Aggarwal S, Gollapudi S, Gupta S. Increased TNF-alpha-induced apoptosis in lymphocytes from aged humans: changes in TNF-alpha receptor expression and activation of caspases. *J Immunol.* 1999;162(4):2154–2161.
183. Gupta S, Bi R, Kim C, Chiplunkar S, Yel L, Gollapudi S. Role of NF-kappaB signaling pathway in increased tumor necrosis factor-alpha-induced apoptosis of lymphocytes in aged humans. *Cell Death Differ.* 2005; 12(2):177–183.
184. Gabay C. Interleukin-6 and chronic inflammation. *Arthritis Res Ther.* 2006;8(Suppl 2):S3.
185. Jones SA, Jenkins BJ. Recent insights into targeting the IL-6 cytokine family in inflammatory diseases and cancer. *Nat Rev Immunol.* 2018;18(12):773–789.
186. Wan S, Yi Q, Fan S, et al. Characteristics of lymphocyte subsets and cytokines in peripheral blood of 123 hospitalized patients with 2019 novel coronavirus pneumonia (NCP). *medRxiv.* 2020. https://doi.org/10.1101/2020.02.1 0.20021832.
187. Tveito K. Cytokine storms in COVID-19 cases? *Tidsskr Nor Laegeforen.* 2020;140.
188. Zhang C, Wu Z, Li JW, Zhao H, Wang GQ. Cytokine release syndrome in severe COVID-19: interleukin-6 receptor antagonist tocilizumab may be the key to reduce mortality. *Int J Antimicrob Agents.* 2020;55(5):105954.
189. Qin C, Zhou L, Hu Z, et al. Dysregulation of immune response in patients with COVID-19 in Wuhan, China. *Clin Infect Dis.* 2020;71(15):762–768.
190. Abdennour L, Zeghal C, Deme M, Puybasset L. Interaction brain-lungs. *Ann Fr Anesth Reanim.* 2012; 31(6):e101–e107.
191. Tu H, Tu S, Gao S, Shao A, Sheng J. Current epidemiological and clinical features of COVID-19; a global perspective from China. *J Infect.* 2020;81(1):1–9.
192. Guo YR, Cao QD, Hong ZS, et al. The origin, transmission and clinical therapies on coronavirus disease 2019 (COVID-19) outbreak - an update on the status. *Mil Med Res.* 2020;7(1):11.
193. Montalvan V, Toledo JD, Nugent K. Mechanisms of stroke in coronavirus disease 2019. *J Stroke.* 2020;22(2):282–283.
194. Tang N, Li D, Wang X, Sun Z. Abnormal coagulation parameters are associated with poor prognosis in patients with novel coronavirus pneumonia. *J Thromb Haemost.* 2020;18(4):844–847.
195. Zhang Y, Xiao M, Zhang S, et al. Coagulopathy and Antiphospholipid Antibodies in Patients with Covid-19. *N Engl J Med.* 2020;382(17), e38.
196. Divani AA, Andalib S, Di Napoli M, et al. Coronavirus disease 2019 and stroke: clinical manifestations and pathophysiological insights. *J Stroke Cerebrovasc Dis.* 2020;29(8):104941.
197. Arbour N, Cote G, Lachance C, Tardieu M, Cashman NR, Talbot PJ. Acute and persistent infection of human neural cell lines by human coronavirus OC43. *J Virol.* 1999;73(4):3338–3350.
198. Lahiri D, Ardila A. COVID-19 pandemic: a neurological perspective. *Cureus.* 2020;12(4), e7889.
199. Willison HJ, Jacobs BC, van Doorn PA. Guillain-Barre syndrome. *Lancet.* 2016;388(10045):717–727.
200. Toscano G, Palmerini F, Ravaglia S, et al. Guillain-Barre syndrome associated with SARS-CoV-2. *N Engl J Med.* 2020;382(26):2574–2576.

FURTHER READING

201. Benussi A, Pilotto A, Premi E, et al. Clinical characteristics and outcomes of inpatients with neurologic disease and COVID-19 in Brescia, Lombardy, Italy. *Neurology.* 2020;95(7):e910–e920.
202. Vonck K, Garrez I, De Herdt V, et al. Neurological manifestations and neuro-invasive mechanisms of the severe acute respiratory syndrome coronavirus type 2. *Eur J Neurol.* 2020;27(8):1578–1587.

CHAPTER 3

Neurological Presentations of COVID-19

ELISSA FORY[a] • CHANDAN MEHTA[b] • KAVITA M. GROVER[c] • RITIKA SURI[b]
[a]Department of Neurology, The Icahn School of Medicine at Mount Sinai, New York, NY, United States, [b]Department of Neurology, Henry Ford Hospital, Detroit, MI, United States, [c]Wayne State University, Henry Ford Hospital, Detroit, MI, United States

INTRODUCTION

The acute manifestations of SARS-CoV-2 on the nervous system are protean, affecting both the central and peripheral nervous systems (Table 3.1). As detailed in Chapter 2, SARS-CoV-2 can interact with the nervous system by multiple pathophysiologic mechanisms, including direct viral effects, cytokine-mediated effects, increasing inflammation and/or hypercoagulable states, para- or postinfectious autoimmune effects, and downstream effects from critical illness or treatments. Neurologic symptoms can define or accompany an acute SARS-CoV-2 presentation or may appear later in the clinical course . This chapter presents a brief overview of the noted neurologic manifestations of COVID-19.

A simple way to think about the neurologic complications of COVID-19 is in terms of their relative occurrence: very common, less common, and rare or uncommon (Table 3.2). Very common neurological symptoms of COVID-19 infection include anosmia, ageusia, headache, generalized encephalopathy, and muscle pain and weakness.

The first reports of neurologic involvement from COVID-19 came out of Wuhan, China, where the pandemic started. In a case series of 214 hospitalized patients with laboratory confirmation of SARS-CoV-2, more than one-third had neurologic symptoms, and this was more common in patients with severe systemic disease. The most common symptoms were dizziness (17%), headache (13%), impairment of consciousness (7%), acute stroke (3%), impaired smell (5%), impaired taste (5%), and skeletal muscle injury defined as muscle pain and high creatine kinase (11%).[1] Mao's landmark paper was the initial crystallization of thoughts regarding neurologic presentations of COVID-19.

BRAIN INVOLVEMENT BY COVID-19

Encephalopathy

Encephalopathy is present in 7%–32% of hospitalized patients with COVID-19.[2, 3] The incidence of encephalopathy is dependent upon the severity of disease, with up to 84% of patients with severe COVID-19 disease displaying encephalopathy at some point during their hospitalization.[3, 4] Older age, a history of neurologic diagnoses, and chronic renal insufficiency are also associated with the presence of encephalopathy.[3] In a French series of 140 intensive care unit patients with COVID-19 and acute respiratory distress syndrome, corticospinal tract signs such as clonus, Babinski sign, and generally increased deep tendon reflexes were seen in 63% of patients, in addition to delirium. These upper motor neuron signs often persisted to discharge.[4] Hyperactive delirium, akinetic mutism, myoclonus, pyramidal and extrapyramidal signs, frontal release signs, and abulia have all been clinically observed in these patients.[3-6]

It should be noted that encephalopathy in this context refers to any alteration in consciousness up to coma, and may ultimately include patients with other well-defined diagnoses such as stroke or encephalitis. Initial publications did not indicate other clinical impressions, nor results of diagnostic or imaging workup.[1] It is this author's opinion that the term encephalitis (and not encephalopathy) should be used if there is imaging, CSF, or biopsy evidence of brain inflammation in the setting of altered mental status, seizures, or focal neurologic deficits.

Brain MRI in patients with neurologic symptoms and COVID-19 admitted to the intensive care unit may be normal in up to half of patients.[7] Abnormal brain

Neurological Care and the COVID-19 Pandemic. https://doi.org/10.1016/B978-0-323-82691-4.00008-X

TABLE 3.1
Acute Neurologic Complications of SARS-CoV-2 Infection.

CENTRAL NERVOUS SYSTEM	
Brain	Acute demyelination/ADEM
	Encephalitis
	Encephalopathy—especially akinetic mutism
	Headache
	Seizures
	Stroke—mostly AIS; also ICH, CVST
Spinal Cord	Acute transverse myelitis
PERIPHERAL NERVOUS SYSTEM	
Cranial nerves	Anosmia, ageusia, Bell's palsy
Nerves	Guillain-Barré syndrome
Neuromuscular Junction	Myasthenia gravis
Muscle	Rhabdomyolysis, muscle pain

AIS, acute ischemic stroke; *ADEM*, acute demyelinating encephalomyelitis; *CVST*, cerebral venous sinus thrombosis; *ICH*, intracerebral hemorrhage.

imaging may lead to a more specific diagnosis than encephalopathy. Common abnormalities are:

(1) Acute or subacute ischemic stroke. This is the most common brain MRI finding in COVID-19 patients.[8]

(2) A patchy or diffuse, confluent, and symmetrical leukoencephalopathy.[4, 7, 8] Radiographically, there are T2 and FLAIR hyperintensities with restricted diffusion in the deep and subcortical white matter, with or without contrast enhancement. In confluent cases, there is a predilection for the precentral gyrus and posterior cerebral white matter.

(3) Microhemorrhages on gradient echo (GRE) or susceptibility-weighted imaging (SWI) sequences. These are often in the juxtacortical white matter and corpus callosum and may be seen alone or accompanying a confluent leukoencephalopathy.[9]

(4) Multifocal linear cortical signal change, manifested by T2 and FLAIR hyperintensity of the cortical ribbon with hyperintensity on diffusion-weighted imaging, with or without changes on the apparent diffusion coefficient (ADC) map.[7]

(5) Contrast enhancement of the subarachnoid space or leptomeninges.[4, 7, 8]

The individual patient's clinical context must be considered when interpreting MRI findings. Imaging abnormalities may not be specific to SARS-CoV-2 infection and can be seen in critically ill patients due to systemic derangements. Restricted diffusion and FLAIR hyperintensity of the cortical ribbon, leptomeningeal enhancement, and cortical microhemorrhages by SWI or GRE sequences can be seen with hypoxia, hypoglycemia, encephalitis, or seizures.[7, 8] Confluent leukoencephalopathy with or without microhemorrhages has been described in comatose COVID-19 patients following several weeks of mechanical ventilation. This imaging pattern can be seen in encephalitis or delayed posthypoxic leukoencephalopathy; given the overall clinical scenario, the latter mechanism has been proposed as more likely.[9]

In COVID-19-related encephalopathy, EEG is typically abnormal and nonspecific. However, a pattern of frontal abnormalities has emerged as potentially characteristic of COVID-19. The most common background abnormality is diffuse slowing (69% of EEGs); many fewer patients have focal slowing (which is frontal in half of cases) or the absence of the posterior dominant rhythm (10%).[10] Other electrographic patterns seen in patients with COVID-19 encephalopathy are frontal intermittent rhythmic delta activity and triphasic waves. Many EEGs are nonreactive.[8] Importantly, when the

TABLE 3.2
Relative Occurrence of Acute Neurologic Complications of SARS-CoV-2 Infection.

Very Common	Less Common	Rare or Uncommon
Anosmia	Acute ischemic stroke	Acute demyelination
Encephalopathy	Intracerebral Hemorrhage	ADEM
Headache	Rhabdomyolysis	Myelitis
Myalgias		Encephalitis
		Meningoencephalitis
		Myasthenia Gravis
		Seizures

clinical indication for an EEG was encephalopathy or coma without a preceding history of seizure, epilepsy, or acute or chronic brain injury, seizures are rarely if ever found.[4, 11, 12] This finding is different than that of the previous studies of patients with sepsis and it has important implications for EEG ordering and triage during a pandemic of an airborne infectious disease.[11]

CSF analysis of patients with COVID-19 encephalopathy reveals a normal cell count or a mild pleocytosis, a normal to elevated protein, and is typically negative for SARS-CoV-2 PCR and other infectious etiologies. Serologic profiles for autoimmune antibodies are normal. Inflammatory cytokines such as IL-6, IL-8, and TNF-alpha may be elevated in the CSF.[4, 13]

Treatment of COVID-19 encephalopathy is not standardized. Supportive medical care, avoidance of iatrogenic causes of delirium, and tincture of time are pillars of treatment for all patients. Over the first few months of the SARS-CoV-2 pandemic, the dramatic role of systemic cytokines and autoimmunity in the pathogenesis of COVID-19 was increasingly appreciated. As such, treatments dedicated toward suppressing the systemic inflammatory response were tried in individuals or small groups of patients with severe encephalopathy. High-dose corticosteroids,[13] intravenous immunoglobulin (IVIg),[6] and plasmapheresis (PLEX)[14] have all been used, with reported quick and dramatic improvement in the patients' clinical syndromes (including coma) over days.[6, 10, 13] Whether these treatments led to improvement, or the improvement was the natural history of the disease, is an open question.

Encephalopathy in COVID-19 is associated with longer hospitalizations,[3] longer mechanical ventilation,[4] and worse discharge functional outcomes.[3] After adjusting for age and severe COVID-19 disease, patients with encephalopathy have a higher risk of mortality at 30 days than those without encephalopathy (OR 2.92).[3] Following discharge, about one-third of patients continued to have cognitive dysfunction, manifesting as poor attention and orientation and difficulty with movements to command.[15] More on COVID-19-related encephalopathy can be found in Chapter 10.

Neuroinflammatory Syndromes
Encephalitis and meningoencephalitis
There are multiple reports of meningoencephalitis associated with SARS-CoV-2 infection, but only rare reports of isolated viral meningitis with COVID-19.[16] Patients described in the literature as having COVID-19 "encephalopathy" have a wide range of underlying conditions, including COVID-19-related meningoencephalitis, and the presentation and treatment were discussed in the previous section. Evidence indicates that most or all of COVID-19-related encephalitis are cytokine- or autoimmune-mediated,[14] rather than due to direct viral invasion of the brain.

Acute necrotizing encephalopathy
Although rare, acute necrotizing encephalopathy (ANE) has been described several times in association with acute SARS-CoV-2 infection.[17] ANE was first described in association with febrile illness in children of Asian descent; in some cases, there is a familial predisposition from a mutation in the RAN-binding protein 2 (RANBP2). Patients often present with a depressed level of consciousness, focal neurologic deficits, or seizures. Radiographically, there are relatively symmetrical T2 and FLAIR hyperintensities in bilateral thalami, temporal lobes, and/or the pons, often hypointense on T1 sequences and with restricted diffusion (Fig. 3.1). There may be internal necrosis or hemorrhage of the lesions. CSF is sterile, with cytoalbuminologic dissociation; viral studies in CSF are typically negative.[18] The exact causative mechanisms for ANE are unknown, but common hypotheses include effects of cytokine storm and increased blood-brain barrier permeability due to antibodies against, or energy failure to maintain, cerebral microvascular endothelial cells.[19]

Treatment for ANE is high-dose intravenous steroids, and is associated with improved outcomes. Prognosis is highly variable, ranging from complete recovery to death. In traditional ANE cohorts, mortality is approximately 30%[18]; mortality of reported COVID-19-associated cases appears similar.[17]

Central nervous system demyelination
Acute disseminated encephalomyelitis (ADEM) is typically a monophasic, postinfectious, multifocal, inflammatory demyelinating syndrome with encephalopathy. Symptoms develop over days, usually several weeks after a systemic infection. Brain MRI shows diffuse, bilateral, poorly demarcated, T2-hyperintense, asymmetrical lesions mostly in the white matter, often greater than 1 cm in diameter. Deep gray matter and cortical lesions may also be present. Lesions enhance in 30% of patients. CSF is bland, with elevated protein, and oligoclonal bands are typically absent. Pathologic evaluation reveals perivenous demyelination and perivascular infiltration of macrophages and lymphocytes. Treatment is high-dose intravenous corticosteroids followed by an oral prednisone taper over 1 month or more, and IVIg or PLEX can be used for refractory cases. Recovery is often complete and quick, over weeks.[20]

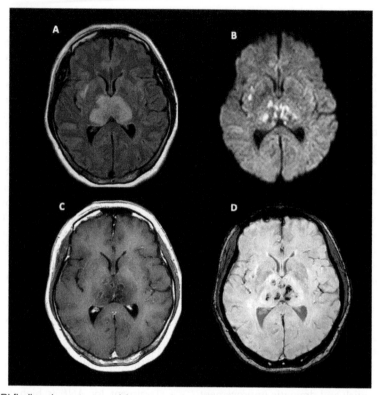

FIG. 3.1 MRI findings in acute necrotizing encephalopathy associated with SARS-CoV-2 infection. MRI brain images from a middle-aged woman with acute SARS-CoV-2 infection and altered mental status. These were obtained on day 7 of her febrile illness. (A) Axial T2-weighted FLAIR image of hyperintense signal involving both thalami, with smaller foci of involvement bilateral insula. (B) Diffusion-weighted jimage demonstrating smaller, scattered foci of restricted diffusion within the thalami and insula. (C) Postcgadolinium T1-weighted image showing that the regions of restricted diffusion in the thalami correspond to T1 hypointense lesions with faint rim enhancement, consistent with necrosis. (D) Susceptibility-weighted image revealing the presence of microhemorrhage within the areas of restricted diffusion. (Images and case courtesy Dr. Elissa Fory.)

It is perhaps not surprising that cases of ADEM have been described following SARS-CoV-2 infection, with typical onset several weeks after recovery from systemic viral symptoms. The largest series of ADEM cases associated with COVID-19 is from Queens Square, London, with nine patients. Some patients in this series presented for hospitalization due to neurologic symptoms, and other patients were diagnosed after a prolonged intensive care stay with difficulty awakening from sedation. One patient with acute hemorrhagic leukoencephalopathy required hemicraniectomy due to mass effect and herniation. A brain biopsy done on this patient was consistent with ADEM, and SARS-CoV-2 PCR was negative in biopsied brain tissue. The patients were treated with high-dose steroids and/or IVIg. Of these nine patients, one died, one made a full

recovery, and the rest had made a partial recovery at the time of series publication.[21] There are other case reports of classic ADEM presentations after COVID-19,[22, 23] and some reports with an ADEM diagnosis where the presentation may be better characterized as encephalitis or COVID-19 encephalopathy, depending on the final common terminology.

Although rare, acute myelitis has been reported in association with COVID-19. As of December 2020, this author counted 18 indexed case reports in PubMed of acute myelitis concurrent with or following COVID-19 infection. Many patients have typical systemic symptoms of COVID-19 in the days or weeks preceding the onset of myelopathic symptoms. MRI findings include longitudinally extensive transverse myelitis, multifocal well-circumscribed T2 signal hyperintensities, or diffuse patchy T2 signal hyperintensity, with or without contrast enhancement[24]; some had concurrent brain involvement. Similar to ADEM, CSF analysis is either normal or with elevated protein and mild lymphocytic pleocytosis. Again, SARS-CoV-2 PCR in the CSF is negative. Many patients have extensive autoimmune and antibody serum and CSF testing with negative results. However, isolated cases of post-COVID-19 inflammatory diseases with classic autoimmune antibodies are now being reported—including anti-GD1b antibodies associated with acute motor axonal neuropathy and C7-T1 posterior myelitis,[25] MOG-antibody-associated neuromyelitis optica spectrum disorder (NMOSD),[26] and aquaporin-4 antibodies in NMOSD.[27]

Both high-dose intravenous steroids and immunotherapies such as plasmapheresis and IVIg have been reported in treatment of COVID-19-associated myelopathy. Good recovery is common with such treatments.[24] COVID-19-related demyelination is further detailed in Chapter 6.

Stroke

Stroke in patients with COVID-19 may occur through any number of pathophysiologic processes: direct inflammatory or hypercoagulable processes on the cerebral vasculature; accrued cardiotoxicity leading to arrhythmias or heart failure from cytokine storming; and from myocardial infarction.[28-32] A generalized inflammatory state in COVID-19 is reflected by elevated serum inflammatory markers such as C-reactive protein (CRP), erythrocyte sedimentation rate (ESR), and interleukin-6 (IL-6).[33] COVID-19-related hypercoagulability may be indicated by elevated D-dimers or antiphospholipid antibodies. Clinical, laboratory, and autopsy evidence of hypercoagulable states in the pathophysiology of COVID-19 has been well described.[33] Both large vessel thrombosis and cerebral intravascular microthrombosis have been reported.[28, 34]

The severity of COVID-19 infection is related to stroke risk. In Mao's seminal paper of the neurologic manifestations of SARS-CoV-2, 41% of the 214 hospitalized patients were described as having severe COVID-19 infections, using the American Thoracic Society (ATS) criteria for defining severe community-acquired pneumonia.[1] The disease is defined as severe if the patient needs vasopressors due to shock, needs mechanical ventilation, or meets three other "minor" physiologic criteria, including confusion.[35] Of the six patients with stroke, five (83%) had severe COVID-19 infection as defined by these criteria. Other series reported similar findings of a correlation between severity of COVID-19 illness and higher incidence of cerebrovascular events.[31, 32, 36, 37] Not only

does severe COVID-19 infection predispose to stroke, but stroke also may increase the risk of in-hospital mortality from COVID-19 compared to matched controls, with an odds ratio for death of 3.[38]

There are certainly limitations in evaluating these often critically ill patients for potential stroke, especially in patients who are already hospitalized. Especially at the height of a local pandemic surge, each diagnostic test must be ordered while considering its effect on the use of PPE, the patient's isolation requirements, and the timing of tests due to the need for the terminal cleaning of the environment following testing for a COVID-positive patient. It may be challenging or not feasible to safely transport patients with high ventilator support settings or who are hemodynamically unstable. Finally, one must consider whether the information gathered would potentially change the patient's treatment or outcome. The frequency of COVID-19-associated cerebrovascular events may be underestimated due to these constraints, particularly in patients with severe systemic illness.

Ischemic stroke occurs in 0.9%–2.7% of patients hospitalized with COVID-19.[1, 31, 37] Comparatively, in a series of patients hospitalized with influenza, only 0.2% had concurrent acute ischemic strokes, even after adjusting for confounding variables.[32] There does seem to be something unique about COVID-19 and stroke predisposition in that "cryptogenic" stroke etiologies are significantly more prevalent in those with COVID-19 infections.[31] Most patients with ischemic stroke and COVID-19 (56%–74%) are diagnosed during their hospitalization for systemic symptoms. The remaining patients (26%–44%) present initially to the hospital for evaluation of stroke symptoms; they are either diagnosed with COVID-19 on admission or had known diagnosis but did not previously require hospitalization.[1, 31, 32]

Rates of ischemic events with COVID-19 are higher than hemorrhage events, and many retrospective reviews hypothesize that intraparenchymal hemorrhages are secondary to hemorrhagic conversion of ischemic strokes. The largest series of COVID-19 patients with spontaneous intracerebral hemorrhage (ICH) was described from the NYU Langone Hospitals; the overall diagnosis of ICH occurred in 0.9% (33 of 3824 patients).[36] This is similar to the pooled incidence rate of 0.7% for ICH in COVID-19 patients from a systematic review of the topic.[39] In the NYU series, ICH was defined as any acute intraparenchymal brain hemorrhage, whether due to primary ICH or to the hemorrhagic conversion of an ischemic infarct. Only four patients (or 0.1% of the overall cohort) had ICH on admission to the hospital, and half of those patients were on therapeutic anticoagulation at home. For most, ICH was diagnosed between hospital days 8 and 23; two-thirds were anticoagulated. In fact, therapeutic anticoagulation carries an odds ratio of 5 for ICH in the setting of acute SARS-CoV-2 infection.[34]

Most of the intraparenchymal hemorrhages were punctate or small, and were interpreted as hemorrhagic conversion of ischemic strokes. However, 15% ($n=5$) of patients with ICH in the NYU series had massive primary parenchymal hemorrhage with herniation. All of these patients also had diffuse hypoxic ischemic injury on imaging, all had been treated with full-dose anticoagulation, and all five patients died.[36] Overall mortality in patients with ICH and COVID-19 is appropriately 50%.[34, 36, 39]

Cerebral venous sinus thrombosis (CVST) and venous infarction have also been described in patients with active COVID-19 infection, although the exact incidence is unknown given its rare occurrence. Publications have been limited to case reports and a 13 patient multicenter, multinational case series.[40] Despite this, the consideration of CVST in the differential diagnosis of stroke with or without hemorrhage remains important, as the treatments of therapeutic anticoagulation and venous thrombectomy are unique to its underlying pathophysiology and may be lifesaving.

Aside from stroke as a manifestation of SARS-CoV-2, it is important to note that patients with a history of stroke who contract COVID-19 have increased morbidity and mortality compared to similar patients without a history of stroke.[1, 29, 41] Qin et al.[41] reviewed 1875 patients with COVID-19 patients from Wuhan, China over the period of late January to early March 2020. About 3% of these patients ($n=50$) had a history of stroke, most ischemic. Although patients with and without a previous stroke had similar severity of COVID-19 infection on hospital admission, patients with a stroke history were more likely to develop acute respiratory distress syndrome (ARDS) and had higher mortality. Other series have similarly reported a higher rate of debility and death in patients with COVID-19 and a history of stroke.[30, 31, 37] Finally, the patient with COVID-19 and a history of stroke also displayed greater derangement of "COVID labs"—higher levels of cardiac troponin I, D-Dimer, pro-BNP, IL-6, and more significant lymphopenia and thrombocytopenia—than patients without a history of stroke, perhaps reflecting the greater disease intensity or greater immune response to infection in this patient population.[41] Chapter 4 focuses on the cerebrovascular manifestations of COVID-19.

Seizures

Worldwide, seizures are reported in approximately 0.7%–2% of the total COVID-19 patient population.[42–44] Patients who are older have preexisting comorbidities, and have severe SARS-CoV-2 infection are more likely to have seizures with COVID-19,[43, 44] and are more susceptible to develop hypoxia, metabolic derangements, or electrolyte abnormalities, which can trigger seizures.[42, 45] Inflammatory markers such as CPK or CRP may be more greatly elevated in patients with seizures than in those without.[43]

With COVID-19, both generalized and focal-onset seizures have been reported, and they may occur de novo or in patients with preexisting epilepsy.[46, 47] In most patients with generalized, de novo seizures, metabolic derangements such as hyponatremia, uremia, or hypoxia are present.[47] Clinicians should be aware that de novo status epilepticus can be an initial presentation of COVID-19, prior to other systemic symptoms[48]; treatment is the same as that for other causes of status epilepticus. Seizures may also be a part of a broader neurologic syndromes caused by COVID-19 such as posterior reversible encephalopathy syndrome or stroke.[49, 50] Finally, patients with epilepsy are at risk of developing breakthrough seizures due to severe systemic infection.

A systematic review was performed on EEG findings in 617 patients with COVID-19. The indications for EEG were encephalopathy or coma in two-thirds of patients and seizure-like events in approximately one-third. In all, 114 patients (18%) had epileptiform discharges on EEG, while 138 (22%) had periodic or rhythmic patterns. Status epilepticus was found in 3.6% of patients who had an EEG ordered, and isolated seizures in an additional 1.9% of patients.[10] Many series have noted that in SARS-CoV-2 infection, electrographic seizures are seen only in patients with a history of epilepsy, clinical seizure-like events, or acute or chronic brain injury.[4, 11, 12, 51] Finally, in patients with seizures and COVID-19, prognosis is variable but seizures do not seem to increase mortality.[39] A detailed account of seizures in COVID-19 can be found in Chapter 5.

NEUROMUSCULAR COMPLICATIONS

Neuromuscular complications were uncommon with earlier SARS-CoV and MERS infections, manifesting mostly as axonal neuropathy or myopathy, and at times due to critical illness neuromyopathy. In contrast, SARS-CoV-2 infection is frequently associated with neuromuscular symptoms. Cranial neuropathy, peripheral neuropathy, myopathy, and rhabdomyolysis are all associated with COVID-19. These neuromuscular effects may be related to proinflammatory cytokines, direct viral effects, or para- or postinfectious autoimmunity.

Cranial Neuropathies

Loss of smell and taste were among the first neurologic symptoms described with SARS-CoV-2 infection.[1] Smell dysfunction is an early sign of infection, is not necessarily associated with rhinorrhea or nasal obstruction, and may precede systemic symptoms by several days.[52] Anosmia may be caused by olfactory nerve involvement through the ensheathing glial cells, which transfer virus independent of ACE2 receptors.[53] Taste dysfunction is secondary to poor olfaction rather than involvement of taste buds or other cranial nerves. The Wuhan retrospective series reported taste and smell impairment in 5.6% and 5.1% of hospitalized patients, respectively.[1] Later studies have reported smell dysfunction in 47%–98% of all patients with COVID-19.[52, 54–56] Complete olfactory recovery occurs in 44%–72% of patients, usually within 8–15 days of the onset.[56–59] A detailed account of anosmia and ageusia in COVID-19 is found in Chapter 10.

Facial nerve palsy has been well described in the context of active or recent SARS-CoV-2 infection,[60] and in the setting of acute COVID-19 may be accompanied by other cranial neuropathies such as olfactory dysfunction,[61] abducens nerve palsy,[62] and acute labyrinthitis.[61] There is a higher incidence of lower motor neuron facial nerve palsies during the COVID-19 pandemic, even in patients without known COVID-19, with cases increased by 1.7–2.7 times in 2020 compared to 2019.[60, 61] As per usual treatment of Bell's palsy, most of the patients were treated with oral corticosteroids. Recovery is complete in the majority of patients, with a lesser percent having partial recovery, and even fewer no recovery.[61, 62] There are also individual reports of acute oculomotor nerve palsy,[63] and abducens nerve palsy.[64] Finally, patients with any cranial nerve deficit should be thoroughly examined for other neurologic signs that might point to a central nervous system process or broader neuropathic process such as Miller-Fisher syndrome or polyneuritis cranialis.

Peripheral Neuropathies

Early in the pandemic, persistent flaccid paralysis was noted in 5% of critically ill patients with SARS-CoV-2 after withdrawal of sedation, but no other description of examination findings or supportive data were available, making this information hard to interpret.[2]

Guillain-Barre syndrome (GBS) and its variants can develop during the course of, or manifest as the initial presentation of, COVID-19.[33, 65] In the classic GBS variant of acute inflammatory demyelinating polyradiculoneuropathy (AIDP), patients present with ascending weakness and paresthesias developing over days and areflexia. Generally, GBS is preceded by a systemic infection or vaccination. In COVID-19-associated GBS, most patients had systemic symptoms of SARS-CoV-2 infection starting an average of 11 days prior to the onset of neurologic symptoms. CSF analysis revealed albuminocytological dissociation in a majority of patients, with none that were tested positive for SARS-CoV-2 PCR in the CSF. Where nerve conduction studies were reported, two-thirds were interpreted as AIDP and 15% as acute motor sensory axonal neuropathy (AMSAN).[65] The Miller-Fisher variant of GBS, characterized by ophthalmoplegia, ataxia, and areflexia, and polyneuritis cranialis, characterized by multiple cranial neuropathies, have also been associated with SARS-CoV-2 infection.[65, 66]

Treatments reported for these patients are standard for GBS, that is, IVIg at a dose of 0.4 g/kg/day for 5 days, or PLEX. Treatment of any concurrent SARS-CoV-2 infection has varied based on contemporary or local trends during the pandemic. Overall outcomes are hard to extrapolate due to varying reporting and timing of follow-up in these case reports and series; however, improvement is reported in about three quarters of patients.[33, 65]

The occurrence rate of GBS with SARS-CoV-2 in the United Kingdom is 0.82 cases per 1000 COVID-19 infections, using PCR-confirmed COVID-19 infections as the denominator. This occurrence rate is similar to that seen with other infectious agents that trigger GBS, such as cytomegalovirus and *Campylobacter jejuni*, of 0.2–2.2 cases per 1000 infections.[67] Importantly, the incidence of reported GBS cases during the COVID-19 pandemic has been similar to or lower than the incidence in other years of 1–2 per 100,000 persons/year.[67–69] While some conclude that there is "no association between COVID-19 and GBS,"[67] clinicians caring for patients who have GBS with a concurrent or preceding febrile illness and a positive SARS-CoV-2 PCR test may disagree. Indeed, some series have reported that half of patients presenting with GBS during the early phase of the pandemic had a serologic or clinical evidence of SARS-CoV-2 infection.[69] Certainly, COVID-19 does not seem to be a more potent trigger for GBS than other infectious agents. It seems likely that social distancing, mask wearing, and increased hand hygiene are limiting the spread of other infectious agents associated with

GBS,[67, 68] leading to lower rates of infections such as seasonal influenza in 2020–2021,[68] and therefore stabilizing or lowering overall rates of GBS.

Neuromuscular Junction Disorders

While not common, isolated cases of myasthenia gravis due to both acetylcholine receptor antibodies[70–72] and muscle-specific kinase (MuSK) antibodies[73] have been reported as developing in the weeks following acute COVID-19 infection. In the former, symptoms developed in four patients approximately 1–4 weeks following the onset of fever due to COVID-19; in the latter, fatigable weakness occurred 4 weeks after SARS-CoV-2 infection. Patients were treated with various combinations of PLEX, IVIg, pyridostigmine, and corticosteroids, and all experienced improvement.[70–73]

Muscle Involvement

Malaise, body aches, and generalized fatigue are common symptoms of febrile illnesses. Mao and colleagues first described the finding of skeletal muscle injury [defined as skeletal muscle pain and a serum creatine kinase (CK) level of greater than 200 U/L] in 11% of the initial cohort of hospitalized patients with SARS-CoV-2 infection.[1] The incidence of body aches, myalgias, and arthralgias in COVID-19 varies between 15% and 74%,[74–76] and seems to be more prevalent in outpatients than in hospitalized patients.[76, 77] Body aches last an average of 5 and 11 days in outpatients and inpatients, respectively.[76]

Mild elevations of serum CK are seen in many patients with COVID-19[1, 74, 75]; indeed, it has become part of the "COVID labs" in many institutions. True rhabdomyolysis—with muscle weakness, pain, and markedly elevated CK due to skeletal muscle necrosis—has been reported in a handful of patients, either as part of their presenting symptoms or later in the disease.[78]

Finally, critically ill patients with COVID-19 may experience acute flaccid quadriplegia or intensive care unit acquired weakness[2, 79]; this has been observed since early in the pandemic.[2] Critical illness myopathy has been reported in a series of six patients with COVID-19 respiratory failure upon attempted liberation from mechanical ventilation. These patients all had flaccid quadriplegia save for minimal hand movement, decreased but present deep tendon reflexes, and normal to mildly elevated CKs. Neurophysiologic studies were consistent with myopathy, with fibrillation potentials and small polyphasic motor units in proximal muscles, markedly reduced compound muscle action potential amplitudes, and normal sensory nerve action potentials. Five patients had marked improvement in

2–3 weeks, and unfortunately the sixth patient died of systemic complications.[79] Neuromuscular complications of COVID-19 are further detailed in Chapter 7.

CONCLUSION

To know COVID-19 is to know medicine, and to know neurologic complications of COVID-19 is to know neurology.

REFERENCES

1. Mao L, Jin H, Wang M, et al. Neurologic manifestations of hospitalized patients with coronavirus disease 2019 in Wuhan, China [published online ahead of print, 2020 Apr 10]. *JAMA Neurol.* 2020;77(6):1–9. https://doi.org/10.1001/jamaneurol.2020.1127.
2. Fan S, Xiao M, Han F, et al. Neurological manifestations in critically Ill patients with COVID-19: a retrospective study. *Front Neurol.* 2020;11:806. Published 2020 Jul 10 https://doi.org/10.3389/fneur.2020.00806.
3. Liotta EM, Batra A, Clark JR, et al. Frequent neurologic manifestations and encephalopathy-associated morbidity in Covid-19 patients. *Ann Clin Transl Neurol.* 2020;7(11):2221–2230. https://doi.org/10.1002/acn3.51210.
4. Helms J, Kremer S, Merdji H, et al. Delirium and encephalopathy in severe COVID-19: a cohort analysis of ICU patients. *Crit Care.* 2020;24(1):491. Published 2020 Aug 8 https://doi.org/10.1186/s13054-020-03200-1.
5. Beach SR, Praschan NC, Hogan C, et al. Delirium in COVID-19: a case series and exploration of potential mechanisms for central nervous system involvement. *Gen Hosp Psychiatry.* 2020;65:47–53. https://doi.org/10.1016/j.genhosppsych.2020.05.008.
6. Muccioli L, Pensato U, Bernabè G, et al. Intravenous immunoglobulin therapy in COVID-19-related encephalopathy [published online ahead of print, 2020 Oct 8]. *J Neurol.* 2020;1–5. https://doi.org/10.1007/s00415-020-10248-0.
7. Kandemirli SG, Dogan L, Sarikaya ZT, et al. Brain MRI findings in patients in the intensive care unit with COVID-19 infection [published online ahead of print, 2020 May 8]. *Radiology.* 2020;201697. https://doi.org/10.1148/radiol.2020201697.
8. Gulko E, Oleksk ML, Gomes W, et al. MRI brain findings in 126 patients with COVID-19: initial observations from a descriptive literature review. *AJNR Am J Neuroradiol.* 2020;41(12):2199–2203. https://doi.org/10.3174/ajnr.A6805.
9. Radmanesh A, Derman A, Lui YW, et al. COVID-19-associated diffuse leukoencephalopathy and microhemorrhages [published online ahead of print, 2020 May 21]. *Radiology.* 2020;202040. https://doi.org/10.1148/radiol.2020202040.
10. Antony AR, Haneef Z. Systematic review of EEG findings in 617 patients diagnosed with COVID-19. *Seizure.* 2020;83:234–241. https://doi.org/10.1016/j.seizure.2020.10.014.

11. Pellinen J, Carroll E, Friedman D, et al. Continuous EEG findings in patients with COVID-19 infection admitted to a New York academic hospital system. *Epilepsia.* 2020;61(10):2097–2105. https://doi.org/10.1111/epi.16667.

12. Pasini E, Bisulli F, Volpi L, et al. EEG findings in COVID-19 related encephalopathy. *Clin Neurophysiol.* 2020;131(9):2265–2267. https://doi.org/10.1016/j.clinph.2020.07.003.

13. Pilotto A, Odolini S, Masciocchi S, et al. Steroid-responsive encephalitis in coronavirus disease 2019. *Ann Neurol.* 2020;88(2):423–427. https://doi.org/10.1002/ana.25783.

14. Dogan L, Kaya D, Sarikaya T, et al. Plasmapheresis treatment in COVID-19-related autoimmune meningoencephalitis: case series. *Brain Behav Immun.* 2020;87:155–158.

15. Helms J, Kremer S, Merdji H, et al. Neurologic features in severe SARS-CoV-2 infection. *N Engl J Med.* 2020;382(23):2268–2270. https://doi.org/10.1056/NEJMc2008597.

16. Khodamoradi Z, Hosseini SA, Gholampoor Saadi MH, Mehrabi Z, Sasani MR, Yaghoubi S. COVID-19 meningitis without pulmonary involvement with positive cerebrospinal fluid PCR. *Eur J Neurol.* 2020;27(12):2668–2669. https://doi.org/10.1111/ene.14536.

17. Bansal P, Fory EK, Malik S, Memon AB. Clinical course of a patient with radiographically described acute necrotizing encephalopathy. *Radiology.* 2020;297(2):E278–E280. https://doi.org/10.1148/radiol.2020203132.

18. Levine JM, Ahsan N, Ho E, Santoro JD. Genetic acute necrotizing encephalopathy associated with RANBP2: clinical and therapeutic implications in pediatrics. *Mult Scler Relat Disord.* 2020;43:102194. https://doi.org/10.1016/j.msard.2020.102194.

19. Wu X, Wu W, Pan W, Wu L, Liu K, Zhang HL. Acute necrotizing encephalopathy: an underrecognized clinicoradiologic disorder. *Mediat Inflamm.* 2015;2015:792578. https://doi.org/10.1155/2015/792578.

20. Pohl D, Alper G, Van Haren K, et al. Acute disseminated encephalomyelitis: updates on an inflammatory CNS syndrome. *Neurology.* 2016;87(9 Suppl 2):S38–S45. https://doi.org/10.1212/WNL.0000000000002825.

21. Paterson RW, Brown RL, Benjamin L, et al. The emerging spectrum of COVID-19 neurology: clinical, radiological and laboratory findings. *Brain.* 2020;143(10):3104–3120. https://doi.org/10.1093/brain/awaa240.

22. Novi G, Rossi T, Pedemonte E, et al. Acute disseminated encephalomyelitis after SARS-CoV-2 infection [published correction appears in Neurol Neuroimmunol Neuroinflamm. 2020 Dec 15;8(1):]. *Neurol Neuroimmunol Neuroinflamm.* 2020;7(5):e797. Published 2020 Jun 1 https://doi.org/10.1212/NXI.0000000000000797.

23. Langley L, Zeicu C, Whitton L, Pauls M. Acute disseminated encephalomyelitis (ADEM) associated with COVID-19. *BMJ Case Rep.* 2020;13(12):e239597. Published 2020 Dec 13 https://doi.org/10.1136/bcr-2020-239597.

24. Keyhanian K, Umeton RP, Mohit B, Davoudi V, Hajighasemi F, Ghasemi M. SARS-CoV-2 and nervous system: from pathogenesis to clinical manifestation [published online ahead of print, 2020 Nov 7]. *J Neuroimmunol.* 2020;350:577436. https://doi.org/10.1016/j.jneuroim.2020.577436.

25. Masuccio FG, Barra M, Claudio G, Claudio S. A rare case of acute motor axonal neuropathy and myelitis related to SARS-CoV-2 infection [published online ahead of print, 2020 Sep 17]. *J Neurol.* 2020;1–4. https://doi.org/10.1007/s00415-020-10219-5.

26. Zhou S, Jones-Lopez EC, Soneji DJ, Azevedo CJ, Patel VR. Myelin oligodendrocyte glycoprotein antibody-associated optic neuritis and myelitis in COVID-19. *J Neuroophthalmol.* 2020;40(3):398–402. https://doi.org/10.1097/WNO.0000000000001049.

27. Ghosh R, De K, Roy D, et al. A case of area postrema variant of neuromyelitis optica spectrum disorder following SARS-CoV-2 infection [published online ahead of print, 2020 Nov 11]. *J Neuroimmunol.* 2020;350:577439. https://doi.org/10.1016/j.jneuroim.2020.577439.

28. Fabbri VP, Foschini MP, Lazzarotto T, et al. Brain ischemic injury in COVID-19-infected patients: a series of 10 post-mortem cases [published online ahead of print, 2020 Oct 1]. *Brain Pathol.* 2020. https://doi.org/10.1111/bpa.12901, e12901.

29. Zubair AS, McAlpine LS, Gardin T, Farhadian S, Kuruvilla DE, Spudich S. Neuropathogenesis and neurologic manifestations of the coronaviruses in the age of coronavirus disease 2019: a review. *JAMA Neurol.* 2020. https://doi.org/10.1001/jamaneurol.2020.2065.

30. Pérez CA. Looking ahead. *Neurol: Clin Pract.* 2020;10(4):371–374. https://doi.org/10.1212/cpj.0000000000000836.

31. Yaghi S, Ishida K, Torres J, et al. SARS-CoV-2 and stroke in a New York healthcare system. *Stroke.* Jul 2020;51(7):2002–2011. https://doi.org/10.1161/STROKEAHA.120.030335.

32. Merkler AE, Parikh NS, Mir S, et al. Risk of ischemic stroke in patients with coronavirus disease 2019 (COVID-19) vs patients with influenza. *JAMA Neurol.* 2020. https://doi.org/10.1001/jamaneurol.2020.2730.

33. Ellul MA, Benjamin L, Singh B, et al. Neurological associations of COVID-19. *Lancet Neurol.* Sep 2020;19(9):767–783. https://doi.org/10.1016/S1474-4422(20)30221-0.

34. Melmed KR, Cao M, Dogra S, et al. Risk factors for intracerebral hemorrhage in patients with COVID-19. [published online ahead of print, 2020 Sept 24]. *J Thromb Thrombolysis.* 2020;1–8. doi:10.100y7/s11239-020-02288-0.

35. Metlay JP, Waterer GW, Long AC, et al. Diagnosis and treatment of adults with community-acquired pneumonia. An official clinical practice guideline of the American Thoracic Society and Infectious Diseases Society of America. *Am J Respir Crit Care Med.* 2019;200(7):e45–e67. https://doi.org/10.1164/rccm.201908-1581ST.

36. Dogra S, Jain R, Cao M, et al. Hemorrhagic stroke and anticoagulation in COVID-19. *J Stroke Cerebrovasc Dis.* 2020;29(8):104984. https://doi.org/10.1016/j.jstrokecerebrovasdis.2020.104984.

37. Tsivgoulis G, Katsanos AH, Ornello R, Sacco S. Ischemic stroke epidemiology during the COVID-19 pandemic: navigating uncharted waters with changing tides. *Stroke.* 2020;51(7):1924–1926. https://doi.org/10.1161/STROKEAHA.120.030791.

38. Eskandar EN, Altschul DJ, de La Garza RR, et al. Neurologic syndromes predict higher in-hospital mortality in COVID-19 [published online ahead of print, 2020 Dec 18]. *Neurology.* 2020. https://doi.org/10.1212/WNL.0000000000011356.

39. Cheruiyot I, Sehmi P, Ominde B, et al. Intracranial hemorrhage in coronavirus disease 2019 (COVID-19) patients [published online ahead of print, 2020 Nov 3]. *Neurol Sci.* 2020;1–9. https://doi.org/10.1007/s10072-020-04870-z.

40. Mowla A, Shakibajahromi B, Shahjouei S, et al. Cerebral venous sinus thrombosis associated with SARS-CoV-2; a multinational case series. *J Neurol Sci.* 2020;419:117183. https://doi.org/10.1016/j.jns.2020.117183.

41. Qin C, Zhou L, Hu Z, et al. Clinical characteristics and outcomes of COVID-19 patients with a history of stroke in Wuhan, China. *Stroke.* 2020;51(7):2219–2223. https://doi.org/10.1161/STROKEAHA.120.030365.

42. Lu L, Xiong W, Liu D, et al. New onset acute symptomatic seizure and risk factors in coronavirus disease 2019: a retrospective multicenter study. *Epilepsia.* 2020;61(6):e49–e53.

43. Romero-Sanchez CM, Diaz-Maroto I, Fernandez-Diaz E, et al. Neurologic manifestations in hospitalized patients with COVID-19: the ALBACOVID registry. *Neurology.* 2020;1. https://doi.org/10.1212/WNL.0000000000009937.

44. Pinna P, Grewal P, Hall JP, et al. Neurological manifestations and COVID-19: experiences from a tertiary Care Center at the frontline. *J Neurol Sci.* 2020;415:116969. https://doi.org/10.1016/j.jns.2020.116969.

45. Hepburn M, Mullaguri N, George P, et al. Acute symptomatic seizures in critically ill patients with COVID-19: is there an association? *Neurocrit Care.* 2020;1–5. https://doi.org/10.1007/s12028-020-01006-1.

46. Sohal S, Mossammat M. COVID-19 presenting with seizures. *IDCases.* 2020;20. https://doi.org/10.1016/j.idcr.2020.e00782, e00782.

47. Anand P, Al-Faraj A, Sader E, et al. Seizure as the presenting symptom of COVID-19: a retrospective case series. *Epilepsy Behav.* 2020;112:107335. https://doi.org/10.1016/j.yebeh.2020.107335.

48. Somani S, Pati S, Gaston T, Chitlangia A, Agnihotri S. De novo status epilepticus in patients with COVID-19. *Ann Clin Transl Neurol.* 2020;7(7):1240–1244. https://doi.org/10.1002/acn3.51071.

49. Klein D, Libman R, Kirsch C, Arora R. Cerebral venous thrombosis: a typical presentation of COVID-19 in the young. *J Stroke Cerebrovasc Dis.* 2020;29(8):104989. https://doi.org/10.1016/j.jstrokecerebrovasdis.2020.104989.

50. Enjuto SG, Requejo VH, Motilva JL, et al. Verapamil as treatment for refractory status epilepticus secondary to PRES syndrome on a SARS-Cov-2 infected patient. *Seizure.* 2020;80:157–158. https://doi.org/10.1016/j.seizure.2020.06.008.

51. Louis S, Dhawan A, Newey C, et al. Continuous electroencephalography characteristics and acute symptomatic seizures in COVID-19 patients. *Clin Neurophysiol.* 2020;131(11):2651–2656. https://doi.org/10.1016/j.clinph.2020.08.003.

52. Lechien JR, Chiesa-Estomba CM, De Siati DR, et al. Olfactory and gustatory dysfunctions as a clinical presentation of mild-to-moderate forms of the coronavirus disease (COVID-19): a multicenter European study. *Eur Arch Otorhinolaryngol.* 2020;277(8):2251–2261. https://doi.org/10.1007/s00405-020-05965-1.

53. Fantini J, Di Scala C, Chahinian H, Yahi N. Structural and molecular modelling studies reveal a new mechanism of action of chloroquine and hydroxychloroquine against SARS-CoV-2 infection. *Int J Antimicrob Agents.* 2020;55(5):105960. https://doi.org/10.1016/j.ijantimicag.2020.105960.

54. Spinato G, Fabbris C, Polesel J, et al. Alterations in smell or taste in mildly symptomatic outpatients with SARS-CoV-2 infection. *JAMA.* 2020. https://doi.org/10.1001/jama.2020.6771. Published online April 22.

55. Moein ST, Hashemian SM, Mansourafshar B, Khorram-Tousi A, Tabarsi P, Doty RL. Smell dysfunction: a biomarker for COVID-19. *Int Forum Allergy Rhinol.* 2020;10(8):944–950. https://doi.org/10.1002/alr.22587.

56. Cho RHW, To ZWH, Yeung ZWC, et al. COVID-19 viral load in the severity of and recovery from olfactory and gustatory dysfunction. *Laryngoscope.* 2020;130(11):2680–2685. https://doi.org/10.1002/lary.29056.

57. Whitcroft KL, Hummel T. Olfactory dysfunction in COVID-19: diagnosis and management. *JAMA.* 2020;323(24):2512–2514. https://doi.org/10.1001/jama.2020.8391.

58. Chary E, Carsuzaa F, Trijolet JP, et al. Prevalence and recovery from olfactory and gustatory dysfunctions in Covid-19 infection: a prospective multicenter study. *Am J Rhinol Allergy.* 2020;34(5):686–693. https://doi.org/10.1177/1945892420930954.

59. Gorzkowski V, Bevilacqua S, Charmillon A, et al. Evolution of olfactory disorders in COVID-19 patients. *Laryngoscope.* 2020;130(11):2667–2673. https://doi.org/10.1002/lary.28957.

60. Codeluppi L, Venturelli F, Rossi J, et al. Facial palsy during the COVID-19 pandemic. *Brain Behav.* 2021;11(1). https://doi.org/10.1002/brb3.1939, e01939.

61. Zammit M, Markey A, Webb C. A rise in facial nerve palsies during the coronavirus disease 2019 pandemic [published online ahead of print, 2020 Oct 1]. *J Laryngol Otol.* 2020;1–4. https://doi.org/10.1017/S0022215120002121.

62. Lima MA, Silva MTT, Soares CN, et al. Peripheral facial nerve palsy associated with COVID-19. *J Neurovirol.* 2020;26(6):941–944. https://doi.org/10.1007/s13365-020-00912-6.

63. Belghmaidi S, Nassih H, Boutgayout S, et al. Third cranial nerve palsy presenting with unilateral diplopia and strabismus in a 24-year-old woman with COVID-19. *Am J Case Rep.* 2020;21:e925897. Published 2020 Oct 15 10.12659/AJCR.925897.

64. Dinkin M, Gao V, Kahan J, et al. COVID-19 presenting with ophthalmoparesis from cranial nerve palsy. *Neurology.* 2020;95(5):221–223. https://doi.org/10.1212/WNL.0000000000009700.

65. Caress JB, Castoro RJ, Simmons Z, et al. COVID-19-associated Guillain-Barré syndrome: the early pandemic experience. *Muscle Nerve.* 2020;62(4):485–491. https://doi.org/10.1002/mus.27024.

66. Gutiérrez-Ortiz C, Méndez-Guerrero A, Rodrigo-Rey S, et al. Miller fisher syndrome and polyneuritis cranialis in COVID-19. *Neurology.* 2020;95(5):e601–e605. https://doi.org/10.1212/WNL.0000000000009619.

67. Keddie S, Pakpoor J, Mousele C, et al. Epidemiological and cohort study finds no association between COVID-19 and Guillain-Barré syndrome [published online ahead of print, 2020 Dec 14]. *Brain.* 2020;awaa433. https://doi.org/10.1093/brain/awaa433.

68. Centers for Disease Control and Prevention. *Weekly U.S. influenza surveillance report*; 2021. January 29 https://www.cdc.gov/flu/weekly/. Accessed 31 January 2021.

69. Fragiel M, Miró Ò, Llorens P, et al. Incidence, clinical, risk factors and outcomes of Guillain-Barré in Covid-19 [published online ahead of print, 2020 Dec 9]. *Ann Neurol.* 2020. https://doi.org/10.1002/ana.25987.

70. Restivo DA, Centonze D, Alesina A, Marchese-Ragona R. Myasthenia gravis associated with SARS-CoV-2 infection. *Ann Intern Med.* 2020;173(12):1027–1028. https://doi.org/10.7326/L20-0845.

71. Huber M, Rogozinski S, Puppe W, et al. Postinfectious onset of myasthenia gravis in a COVID-19 patient. *Front Neurol.* 2020;11:576153. Published 2020 Oct 6 https://doi.org/10.3389/fneur.2020.576153.

72. Sriwastava S, Tandon M, Kataria S, Daimee M, Sultan S. New onset of ocular myasthenia gravis in a patient with COVID-19: a novel case report and literature review [published online ahead of print, 2020 Oct 12]. *J Neurol.* 2020;1–7. https://doi.org/10.1007/s00415-020-10263-1.

73. Muhammed L, Baheerathan A, Cao M, Leite MI, Viegas S. MuSK antibody-associated myasthenia gravis with SARS-CoV-2 infection: a case report [published online ahead of print, 2021 Jan 12]. *Ann Intern Med.* 2021;L20–1298. https://doi.org/10.7326/L20-1298.

74. Guan W, Ni Z, Hu Y, et al. Clinical characteristics of coronavirus disease 2019 in China. *N Engl J Med.* 2020;382:1708–1720.

75. Huang C, Wang Y, Li X, et al. Clinical features of patients infected with 2019 novel coronavirus in Wuhan, China. *Lancet.* 2020;395:497–506.

76. Vahey GM, Marshall KE, McDonald E, et al. Symptom profiles and progression in hospitalized and nonhospitalized patients with coronavirus disease, Colorado, USA, 2020. *Emerg Infect Dis.* 2021;27(2):385–395. https://doi.org/10.3201/eid2702.203729.

77. Lapostolle F, Schneider E, Vianu I, et al. Clinical features of 1487 COVID-19 patients with outpatient management in the Greater Paris: the COVID-call study. *Intern Emerg Med.* 2020;15(5):813–817. https://doi.org/10.1007/s11739-020-02379-z.

78. Paliwal VK, Garg RK, Gupta A, Tejan N. Neuromuscular presentations in patients with COVID-19. *Neurol Sci.* 2020;41(11):3039–3056. https://doi.org/10.1007/s10072-020-04708-8.

79. Madia F, Merico B, Primiano G, Cutuli SL, De Pascale G, Servidei S. Acute myopathic quadriplegia in patients with COVID-19 in the intensive care unit. *Neurology.* 2020;95(11):492–494. https://doi.org/10.1212/WNL.0000000000010280.

CHAPTER 4

COVID-19 and Cerebrovascular Diseases

PANAYIOTIS D. MITSIAS[a,b,c,d,e] • HASSAN ABOUL NOUR[b] •
ALI MOHAMUD[b] • GEORGE VOURAKIS[d,e] • ALEX ABOU CHEBL[a,b] •
OWAIS KHADEM ALSROUJI[a,b]
[a]Comprehensive Stroke Center, Henry Ford Hospital, Detroit, MI, United States, [b]Department of Neurology, Henry Ford Hospital, Detroit, MI, United States, [c]School of Medicine, Wayne State University, Detroit, MI, United States, [d]School of Medicine, University of Crete, Heraklion, Greece, [e]Department of Neurology, University General Hospital, Heraklion, Greece

INTRODUCTION

Coronavirus disease 2019 (COVID-19) is the result of infection by the severe acute respiratory syndrome coronavirus 2 (SARS-CoV-2). Between the start of the outbreak in the last quarter of 2019 and January 25, 2021, there have been 97,831,595 confirmed cases of COVID-19 and 2,120,877 deaths reported to the World Health Organization in 237 countries, areas, and territories.[1]

COVID-19 typically affects the respiratory system, resulting in a wide variety of manifestations, from mild upper airway symptoms to pneumonia and severe acute respiratory distress syndrome.[2] The central nervous system is increasingly recognized as a target for the SARS-CoV-2; it can be invaded via the olfactory route, hematogenously, and also through the lymphatic tissue and CSF.[3] Clinically, headache, dizziness, confusion, seizures, delirium, and coma have been reported.

Cerebrovascular complications of COVID-19 were initially reported with a rather high prevalence in patients who developed more serious disease.[4] Since then, multiple published reports have argued whether the link between COVID-19 and stroke is a mere coincidence or directly causal. Despite this vivid argument, the ongoing COVID-19 pandemic has resulted in decreasing numbers of stroke admissions throughout the world[5,6] and the emergence of more severe strokes linked with the infection.[7]

In this chapter, we review the possible pathogenetic mechanisms of stroke in the context of COVID-19 infection, the clinical syndromes, and the possible therapeutic options for stroke in this setting, as well as the change in the delivery of care for acute stroke patients during the pandemic.

STROKE PATHOGENESIS IN COVID-19

In the setting of COVID-19, stroke can occur in the absence of any known stroke risk factors. However, patients with severe COVID-19 usually harbor common stroke risk factors such as hypertension, diabetes mellitus, smoking, dyslipidemia, prior stroke, or underlying cardiovascular disease,[8] making the association between COVID-19 and stroke range between direct causation and mere coincidence. However, in the setting of COVID-19, certain pathogenic mechanisms for cerebrovascular disease appear to play a more distinct role. These are summarized in Table 4.1.

Angiotensin-Converting Enzyme 2 (ACE2) Dysregulation

The proposed mechanism of entry of SARS-CoV into the epithelial cells of the respiratory system relates to the expression of the metallopeptidase ACE2[9] indicating that ACE2 is a functional receptor for the virus. Hamming et al. investigated the localization of ACE2 protein in various human organs (oral and nasal mucosa, nasopharynx, lung, stomach, small intestine, colon, skin, lymph nodes, thymus, bone marrow, spleen, liver, kidney, and brain) and found that there was a surface expression of ACE2 protein not only on lung alveolar epithelial cells and enterocytes of the small intestine, but also in arterial and venous endothelial cells, and arterial smooth muscle cells in all organs studied.[10] This epithelial expression in the lung and small intestine, together with the presence of ACE2 in vascular endothelium, provided a first step in understanding the pathogenesis of the main disease manifestations. Evidence also exists that ACE2 is present in glial cells and neurons.[11]

Neurological Care and the COVID-19 Pandemic. https://doi.org/10.1016/B978-0-323-82691-4.00008-X

TABLE 4.1
Pathophysiological States Contributing to Stroke in COVID-19.

	Ischemic Stroke	Cerebral Venous Thrombosis	Intracerebral Hemorrhage
ACE2 dysregulation	• Vasoconstriction • Neuroinflammation • Oxidative stress • Thrombogenesis • Tissue hypoperfusion		• Blood pressure elevation • Vasodilation
Coagulation disorders	• Cerebral arterial thrombosis • Paradoxical embolism (patent foramen ovale and pulmonary arteriovenous shunts) • Microcirculation thromboses	• Extensive dural sinus and cortical vein thromboses	• Severe derangement of hemostasis (decreased platelet count, increased fibrin degradation products, low fibrinogen, prolonged PT) • Therapeutic anticoagulation
CNS endotheliitis and vasculitis	• Endothelial dysfunction • In situ thrombosis • Vessel stenosis		• Microvascular fragility
Cardiac dysfunction	• Ventricular dysfunction • Myocarditis • Myocardial ischemia • Cardiac arrhythmias		
Critical illness	• Hypotension • Hypoxia/anoxia		• Cerebral microhemorrhages • Therapeutic anticoagulation

Binding of the SARS-CoV-2 virus to the ACE2 causes inactivation of the receptor, resulting in reduced conversion of Angiotensin II (Ang II), a potent vasoconstrictor and angiogenic factor, to Angiotensin (1–7) (Ang 1–7), a factor with vasodilatory and several antiinflammatory properties. This imbalance in turn leads to overactivation of the classical renin-angiotensin-aldosterone system (RAAS) axis, as well as underactivation of the alternative RAAS signaling in the brain. The downstream effects are enhanced vasoconstriction, neuroinflammation, blood–brain barrier permeability, oxidative stress, and thrombogenesis, all of which can contribute to stroke pathophysiology during SARS-CoV-2 infection[12] (Fig. 4.1). Blood pressure elevations can occur, which can be particularly important in the pathogenesis of intracerebral hemorrhage (ICH), although data available to date suggest that patients with ICH in the context of COVID-19 present with lower blood pressure levels compared to those with spontaneous, non-COVID-19 related ICH.[13]

ACE2 inactivation may also result in endothelial dysfunction of the brain arteries and has been considered important in the pathogenesis of stroke, ischemic, and hemorrhagic.[14-16] ACE2 dysregulation can also play a major role in the inflammation cascade after acute ischemia, which in turn can result in larger infarct volumes as a result of decreased perfusion.[17]

Coagulation Disorders and the Hypercoagulable States

Several studies have addressed the issue of hypercoagulability associated with severe COVID-19 illness, which may be associated with several diverse factors,[18-21] including dehydration, inflammation, hyperfibrinogenemia, endothelial cell injury, and platelet activation.

The severe inflammatory state secondary to COVID-19 leads to a severe derangement of hemostasis that has been recently described as a state of disseminated intravascular coagulation (DIC) and consumption coagulopathy, defined as decreased platelet count, increased fibrin degradation products such as D-dimer, as well as low fibrinogen.[22] Often, however, this coagulation disorder does not meet the criteria for DIC.[23]

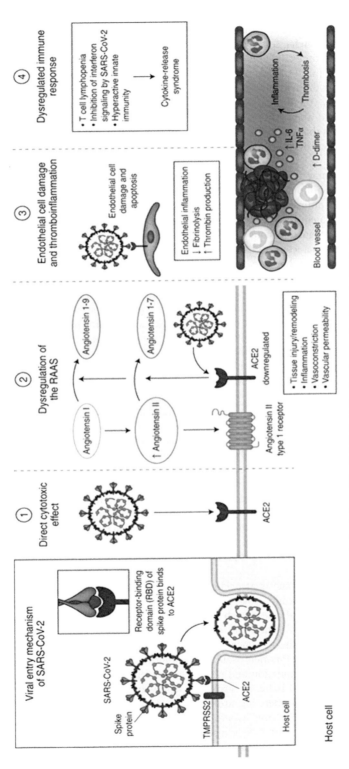

FIG. 4.1 Schematic depicting of the SARS-CoV-2 cell entry mechanism via ACE2, the resulting RAAS dysregulation and its complications. (Reproduced with permission from Gupta A, Madhavan MV, Sehgal K. et al. Extrapulmonary manifestations of COVID-19. Nat Med, 2020;26:1017–1032.)

In a study of thromboelastrography in patients with severe COVID-19, the parameters were consistent with a state of hypercoagulability. Platelet count was normal or increased, prothrombin time (PT) and activated partial thromboplastin time (aPTT) were near normal, fibrinogen, D-dimer was dramatically increased, C-reactive protein, factor VIII, von Willebrand factor, and protein C were all increased, and antithrombin was marginally decreased,[24] results that were in support of hypercoagulability in the context of a severe inflammatory state.

COVID-19 coagulopathy may also manifest with the development of antiphospholipid antibodies, usually the lupus anticoagulant, anticardiolipin IgA and antibodies against β2-glycoprotein-I.[18, 25] Often these antibodies can cause a hypercoagulable state, but they can also appear in conditions characterized by intense immune activation where they may have no apparent pathogenic role.

Another important part of the pathogenicity of the hypercoagulable state in COVID-19 is the development of a potent cytokine storm. This is not unique to COVID-19 and has been described in MERS and SARS, both of which are closely related coronaviruses. IL-6, TNF, and IL-1β, all proinflammatory cytokines, are central in this process. The inflammatory state seen in COVID-19 is closely associated with a procoagulant state, caused by consumption of anticoagulant factors, overproduction of prothrombotic factors, and endothelial injury. This leads to microthrombosis, DIC, and venothrombotic events frequently seen in COVID-19 patients and is associated with a worse prognosis. Thrombin and Factor Xa have proinflammatory properties via activation of proteinase-activated receptors (PARs) and, therefore, their antagonists, such as Factor Xa inhibitors (e.g., apixaban and rivaroxaban) and low-molecular-weight heparins (LMWH) (e.g., enoxaparin), could not only have anticoagulant properties but antiinflammatory ones as well.[26]

The COVID-19 hypercoagulable state is associated with an increased risk of arterial ischemic stroke or cerebral venous thrombosis,[20, 27, 28] and also a high incidence of deep vein thrombosis.[29, 30] The latter can result in paradoxical embolism in the presence of a right-to-left circulation shunt. Patent foramen ovale is a common finding in the general population and it is important in the etiopathogenesis of ischemic stroke especially in young patients with no underlying stroke risk factors, especially when an underlying hypercoagulable state is present, such as the one associated with COVID-19. Right-to-left circulation shunts can also occur at the pulmonary level, usually related to pulmonary arteriovenous malformations or vascular dilatations. In a recent very important study in mechanically ventilated COVID-19 patients, contrast-enhanced transcranial Doppler detected microembolic signals in 83% of patients, the $PaO_2:FIO_2$ ratio was inversely correlated with the number of microbubbles, and the number of microbubbles was inversely correlated with lung compliance.[31] The authors suggested that pulmonary microvascular dilatations were the culprit for right-to-left circulation shunt and that these explain the disproportionate degree of hypoxemia in some patients with COVID-19 lung injury. However, the presence or absence of PFO was not assessed in this study.

The other face of coagulopathy, especially in the setting of severe COVID-19, is that of dysfunctional hemostasis, prolonged coagulation parameters, and a bleeding disorder. As already mentioned, the COVID-19 coagulopathy shares some features with DIC, but the overall combination of hematological findings suggests a different form of coagulation disorder.[23] Nevertheless, it can result in an increased risk of intracranial hemorrhage, especially given the frequent use of therapeutic anticoagulation in this setting.

Endotheliitis and Vasculitis of the central nervous system (CNS)

In a postmortem study of patients with COVID-19, viral elements were found within endothelial cells of various organs, including the kidney, heart, lungs, and small bowel in postmortem studies.[32] The investigators of this study found no evidence of myocarditis or inflammatory changes of the other organs. In one case, in particular, the patient developed acute reduction of the cardiac ejection fraction with mesenteric ischemia and histological evidence of endotheliitis of the submucosal vessels. In another patient, there was histological evidence of myocardial infarction without evidence of lymphocytic myocarditis.[32] These findings suggested that SARS-CoV-2 can cause widespread endotheliitis, without necessary associated vasculitis or myocarditis. Since then, similar observations have been made at postmortem examination of frontal lobe tissue from a patient who died from COVID-19, where the virus was found in neural and capillary endothelial cells.[33] In another series, brain biopsies showed signs of thrombotic microangiopathy, endothelial injury, and resulting hemorrhagic predisposition.[34] These findings support the notion that SARS-Cov-2 is a neurotropic and endotheliotropic virus that causes major endothelial dysfunction and subsequent degeneration (Fig. 4.2).

SARS-CoV-2 has been implicated in triggering a CNS vasculitis, which is often the case with several other

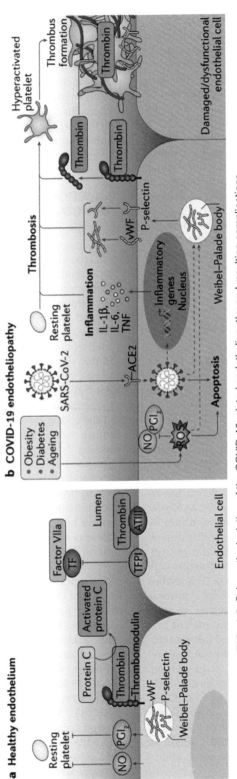

FIG. 4.2 Schematic depiction of the COVID-19 related endotheliopathy and resulting complications. (Reproduced with permission from Gu SX, Tyagi T, Jain K. et al. Thrombocytopathy and endotheliopathy: crucial contributors to COVID-19 thromboinflammation. Nat Rev Cardiol. 2020;1–16. doi: 10.1038/s41569-020-00469-1.)

viral infections, such as varicella zoster, hepatitis C, cytomegalovirus, human immunodeficiency virus and others, presumably due to the severe inflammatory response related to the cytokine storm. However, most reports do not refer to solid histological evidence from biopsy or autopsy specimens but rather to combinations of clinical and imaging findings, which do not establish the diagnosis of definite vasculitis.[34–36] It is possible that some of the reported cases were due to brain vasculitis, given the evidence of multiple coincidental ischemic and hemorrhagic strokes, but the lack of histological confirmation could still lend support to the possibility that most of these cases were actually related to endotheliitis.

Reversible cerebral vasoconstriction syndrome has also been reported in the context of COVID-19.[37, 38] This can mimic primary angiitis of the central nervous system, and typically presents with recurrent thunderclap headaches, and small subarachnoid bleeds in the brain convexities.[39]

Cardiac Dysfunction and Cardiogenic Embolism

Although COVID-19 clinical manifestations are mainly respiratory, virus-related cardiac injury leading to major cardiac complications are being reported. Proposed mechanisms of SARS-CoV-2 cardiac injury include direct viral injury, up- and downregulation of ACE2, cytokine release syndrome, hypoxia, aggravation of the underlying cardiac disease, and drug-induced toxicity.[40] Specifically, COVID-19 can be complicated with myocarditis, coronary artery disease, and acute coronary syndromes, as well as cardiac arrhythmias, including atrial fibrillation.[40–42] Autopsies have indeed revealed infiltration of myocardium by interstitial mononuclear inflammatory cells, providing strong evidence for COVID-19-induced myocarditis.[43] Additionally, in a small review, 38 patients with COVID-19 met clinical criteria for stress (Takotsubo) cardiomyopathy but the prevalence of the syndrome was not thought to be necessarily higher than in pre-COVID-19 times.[44] In one case, the patient presented with an acute ischemic stroke and Takotsubo.[45] Whether the cardiomyopathy was the cause, the result or a mere coincidence is subject to speculation. Cardiac imaging, and more specifically cardiac MRI, plays a major role in the diagnosis of COVID-19-related myocarditis.[42] Cardiac wall motion abnormalities and reduced cardiac output have the potential to be pathogenetic mechanisms for ischemic stroke in patients with COVID-19 through cardiogenic embolism and cerebral hypoperfusion.

Critical Illness Due to COVID-19

A significant fraction of patients with COVID-19, in some series up to approximately 30%, present with severe manifestations requiring intensive care unit management, which may include intubation and mechanical ventilation, resulting in prolonged hospitalizations. In this set of patients, systemic hypotension and hypoxia can result in additional cerebral ischemic complications, such as hypoxic/anoxic encephalopathy and hypoperfusion-induced brain ischemia.[46]

CEREBROVASCULAR COMPLICATIONS OF SARS-COV-2 INFECTION
Ischemic Stroke

In the first original study on stroke in COVID-19, Li et al. reported 219 cases presenting with acute neurological symptoms, 5% of which presented with acute ischemic stroke (AIS).[47] In another retrospective study, of the reported 214 cases with COVID-19, 5.7% had AIS,[4] and they mostly occurred in patients with severe infection. A recent prospective multinational study reported that of 17,799 patients, 123 patients had an AIS and that the need for mechanical ventilation and the presence of ischemic heart disease were independent predictors of stroke. A very interesting observation was also the fact that AIS could be the initial manifestation and the reason for hospital admission in a significant number, 26%, of patients with confirmed SARS-CoV-2 infection.[48]

In another study, patients who had a history of stroke and sustained COVID-19 infection were more likely to be admitted to the ICU and require mechanical ventilation. They were less likely to be discharged from the hospital and more likely to die in the hospital (22.4% vs 42.2%, 14.3%, vs 13.0%, respectively),[49] indicating that prior stroke results in a more severe clinical syndrome and poorer outcomes of COVID-19.

The matter of ischemic stroke subtype, according to the Trial of Org178 in Acute Stroke Treatment (TOAST) criteria, in patients with COVID-19 is of particular interest. COVID-19 has been associated with a higher than usual incidence of cryptogenic strokes.[48, 50] In a study from a Comprehensive Stroke Center in New York, cryptogenic stroke was more common in patients with COVID-19 (65.6%) as compared to contemporary controls (30.4%, $P = 0.003$) and historical controls (25.0%, $P < 0.001$).[51] In a large meta-analysis, compared to non-infected contemporary or historical controls, patients with SARS-CoV-2 infection had increased odds of ischemic stroke (OR = 3.58, 95% CI = 1.43–8.92, $I^2 = 43\%$) and cryptogenic stroke (OR = 3.98, 95% CI = 1.62–9.77,

$I^2 = 0\%$).[52] These findings raise the suspicion that a significant number of COVID-19-related strokes are caused by an acquired hypercoagulable state, or perhaps endotheliitis or paradoxical embolism. In other series, cryptogenic AIS subtype was also diagnosed with high frequency, up to 35%.[50, 53] Interestingly, while cardiogenic embolism has been the underlying stroke mechanisms for an increased proportion of patients with COVID-19 (up to 40%),[51, 53] small vessel disease/lacunar infarction subtype has been underrepresented in this patient population.[51, 53, 54] The latter suggests a lack of etiological association between COVID-19 and small vessel disease.

Another significant observation is that the younger patients without underlying risk factors present with stroke due to emergent large vessel occlusion (LVO).[55] More than half of the LVO stroke patients during the peak time of the New York City's COVID-19 outbreak were COVID-19 positive, and those patients with COVID-19 were younger, more likely to be male, and less likely to be white.[7] Multifocal LVOs is also a very concerning clinical presentation associated with poorer outcomes and is significantly more frequent in COVID-19 positive patients representing approximately 10% of all LVO strokes.[54] Figs. 4.3 and 4.4 illustrate the cases of two patients whose LVO strokes were attributed to SARS-CoV-2. The former occurred in a patient with no notable past medical history and the latter happened to a patient with presenting hypoxia and severe COVID-19 pneumonia.

Cerebral Venous Thrombosis

Venous thromboembolism occurs at a surprisingly high rate in patients with COVID-19 hospitalized in critical care units, and it may occur despite therapeutic anticoagulation treatment.[56] Cerebral venous thrombosis (CVT) likely is no exception, but its association with COVID-19 has not been as well described. The risk of thrombosis associated with COVID-19 is likely responsible for CVT. The majority of current knowledge comes from multiple case reports. One of the earliest cases of cerebral venous thrombosis was reported by Hughes et al. in which a 59-year-old male was presented with worsening headache, dysarthria, and subtle weakness. CT venogram identified thrombosis extending from the superior sagittal sinus through the right transverse and sigmoid sinuses, terminating in the right internal jugular vein.[57] In another report, a 65-year-old male presented with altered mental status, tongue biting, and gaze deviation was ultimately diagnosed with acute hemorrhagic venous infarction involving the right temporal lobe as a complication of right sigmoid

and transverse sinus thrombosis.[58] The patients in both cases were discharged from the hospital in fair condition. In another case, extensive thrombosis of the deep venous system was discovered in a patient presenting with sudden onset of hemiparesis and status epilepticus, with a demonstration of subacute strokes and basal ganglia and subcortical white matter hemorrhage.[59] The patient ultimately progressed to brain death. In a series of extensive CVT in COVID-19 patients, 3 young patients aged 23–41 years developed extensive cerebral venous thromboses, involving the straight sinus, vein of Galen, and internal cerebral veins. Two of them developed acute hemorrhage, and all had a fatal outcome.[60]

In a recent systematic review and meta-analysis, Baldini et al. summarized the clinical, neuroimaging, laboratory, treatment, and outcome features of 57 patients.[61] The mean age at diagnosis of CVT was 53.5 years; only 11/57 patients were under the age of 50 years.[61] The diagnosis of CVT followed the onset of clinical manifestations of COVID-19 in 90% of the patients. All patients had neurological signs or symptoms of CVT; epileptic seizures were reported in 27.8% of patients.[61] In neuroimaging studies, involvement of multiple vessels was more frequent than involvement of a single vessel (29/43 vs 14/43), with the transverse sinus being the most frequently affected vessel (65%) and hemorrhagic lesions developing in 42% of patients.[61] The cerebral deep venous system was also frequently affected, 37% of patients. D-dimer and C-reactive protein levels were almost universally elevated, and hyperfibrinogenemia was found in 54.5% of cases. In a small fraction of patients that had thrombophilia testing, antiphospholipid antibodies were found in 3/12 cases. Cerebrospinal fluid testing for COVID-19 by PCR was universally negative. In-hospital mortality was 40%, with patients having parenchymal hemorrhage having higher mortality (60%).

CVT related to COVID-19 seems to occur in older patients, compared to those with non-COVID-19-related CVT. It is also associated with extensive thrombosis and large clot burdens and results in poor outcomes. Diagnosing this condition is challenging, given the often atypical presentations, especially in critically ill patients. Clinicians should therefore be vigilant and proactive in making this diagnosis as early as possible in the course of the disease in order to improve outcomes.

Intracerebral Hemorrhage

In a retrospective case series of five patients with intracerebral hemorrhage (ICH), COVID-19 patients with ICH were younger than expected (mean age 52 years) and 4/5 (80%) developed lobar ICH with no underlying

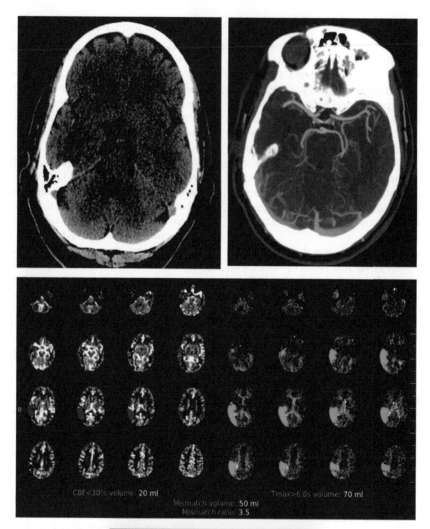

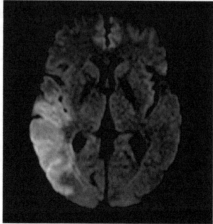

FIG. 4.3 A 58-year-old man with no significant past medical history presented with minor aphasia. The initial NIHSS score was 1. Computed tomography (CT) head revealed a hyperdense M2 segment of the right middle cerebral artery (MCA) (A, *arrow*). CT angiography (CTA) revealed right MCA occlusion (B, *arrow*). CT perfusion images are shown in (C) revealing a large penumbra-ischemic core mismatch. He received treatment with IV alteplase. SARS-CoV-2 PCR was positive. Postthrombolysis diffusion-weighted imaging (DWI) MRI revealed a large right temporoparietal infarct (D).

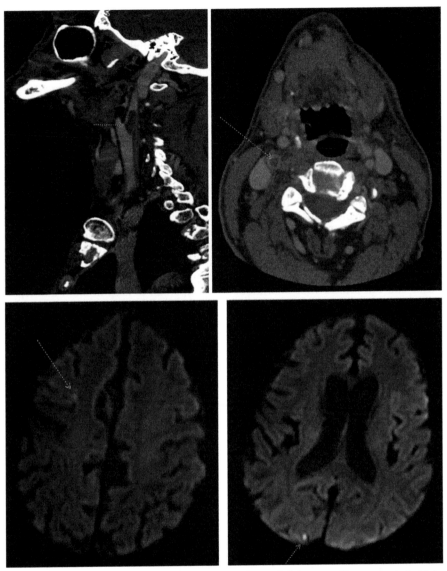

FIG. 4.4 A 75-year-old woman with underlying hypertension and diabetes mellitus presented with hypoxia (SpO2 85%) and altered mental status. Chest X-ray showed multifocal pneumonia. SARS-Cov-2 PCR was positive. CTA head and neck showed right carotid bulb thrombus with near occlusion of right internal carotid artery (ICA) (A and B, *arrows*). DWI revealed small acute ischemic lesions in the right hemisphere (C and D, *arrows*). The patient was initially started on anticoagulation with LMWH and 2 days later, she underwent right carotid endarterectomy with complete resolution of the clot on postoperative imaging.

vascular abnormality,[62] which is in contrast with the general population, where 25%–30% of ICH are of lobar location and are often associated with underlying vascular abnormalities. One of the patients described in this report had multifocal ICH without any underlying vascular abnormality.[62] The other interesting observation in this series was the delay between the time of COVID-19 symptom onset and time of ICH diagnosis, a median of 32 days (range 14–38 days), during which all five patients had evidence of a period of prolonged inflammation, demonstrated by markedly raised D-Dimer values and by severe end organ damage in 4/5 patients requiring multiple organ support. Similar results were reported in another cohort study, in which

19 of 4071 (0.5%) of hospitalized COVID-19 patients were diagnosed with hemorrhagic stroke, mostly related to coagulopathy.[63] In another observational study of hospitalized patients with COVID-19, however, cerebral hemorrhagic events were not more frequent compared to noninfected patients.[64]

It remains undetermined whether COVID-19 is the direct cause of ICH or whether secondary effects of COVID-19 such as renal or hepatic failure or the frequently used therapeutic anticoagulation in a critically ill older population is the culprit. Potential mechanisms that would link COVID-19 with ICH could include ACE2 inactivation, endothelial infection and inflammation, and SARS-CoC-2-induced coagulopathy. The atypical multifocal nature of many of the reported ICH cases to date would suggest some form of underlying vasculopathy which likely acts synergistically with the aforementioned factors in causing ICH.[65] Cerebral microbleeds have also been demonstrated in critically ill COVID-19 patients and can present with or without leukoencephalopathy.[65, 66] The atypical location of cerebral microbleeds in the corpus callosum and juxtacortical region may raise the suspicion of SARS-CoV-2 infection in critically ill patients.[65]

THERAPIES IN STROKE PATIENTS WITH COVID-19

The COVID-19 pandemic has caused challenges to the care of patients with AIS. Protocols have been implemented to help streamline the care process during the pandemic. Stroke has been reported to be the presenting symptom for COVID-19 in a minority of patients.[67] This puts clinicians at risk for contracting the disease although the specific risk has not yet been established. All patients presenting for evaluation of stroke-like symptoms should be screened for COVID-19 signs, symptoms, exposure, and travel within the past 14 days.[67] This can be done in the prehospital phase by emergency medical services (EMS) and results can be communicated to the hospital.[68] Patients who are unable to answer questions due to the stroke should be assumed to have COVID-19 until proven otherwise. Telecommunication should be used to limit physical interaction with the patient. If telecommunication is not present, donning of personal protection equipment (PPE) should be done prior to contact with the patient. A mask should be placed on all patients presenting for stroke evaluation preferably in the prehospital phase. Oxygen can be supplemented via nasal cannula underneath the mask and saturation should be targeted to >94%. All patients should be swabbed for rapid

SARS-CoV2 PCR. COVID-19 status does not change the patient's management but rather triage disposition and provide guidance for the care team and infection control. Timely assessment and hyperacute treatment remain the key to minimize mortality and morbidity of patients with acute stroke.

Intravenous Thrombolysis

After taking appropriate precautions patients should be evaluated for intravenous thrombolysis eligibility as soon as possible following current 2019 American Heart Association/American Stroke Association (AHA/ASA) stroke guidelines.[69] Imaging with CT and CT angiogram (CTA) and in some cases CT perfusion (CTP) should be performed as per pre-COVID-19 protocols. There have been reports of incidentally diagnosing pneumonia on stroke CTA. Careful evaluation of the lung fields shown in CTA head and neck should be undertaken. When considering IV thrombolysis it is important to keep in mind that sepsis can alter the coagulation profile and the patient may be hyper- or hypocoagulable.[70] Certain laboratory levels such as PT, aPTT, and platelet count may be needed to guide the decision to administer thrombolysis in select patients with confirmed or suspected COVID-19. Exclusion criteria for the use of intravenous thrombolysis in AIS remain the same and have not been altered for the patient with COVID-19. The door-to-needle time target should still be set for under 45 min while taking all safety measures to protect health-care providers. It is also very interesting that in a case series of patients with stroke and acute respiratory syndrome (ARDS) due to COVID-19, IV thrombolysis resulted in improved oxygenation in three patients, with one of them manifesting a durable response.[71] Postthrombolysis patients should be admitted and managed in an acute stroke unit

Endovascular Thrombectomy

Patients with large vessel occlusion (LVO)-related strokes who meet the current guidelines criteria[69] should undergo endovascular thrombectomy as soon as possible. Airway and respiratory status should be assessed immediately on the spot. Performing the procedure under conscious sedation should be considered as the initial option. Endotracheal intubation should be reserved for patients who are at risk for airway compromise, including patients with high oxygen demand, agitated and uncooperative and unable to protect their airway, and patients who are vomiting. If endotracheal intubation is deemed necessary, it must be done in a negative-pressure room by an airway expert prior to transfer to the angiography suite.

If possible, the angiography suite should also be set to negative pressure to minimize the airborne spread of the virus.[72] The members of the team caring for the patient should continue to assume full PPE including N95 masks, face shields, double cover gloves, gown and shoe covers, in addition to sterile precautions, until the results of COVID-19 PCR become available. The angiography suite should be emptied from all unnecessary items given possible viral spread from fomite transmission. Before the arrival of the patient, all procedural elements should be prepared including (devices, catheters, medications, and others) to limit breaking scrub, doffing of PPE, as well as personnel getting in and out of the room. Staff must be kept to the minimum to minimize exposure and preserve PPE. Hanging and standing lead shields must be used as a second layer of protection while using fluoroscopy as much as possible. Postprocedure neurological exam and access site check should be done before doffing of PPE.[73] Stable nonintubated patients may be placed in a step-down stroke unit instead of the intensive care unit to preserve resources. If available, telemedicine must be utilized to its full extent to perform frequent postprocedure checks and neurological monitoring. Postprocedure vital signs and neuro checks may be relaxed in an attempt to limit exposure and preserve PPE during the pandemic.

Antithrombotic Medications and Statin Therapy

Treatment with antithrombotic agents and statin medications remains crucial for all patients with ischemic stroke, including patients with concurrent COVID-19 infection. Current guidelines recommend immediate administration of aspirin or aspirin plus clopidogrel for minor strokes and high-risk transient ischemic attacks. Early in the pandemic, a concern was raised about the use of nonsteroidal-antiinflammatory medications (NSAID), and specifically ibuprofen, as they could worsen COVID-19 symptoms. The World Health Organization (WHO) initially recommended against the use of such medications, which are in the same drug class as aspirin. This concern was raised after a published short report indicated that ibuprofen can upregulate ACE2 which is the target receptor for SARS-CoV2, and therefore it was hypothesized that ibuprofen can worsen COVID-19 symptoms.[74] Subsequently, the WHO reversed this recommendation given the lack of true evidence and the risk being theoretical. Patients with COVID-19 and stroke should continue to receive all indicated antiplatelet medications as per current stroke guidelines.

Statins are also crucial for stroke secondary prevention. In addition to their lipid-lowering activity, statins have antiinflammatory, immune-modulatory, and angiogenic properties. Observation studies have shown that statin therapy had a positive effect in reducing all-cause mortality in hospitalized patients with influenza virus infection.[75] However, subsequent studies demonstrated no benefit for statin therapy was in patients with sepsis,[76] or in patients with ARDS.[77] In the absence of any reliable evidence supporting any benefit or harm for statin treatment in stroke patients with COVID-19, this treatment should be continued for secondary stroke secondary prevention, as per secondary stroke prevention guidelines.

Hypertension Management and ACE Inhibitors and Angiotensin Receptor Blockers

Hypertension is the most important risk factor for stroke, and hypertension control remains one of the major effective interventions for both primary and secondary stroke prevention. RAA antagonists, such as ACE inhibitors (ACE-I) and Angiotensin Receptor Blockers (ARBs), represent one of the most common classes of medications used for blood pressure control, and they have gained a special interest during the COVID-19 pandemic. This interest was raised after it was established that ACE2 is a cellular transporter of the SARS-CoV-2 into the host cell.[9, 78] Treatment with ACE-I and ARBs was shown to result in increased expression of ACE2 in animals[79, 80] and therefore a theoretical concern was raised of a possibility of more severe infections and worse outcomes in patients with COVID-19 who are on treatment with ACE-I/ARBs. In a large, population-based study from Italy, the use of ACE-I and ARBs was shown to be more frequent among patients with COVID-19 than among controls because of their higher prevalence of the cardiovascular disease. However, there was no evidence that ACE-I or ARBs affected the risk of COVID-19.[81] A subsequent metaanalysis found that compared with untreated subjects, those using either ACE-I or ARBs had a similar risk of severe or lethal COVID-19.[82] The results did not change when both drugs were considered together, and when death was the outcome. Another cohort analysis of over one million patients using antihypertensive medications in Spain and the US found no association between RAAS antagonists and the risk of contracting COVID-19 or respiratory failure.[83] The evidence to date strongly supports the recommendation of several scientific societies, such as the American College of Cardiology,[84] to continue ARBs or ACE-I for patients already taking them or to initiate them if clinically indicated, unless advised by their physicians against this treatment for non-COVID-19 reasons.

IMPACT OF THE PANDEMIC ON THE CARE OF STROKE PATIENTS
Prehospital Stroke Care During the Pandemic

Emergency medical services (EMS) alert, dispatch, contact, initial assessment, and triage/transport of patients to healthcare facilities are some of the prehospital steps that have been affected by COVID-19. First responders are at substantially higher risk to get infected with COVID-19 while on duty. A report published in JAMA reveals that, as of May 31, 2020, nearly 41% of EMS personnel and 34.5% of firefighters among New York City first responders had been on medical leave for suspected exposure or symptoms.[85] Almost a third of these responders were ultimately confirmed to have been infected. An international group of stroke specialists published a statement on behalf of the American Heart Association (AHA) and American Stroke Association (ASA) Stroke Council Science Subcommittees, recommending, among other things, the proper procurement and donning of PPE by EMS prior to arrival to the patient's location.[68] The statement also recommended the use of COVID-19 screening tools and direct notification of the receiving hospital in case of a positive screen to mobilize staff and isolate patients on arrival in order to contain the potential viral spread. Additionally, routing patients who need intubation and intensive care directly to a comprehensive stroke center (CSC), and the use of telestroke (TS) consultative services between primary stroke centers and CSCs were encouraged as ways to minimize delays in care and optimize resource utilization.

The use of mobile stroke units (MSUs) during COVID-19 was reported by Yamal et al. who found that there was no significant impact of the pandemic on time metrics, interventions, and outcomes as a result of care initiated by the MSU.[86] Specifically, there were no differences in times from initial alert to MSU arrival, thrombolysis or arterial puncture for thrombectomy compared to pre-COVID times.[86] MSU-administered IV alteplase was, however, noted to have decreased during the pandemic due to a decline in eligibility rates.

Stroke Admission Rates

Many stroke centers observed a decrease in the volumes of stroke admissions, IV thrombolysis, and endovascular thrombectomy during the pandemic.[87–90] Data from China showed that the COVID-19 outbreak impacted stroke care significantly, including prehospital and in-hospital care, and resulting in a 26% reduction in thrombolysis cases and 25% in endovascular thrombectomy cases for the month of February 2020 compared to February 2019, while hospital admissions for stroke dropped by about 40% and there was a decline in stroke education efforts to the general public during the same month.[88] Along the same line, data from northeast Ohio showed a 30% decrease in acute stroke presentation to the ER during the pandemic, which resulted in a 52% decrease in the rate of IV thrombolysis treatments, while the endovascular thrombectomy rate remained stable.[89] Another comprehensive stroke center reported that hospital presentations for stroke symptoms decreased during the COVID-19 pandemic, especially for individuals living outside the city of the stroke center, without differences in stroke severity or early outcomes.[90]

The pandemic had a negative effect on stroke admission rates. It is uncertain whether this represents a true decline in stroke incidence, but it seems more likely that this represents the unintended consequence of confinement efforts in effect in many areas around the world and the fear of exposure by the public, resulting in the avoidance of emergency rooms and healthcare settings, especially by patients with minor or resolving symptoms. Public health initiatives focusing on increasing awareness for non-COVID-19 medical emergencies such as stroke during the pandemic are critical.

Telestroke During the Pandemic

Several stroke centers have reported their observations on the utilization of TS services during the pandemic. In a cross-sectional analysis of TS activations in the 30 days before and after the declaration of the COVID-19 pandemic, one stroke center found a 50% reduction in total TS activations between the predeclaration group (142 patients) and the postdeclaration group (71 patients), with no differences in age, sex, diagnosis, or regional variations in activation volumes. This resulted in reductions in IV thrombolysis and endovascular thrombectomy recommendations of 44% and 33%, respectively.[91] Another center reported a 49% decline in TS activations from the prepandemic year (59 vs 148 patient monthly), with an accompanying mobile stroke unit consults decrease of 72%.[92] Despite these declines, the investigators found that the mean percentage of patients receiving IV thrombolysis was 16% in the prepandemic year and increased to 31% after the declaration of the pandemic; a similar change was noted in the mean percentage of patients receiving endovascular therapy, an increase from 10% in the prepandemic year to 19% after the declaration of the pandemic.[92] The reasons for this substantial decrease in TS activations are likely multifactorial. In part, they may relate to patient avoidance to seek emergency stroke care and may have an association to population mobility.[93] They, however, emphasize the importance of continued public health measures to encourage patients and families to seek emergency medical care at the time of symptom onset.[91]

Despite the decline in utilization of TS services in the COVID-19 era, telemedicine technology remains an ideal tool to ensure the safety of hospital staff managing acute stroke patients, when their physical presence is not essential while ensuring the proper delivery of care to acute stroke victims.

Quality and Delivery of Acute Stroke Care During the Pandemic

For patients admitted with acute stroke in the COVID-19 era, with all the associated restrictions, the major concern of the healthcare system is the timely, safe, and effective delivery of reperfusion therapies, and subsequent monitoring and management in the stroke unit or ICU. This may be even more important for patients with LVO who are in need of endovascular thrombectomy. Substantial delays in seeking care have been reported by several stroke centers, including those using TS systems.[88, 89, 94] The AHA/ASA Stroke Council Leadership responded promptly and provided emergency guidance on how to address these issues while securing the delivery of appropriate emergency stroke treatments.[95]

A "protected code stroke" has been recommended and multiple stroke centers have already adopted new or modified their existing acute stroke protocols during the pandemic. These protocols aim to quickly screen for COVID-19 and optimize resources, given the lack of PPE, hospital beds and risk of exposure in addition to providing the best care possible throughout the pandemic. It is possible though that these measures may result in slightly longer door-to-groin times due to precautionary measures, while door-to-needle times are expected to remain stable. The experience of large stroke centers falls along these lines.[96] Hopefully, this approach will contribute to stabilizing the delivery of stroke treatments in the time of this ferocious global health threat.

The multidisciplinary clinical, monitoring, and procedural expertise available in stroke centers can potentially support COVID-19 treatment teams, without sacrificing staff or patient safety.[97] Open lines of communication between stroke center leaders and hospital leadership in a pandemic where policies and procedures can change or evolve rapidly are essential, and support needs may need to be allocated in a way that allows for the continued operation of a fully capable stroke center, with the ability to adjust if stroke center volume or staff attrition requires.[97]

CONCLUDING REMARKS

COVID-19 is an aggressive and merciless global health threat. A significant fraction of patients with COVID-19 develops neurological complications, with stroke being one of the most catastrophic ones. SARS-CoV-2 binding to ACE2 on cellular membranes, especially in the brain, plays a major role in the pathogenesis of cerebrovascular disease, along with the cytokine storm, hypercoagulable states, endotheliitis, cardiac dysfunction, and critical illness and the resulting hypoxia. COVID-19 is mostly associated with ischemic stroke, especially of the cryptogenic subtype, and an increasing frequency of LVO-related stroke in patients without the traditional risk factors. CVT also appears in patients of older age and without the usual risk factors, likely an expression of hypercoagulable states, and is associated with poor outcomes. Every effort should be made so that patients with acute ischemic stroke can receive timely reperfusion therapies, including IV thrombolysis and endovascular thrombectomy. Secondary stroke prevention measures follow the traditional guidelines, and there is no reason to exclude patients from receiving ACE inhibitors or ARBs for hypertension control. A decline in stroke codes and TS codes as well as stroke admissions has been observed during the pandemic, perhaps reflecting the effects of prolonged lockdowns and widespread fear. Major public campaign efforts are needed to reverse this trend. Stroke centers should adopt "protected stroke codes" to ensure the safety of staff and patients while ensuring the prompt delivery of emergency and stroke unit or ICU stroke treatments. SARS-CoV-2 has no similarity to other pathogens that clinicians and scientists have experienced in recent decades. Stroke care protocols should be modified to adapt to the new reality and provide a better and individualized care for stroke patients in the COVID-19 era.

REFERENCES

1. https://covid19.who.int/.
2. Chen N, Zhou M, Dong X, et al. Epidemiological and clinical characteristics of 99 cases of 2019 novel coronavirus pneumonia in Wuhan, China: a descriptive study. *Lancet.* 2020;395:507–513.

3. Lima M, Siokas V, Aloizou AM, et al. Unraveling the possible routes of SARS-CoV-2 invasion into the central nervous system. *Curr Treat Options Neurol.* 2020;22:37.

4. Mao L, Jin H, Wang M, et al. Neurologic manifestations of hospitalized patients with coronavirus disease 2019 in Wuhan, China. *JAMA Neurol.* 2020;77:683–690.

5. Markus HS, Brainin M. COVID-19 and stroke—a global world stroke organization perspective. *Int J Stroke.* 2020;15:361–364.

6. Morelli N, Rota E, Terracciano C, et al. The baffling case of ischemic stroke disappearance from the casualty department in the COVID-19 era. *Eur Neurol.* 2020;83:213–215.

7. Majidi S, Fifi JT, Ladner TR, et al. Emergent large vessel occlusion stroke during New York city's COVID-19 outbreak: clinical characteristics and paraclinical findings. *Stroke.* 2020;51:2656–2663.

8. Kummer BR, Klang E, Stein LK, Dhamoon MS, Jetté N. History of stroke is independently associated with in-hospital death in patients with COVID-19. *Stroke.* 2020;51:3112–3114.

9. Li W, Moore MJ, Vasilieva N, et al. Angiotensin-converting enzyme 2 is a functional receptor for the SARS coronavirus. *Nature.* 2003;426:450–454.

10. Hamming I, Timens W, Bulthuis ML, Lely AT, Navis G, van Goor H. Tissue distribution of ACE2 protein, the functional receptor for SARS coronavirus. A first step in understanding SARS pathogenesis. *J Pathol.* 2004;203:631–637.

11. Baig AM, Khaleeq A, Ali U, Syeda H. Evidence of the COVID-19 virus targeting the CNS: tissue distribution, host-virus interaction, and proposed neurotropic mechanisms. *ACS Chem Nerosci.* 2020;11:995–998.

12. Divani AA, Andalib S, Di Napoli M, et al. Coronavirus disease 2019 and stroke: clinical manifestations and pathophysiological insights. *J Stroke Cerebrovasc Dis.* 2020;29:104941.

13. Hernández-Durán S, Salfelder C, Schaeper J, et al. Mechanical ventilation, sedation and neuromonitoring of patients with aneurysmal subarachnoid hemorrhage in Germany: results of a nationwide survey. *Neurocrit Care.* 2020;1–12.

14. Peña Silva RA, Chu Y, Miller JD, et al. Impact of ACE2 deficiency and oxidative stress on cerebrovascular function with aging. *Stroke.* 2012;43:3358–3363.

15. Pavlov V, Beylerli O, Gareev I, Torres Solis LF, Solís Herrera A, Aliev G. COVID-19-related intracerebral hemorrhage. *Front Aging Neurosci.* 2020;12:600172.

16. Rajdev K, Lahan S, Klein K, Piquette CA, Thi M. Acute ischemic and hemorrhagic stroke in COVID-19: mounting evidence. *Cureus.* 2020;12, e10157.

17. Escalard S, Chalumeau V, Escalard C, et al. Early brain imaging shows increased severity of acute ischemic strokes with large vessel occlusion in COVID-19 patients. *Stroke.* 2020;51:3366–3370.

18. Zhang Y, Xiao M, Zhang S, et al. Coagulopathy and antiphospholipid antibodies in patients with COVID-19. *N Engl J Med.* 2020;382, e38.

19. Becker RC. COVID-19 update: COVID-19-associated coagulopathy. *J Thromb Thrombolysis.* 2020;50:54–67.

20. Klok FA, Kruip M, van der Meer NJM, et al. Incidence of thrombotic complications in critically ill ICU patients with COVID-19. *Thromb Res.* 2020;191:145–147.

21. Klok FA, Kruip M, van der Meer NJM, et al. Confirmation of the high cumulative incidence of thrombotic complications in critically ill ICU patients with COVID-19: an updated analysis. *Thromb Res.* 2020;191:148–150.

22. Ribes A, Vardon-Bounes F, Mémier V, et al. Thromboembolic events and COVID-19. *Adv Biol Regul.* 2020;77:100735.

23. Levi M, Iba T. COVID-19 coagulopathy: is it disseminated intravascular coagulation? *Intern Emerg Med.* 2020;1–4.

24. Panigada M, Bottino N, Tagliabue P, et al. Hypercoagulability of COVID-19 patients in intensive care unit: a report of thromboelastography findings and other parameters of hemostasis. *J Thromb Haemost.* 2020;18:1738–1742.

25. Beyrouti R, Adams ME, Benjamin L, et al. Characteristics of ischaemic stroke associated with COVID-19. *J Neurol Neurosurg Psychiatry.* 2020;91:889–891.

26. Jose RJ, Manuel A. COVID-19 cytokine storm: the interplay between inflammation and coagulation. *Lancet Respir Med.* 2020;8:e46–e47.

27. Kananeh MF, Thomas T, Sharma K, et al. Arterial and venous strokes in the setting of COVID-19. *J Clin Neurosci.* 2020;79:60–66.

28. Helms J, Tacquard C, Severac F, et al. High risk of thrombosis in patients with severe SARS-CoV-2 infection: a multicenter prospective cohort study. *Intensive Care Med.* 2020;46:1089–1098.

29. Ren B, Yan F, Deng Z, et al. Extremely high incidence of lower extremity deep venous thrombosis in 48 patients with severe COVID-19 in Wuhan. *Circulation.* 2020;142:181–183.

30. Zhang L, Feng X, Zhang D, et al. Deep vein thrombosis in hospitalized patients with COVID-19 in Wuhan, China: prevalence, risk factors, and outcome. *Circulation.* 2020;142:114–128.

31. Reynolds AS, Lee AG, Renz J, et al. Pulmonary vascular dilatation detected by automated transcranial Doppler in COVID-19 pneumonia. *Am J Respir Crit Care Med.* 2020;202:1037–1039.

32. Varga Z, Flammer AJ, Steiger P, et al. Endothelial cell infection and endotheliitis in COVID-19. *Lancet.* 2020;395:1417–1418.

33. Paniz-Mondolfi A, Bryce C, Grimes Z, et al. Central nervous system involvement by severe acute respiratory syndrome coronavirus-2 (SARS-CoV-2). *J Med Virol.* 2020;92:699–702.

34. Hernández-Fernández F, Sandoval Valencia H, Barbella-Aponte RA, et al. Cerebrovascular disease in patients with COVID-19: neuroimaging, histological and clinical description. *Brain.* 2020;143:3089–3103.

35. Vaschetto R, Cena T, Sainaghi PP, et al. Cerebral nervous system vasculitis in a COVID-19 patient with pneumonia. *J Clin Neurosci.* 2020;79:71–73.

36. Dixon L, Coughlan C, Karunaratne K, et al. Immunosuppression for intracranial vasculitis associated with SARS-CoV-2: therapeutic implications for COVID-19 cerebrovascular pathology. *J Neurol Neurosurg Psychiatry.* 2021;92:103–104.

37. Dakay K, Kaur G, Gulko E, et al. Reversible cerebral vasoconstriction syndrome and dissection in the setting of COVID-19 infection. *J Stroke Cerebrovasc Dis.* 2020;29:105011.

38. Al-Mufti F, Becker C, Kamal H, et al. Acute cerebrovascular disorders and vasculopathies associated with significant mortality in SARS-CoV-2 patients admitted to the intensive care unit in the New York Epicenter. *J Stroke Cerebrovasc Dis.* 2021;30:105429.

39. Salvarani C, Brown Jr RD, Hunder GG. Adult primary central nervous system vasculitis. *Lancet.* 2012;380:767–777.

40. Yu WL, Toh HS, Liao CT, Chang WT. Cardiovascular complications of COVID-19 and associated concerns: a review. *Acta Cardiol Sin.* 2021;37:9–17.

41. Kochi AN, Tagliari AP, Forleo GB, Fassini GM, Tondo C. Cardiac and arrhythmic complications in patients with COVID-19. *J Cardiovasc Electrophysiol.* 2020;31:1003–1008.

42. Panchal A, Kyvernitakis A, Mikolich JR, Biederman RWW. Contemporary use of cardiac imaging for COVID-19 patients: a three center experience defining a potential role for cardiac MRI. *Int J Cardiovasc Imaging.* 2021;37:1–13.

43. Guo T, Fan Y, Chen M, et al. Cardiovascular implications of fatal outcomes of patients with coronavirus disease 2019 (COVID-19). *JAMA Cardiol.* 2020;5:811–818.

44. Finsterer J, Stöllberger C. SARS-CoV-2 triggered takotsubo in 38 patients. *J Med Virol.* 2020;93:1236–1238.

45. Kariyanna PT, Chandrakumar HP, Jayarangaiah A, et al. Apical takotsubo cardiomyopathy in a COVID-19 patient presenting with stroke: a case report and pathophysiologic insights. *Am J Med Case Rep.* 2020;8:350–357.

46. Fan S, Xiao M, Han F, et al. Neurological manifestations in critically ill patients with COVID-19: a retrospective study. *Front Neurol.* 2020;11:806.

47. Li Y, Li M, Wang M, et al. Acute cerebrovascular disease following COVID-19: a single center, retrospective, observational study. *Stroke Vasc Neurol.* 2020;5:279–284.

48. Merkler AE, Parikh NS, Mir S, et al. Risk of ischemic stroke in patients with coronavirus disease 2019 (COVID-19) vs patients with influenza. *JAMA Neurol.* 2020;77:1–7.

49. Qin C, Zhou L, Hu Z, et al. Clinical characteristics and outcomes of COVID-19 patients with a history of stroke in Wuhan, China. *Stroke.* 2020;51:2219–2223.

50. Siegler JE, Cardona P, Arenillas JF, et al. Cerebrovascular events and outcomes in hospitalized patients with COVID-19: the SVIN COVID-19 multinational registry. *Int J Stroke.* 2021;16:437–447.

51. Yaghi S, Ishida K, Torres J, et al. SARS-CoV-2 and stroke in a New York healthcare system. *Stroke.* 2020;51:2002–2011.

52. Katsanos AH, Palaiodimou L, Zand R, et al. The impact of SARS-CoV-2 on stroke epidemiology and care: a meta-analysis. *Ann Neurol.* 2021;89:380–388.

53. Rothstein A, Oldridge O, Schwennesen H, Do D, Cucchiara BL. Acute cerebrovascular events in hospitalized COVID-19 patients. *Stroke.* 2020;51:e219–e222.

54. Kihira S, Schefflein J, Mahmoudi K, et al. Association of coronavirus disease (COVID-19) with large vessel occlusion strokes: a case-control study. *Am J Roentgenol.* 2021;216:150–156.

55. Oxley TJ, Mocco J, Majidi S, et al. Large-vessel stroke as a presenting feature of COVID-19 in the young. *N Engl J Med.* 2020;382, e60.

56. Llitjos JF, Leclerc M, Chochois C, et al. High incidence of venous thromboembolic events in anticoagulated severe COVID-19 patients. *J Thromb Haemost.* 2020;18:1743–1746.

57. Hughes C, Nichols T, Pike M, Subbe C, Elghenzai S. Cerebral venous sinus thrombosis as a presentation of COVID-19. *Eur J Case Rep Intern Med.* 2020;7, 001691.

58. Hemasian H, Ansari B. First case of COVID-19 presented with cerebral venous thrombosis: a rare and dreaded case. *Rev Neurol (Paris).* 2020;176:521–523.

59. Chougar L, Mathon B, Weiss N, Degos V, Shor N. Atypical deep cerebral vein thrombosis with hemorrhagic venous infarction in a patient positive for COVID-19. *Am J Neuroradiol.* 2020;41:1377–1379.

60. Cavalcanti DD, Raz E, Shapiro M, et al. Cerebral venous thrombosis associated with COVID-19. *Am J Neuroradiol.* 2020;41:1370–1376.

61. Baldini T, Asioli GM, Romoli M, et al. Cerebral venous thrombosis and severe acute respiratory syndrome coronavirus-2 infection: a systematic review and meta-analysis. *Eur J Neurol.* 2021;00:1–13.

62. Benger M, Williams O, Siddiqui J, Sztriha L. Intracerebral haemorrhage and COVID-19: clinical characteristics from a case series. *Brain Behav Immun.* 2020;88:940–944.

63. Kvernland A, Kumar A, Yaghi S, et al. Anticoagulation use and hemorrhagic stroke in SARS-CoV-2 patients treated at a New York healthcare system. *Neurocrit Care.* 2020;1–12.

64. Benussi A, Pilotto A, Premi E, et al. Clinical characteristics and outcomes of inpatients with neurologic disease and COVID-19 in Brescia, Lombardy, Italy. *Neurology.* 2020;95:e910–e920.

65. Tsivgoulis G, Palaiodimou L, Zand R, et al. COVID-19 and cerebrovascular diseases: a comprehensive overview. *Ther Adv Neurol Disord.* 2020;13, 1756286420978004.

66. Kremer S, Lersy F, de Sèze J, et al. Brain MRI findings in severe COVID-19: a retrospective observational study. *Radiology.* 2020;297:E242–e251.

67. Avula A, Nalleballe K, Narula N, et al. COVID-19 presenting as stroke. *Brain Behav Immun.* 2020;87:115–119.

68. Goyal M, Ospel JM, Southerland AM, et al. Prehospital triage of acute stroke patients during the COVID-19 pandemic. *Stroke.* 2020;51:2263–2267.

69. Powers WJ, Rabinstein AA, Ackerson T, et al. Guidelines for the early management of patients with acute ischemic stroke: 2019 update to the 2018 guidelines for the early management of acute ischemic stroke: a guideline for healthcare professionals from the American Heart Association/American Stroke Association. *Stroke.* 2019;50:e344–e418.

70. Müller MC, Meijers JC, Vroom MB, Juffermans NP. Utility of thromboelastography and/or thromboelastometry in adults with sepsis: a systematic review. *Crit Care.* 2014;18:R30.

71. Wang J, Hajizadeh N, Moore EE, et al. Tissue plasminogen activator (tPA) treatment for COVID-19 associated acute respiratory distress syndrome (ARDS): a case series. *J Thromb Haemost.* 2020;18:1752–1755.

72. Smith MS, Bonomo J, Knight WA, et al. Endovascular therapy for patients with acute ischemic stroke during the COVID-19 pandemic: a proposed algorithm. *Stroke.* 2020;51:1902–1909.

73. Nguyen TN, Abdalkader M, Jovin TG, et al. Mechanical thrombectomy in the era of the COVID-19 pandemic: emergency preparedness for neuroscience teams: a guidance statement from the society of vascular and interventional neurology. *Stroke.* 2020;51:1896–1901.

74. Fang L, Karakiulakis G, Roth M. Are patients with hypertension and diabetes mellitus at increased risk for COVID-19 infection? *Lancet Respir Med.* 2020;8, e21.

75. Vandermeer ML, Thomas AR, Kamimoto L, et al. Association between use of statins and mortality among patients hospitalized with laboratory-confirmed influenza virus infections: a multistate study. *J Infect Dis.* 2012;205:13–19.

76. Pertzov B, Eliakim-Raz N, Atamna H, Trestioreanu AZ, Yahav D, Leibovici L. Hydroxymethylglutaryl-CoA reductase inhibitors (statins) for the treatment of sepsis in adults—a systematic review and meta-analysis. *Clin Microbiol Infect.* 2019;25:280–289.

77. Grimaldi D, Durand A, Gleeson J, Taccone FS. Failure of statins in ARDS: the quest for the Holy Grail continues. *Minerva Anestesiol.* 2016;82:1230–1234.

78. Hoffmann M, Kleine-Weber H, Schroeder S, et al. SARS-CoV-2 cell entry depends on ACE2 and TMPRSS2 and is blocked by a clinically proven protease inhibitor. *Cell.* 2020;181:271–280.e278.

79. Soler MJ, Barrios C, Oliva R, Batlle D. Pharmacologic modulation of ACE2 expression. *Curr Hypertens Rep.* 2008;10:410–414.

80. Ferrario CM, Jessup J, Chappell MC, et al. Effect of angiotensin-converting enzyme inhibition and angiotensin II receptor blockers on cardiac angiotensin-converting enzyme 2. *Circulation.* 2005;111:2605–2610.

81. Mancia G, Rea F, Ludergnani M, Apolone G, Corrao G. Renin-angiotensin-aldosterone system blockers and the risk of Covid-19. *N Engl J Med.* 2020;382:2431–2440.

82. Flacco ME, Acuti Martellucci C, Bravi F, et al. Treatment with ACE inhibitors or ARBs and risk of severe/lethal COVID-19: a meta-analysis. *Heart.* 2020;106:1519–1524.

83. Morales DR, Conover MM, You SC, et al. Renin-angiotensin system blockers and susceptibility to COVID-19: an international, open science, cohort analysis. *Lancet Digit Health.* 2021;3:e98–e114.

84. https://www.acc.org/latest-in-cardiology/articles/2020/07/15/13/12/covid-19-and-use-of-drugs-targeting-the-renin-angiotensin-system.

85. Prezant DJ, Zeig-Owens R, Schwartz T, et al. Medical leave associated with COVID-19 among emergency medical system responders and firefighters in New York city. *JAMA Netw Open.* 2020;3, e2016094.

86. Yamal JM, Parker SA, Jacob AP, et al. Successful conduct of an acute stroke clinical trial during COVID. *PLoS One.* 2021;16, e0243603.

87. Rudilosso S, Laredo C, Vera V, et al. Acute stroke care is at risk in the era of COVID-19: experience at a comprehensive stroke center in Barcelona. *Stroke.* 2020;51:1991–1995.

88. Zhao J, Li H, Kung D, Fisher M, Shen Y, Liu R. Impact of the COVID-19 epidemic on stroke care and potential solutions. *Stroke.* 2020;51:1996–2001.

89. Uchino K, Kolikonda MK, Brown D, et al. Decline in stroke presentations during COVID-19 surge. *Stroke.* 2020;51:2544–2547.

90. Jasne AS, Chojecka P, Maran I, et al. Stroke code presentations, interventions, and outcomes before and during the COVID-19 pandemic. *Stroke.* 2020;51:2664–2673.

91. Huang JF, Greenway MRF, Nasr DM, et al. Telestroke in the time of COVID-19: the Mayo Clinic experience. *Mayo Clin Proc.* 2020;95:1704–1708.

92. Shah SO, Dharia R, Stazi J, DePrince M, Rosenwasser RH. Rapid decline in telestroke consults in the setting of COVID-19. *Telemed J E Health.* 2021;27:227–230.

93. Schlachetzki F, Theek C, Hubert ND, et al. Low stroke incidence in the TEMPiS telestroke network during COVID-19 pandemic—effect of lockdown on thrombolysis and thrombectomy. *J Telemed Telecare.* 2020;, 1357633x20943327.

94. Kerleroux B, Fabacher T, Bricout N, et al. Mechanical thrombectomy for acute ischemic stroke amid the COVID-19 outbreak: decreased activity, and increased care delays. *Stroke.* 2020;51:2012–2017.

95. AHA/ASA Stroke Council Leadership. Temporary emergency guidance to us stroke centers during the coronavirus disease 2019 (COVID-19) pandemic: on behalf of the American Heart Association/American Stroke Association Stroke Council Leadership. *Stroke.* 2020;51:1910–1912.

96. Agarwal S, Scher E, Rossan-Raghunath N, et al. Acute stroke care in a New York city comprehensive stroke center during the COVID-19 pandemic. *J Stroke Cerebrovasc Dis.* 2020;29:105068.

97. Wira CR, Goyal M, Southerland AM, et al. Pandemic guidance for stroke centers aiding COVID-19 treatment teams. *Stroke.* 2020;51:2587–2592.

CHAPTER 5

COVID-19 and Seizures

SHELLEY LEE • OMAR A. DANOUN • VIBHANGINI S. WASADE
Department of Neurology, Henry Ford Health System, Detroit, MI, United States

INTRODUCTION

Over time as human civilization has grown, it has faced several pandemics over thousands of years. To name a few, lately, since the beginning of the 21st century, pandemics have included swine flu (H1N1) in 2009 and two novel coronaviruses—severe acute respiratory syndrome (SARS) in 2002 and Middle East respiratory syndrome (MERS) in 2015[1]—before the current novel coronavirus disease 2019 (COVID-19) infection caused by a beta-coronavirus (SARS-CoV-2) in 2019. Other than the common respiratory presentations for COVID-19, neurological presentations such as headaches, dizziness, stroke along with seizures have been described. Seizure occurrence is varied in the published literature, ranging from new onset seizures or new onset status epilepticus to the presence of electrographic seizures or nonepileptic spells.

SEIZURES IN CORONAVIRUS INFECTIONS

Over the last few decades, a variety of viral infections have been associated with neurologic manifestations including seizures and status epilepticus. These have been described in previous coronavirus pandemics such as MERS and the influenza A H1N1 pandemic. Seizures may also be seen in a variety of forms of viral encephalitis associated with upper respiratory infections such as influenza A H3N2 encephalitis. Prior studies have demonstrated that coronaviruses in particular are one of the most common viral respiratory illnesses responsible for febrile seizures in children.[2]

Neurologic manifestations associated with coronavirus infections were first reported in a patient with SARS-CoV infection in 2003.[3] More specifically, this patient presented with seizures. A second patient with documented SARS-CoV infection and seizures was reported in the literature shortly after.[4] Both had SARS-CoV RNA in the cerebrospinal fluid (CSF). Additional studies found that up to 23% of hospitalized children with suspected encephalitis in the setting of the coronavirus infection had seizures.[5] Similar reports of seizures associated with infections were reported with MERS. One study looking at 70 patients with MERS-CoV infection found that 26% of patients had altered mental status and 8.6% of infected patients had seizures.[6]

In the early months of the COVID-19 pandemic, data regarding the incidence of seizures in COVID-19 infections was very scarce. Since then, numerous case reports have been published reporting seizures or status epilepticus associated with the SARS-CoV-2 infection (Table 5.1).[7–18] A study by Mao et al. on neurological presentations revealed that 0.5% of patients (1/214) had seizures,[19] whereas another study reported clinical seizure-like events of concern in 63.3% of patients with COVID-19 infection.[20]

PREDISPOSITION TO SEIZURES IN COVID-19 INFECTION

Similar to other coronaviruses, the SARS-CoV-2 virus has been found to be neurotropic and to have neuroinvasive properties. The SARS-CoV-2 virus has an affinity to the angiotensin-converting enzyme 2 (ACE2) receptor found on the cells of multiple organs, including cells of the central nervous system. Binding of the virus to this receptor allows for entry of the virus into these cells.[21] The specific mechanism responsible for seizure development in infected patients remains unclear; however, it is likely multifactorial in nature. Contributing factors are thought to include direct neuroinvasion leading to focal cerebral injury, breakdown of the blood–brain barrier, and cerebral blood flow dysfunction. Additional factors likely include an inflammatory cascade leading to accumulation of inflammatory mediators, activation of glutamate receptors, and neuronal hyperexcitability. The possibility of a cytokine storm mechanism via activation of the ACE2 signaling pathway has also been hypothesized for seizure occurrence.[13] Given that the SARS-CoV-2 infection can lead to severe organ dysfunction, seizures may also occur with metabolic derangements, in the setting of other associated conditions such as renal, hepatic, and hypoxemic respiratory failure.

Neurological Care and the COVID-19 Pandemic. https://doi.org/10.1016/B978-0-323-82691-4.00009-1

TABLE 5.1
Summary of Patients With COVID-19 Infection Presenting With Seizures Or Status Epilepticus With Relevant Information Including Outcomes.

Author, Publication Month and Year, and Country	Patient Age (Years), Gender, and Presentation	History of Epilepsy	Pertinent Medical History	Presentation of Seizure/Status Epilepticus	COVID-19 Diagnosis	Workup (Imaging, CSF)	EEG Findings	Outcome
Vollono et al., May 2020; Italy[7]	78, F, R face and limb twitching	Yes	Postencephalitic epilepsy (HSV-1)	Myoclonic jerks of R face, upper, and lower extremities	NP (+)	MRI: gliosis and atrophy involving L temporoparietal lobe	Semirhythmic, irregular, high amplitude delta waves in L Fr-C-T regions consistent with SE	Treated with valproic acid, midazolam, lopinavir-ritonavir, hydroxychloroquine. Discharged in stable condition
Somani et al., June 2020; USA[8]	73, F, dyspnea and confusion	No	L frontal skull base encephalocele and hydrocephalus requiring ventriculoperitoneal shunt	Face and arm myoclonus, worsening mentation 1 day after presentation	TA (+)	MRI and CSF deferred	Continuous b/l independent PDs over b/l hemispheres with evolution into recurrent sz from alternating hemispheres consistent with myoclonic SE	EEG improved with levetiracetam, lacosamide, phenytoin, and midazolam. Care was withdrawn due to organ failure
	49, F, altered mentation, witnessed sz	No	Conversion disorder and schizoaffective disorder	R facial twitching and head version to R, followed by GTC sz	NP (−) on admission. After 3 days, repeat NP (+)	MRI unremarkable. CSF deferred	Multiple sz (4–6/h) from midline and L Fr-C regions	Seizures resolved with levetiracetam, multiple doses of lorazepam, and propofol
Hepburn et al., May 2020; USA[9]	82, M, dyspnea and altered mentation × 10 days	No	CKD and COPD	R eyelid and facial twitching on hospital day 5	NP(+)	MRI deferred due to pacemaker, CSF deferred due to coagulopathy	Multiple sz from b/l Fr-T regions (L > R), progressing to focal SE, most were NC	Seizures resolved with levetiracetam. However, care was withdrawn given persistent respiratory failure
	76, M, fever, encephalopathy	No	L3-S1 laminectomy 5 days prior and asthma on benralizumab	Worsening encephalopathy and L upper extremity clonic activity following surgical drainage of epidural abscess	NP(+)	MRI: chronic white matter hyperintensities. CSF deferred	3 focal sz arising from R C-P region × 30 s each	Seizures resolved with levetiracetam

Reference	Comorbid	History	Clinical development	NP	Neuroimaging	EEG	Treatment/Outcome
Pilato et al., July 2020; USA[10]	No	71, M, presyncopal episode, developed fever and URI symptoms after admission	Developed agitation, eye twitching, and rhythmic movements involving head, mouth, and neck	NP(+)	MRI: periventricular white matter hypodensities	Generalized PDs, generalized delta/theta slowing, decreased voltage L hemisphere. After 32 days, EEG-multiple independent b/l Fr-T sz with R face twitching	Seizures controlled with levetiracetam, phenobarbital, and lacosamide. Patient deceased after cardiac arrest
	Yes	57, M, prolonged seizure in the setting of fever	Persistent decreased level of consciousness	NP(+)	Neuroimaging N/A	R posterior quadrant PDs, focal, NC SE. After 18 days, EEG-R posterior-quadrant lateralized PDs	Seizures resolved with propofol infusion and up-titration of home medications
Sohal et al., May 2020; USA[11]	No	72, F, hypoglycemia, shortly after developed respiratory failure and altered mental status	On day 3, developed multiple episodes of tonic clonic movements of all extremities for several minutes	NP (+)	MRI and CSF deferred	6 L T sz, interictal—L T sharp waves	Treated with midazolam infusion, levetiracetam, and valproate. Patient deceased after cardiac arrest
Flamand et al., August 2020; France[12]	No	80, F, respiratory distress, fever x 2 days	Altered mental status and clonic movements of L foot	Initial NP(−), repeat on day 25 NP(+)	MRI and CSF studies normal	days 6 & 8—EEG-repetitive epileptiform discharges with quasi-rhythmic spatiotemporal evolution in bi-frontal regions. Days 18 and 21—EEG periodic triphasic activity	Seizures improved with valproate, lacosamide, and clobazam. Patient deceased on hospital day 25

Continued

TABLE 5.1
Summary of Patients With COVID-19 Infection Presenting With Seizures Or Status Epilepticus With Relevant Information Including Outcomes—cont'd

Author, Publication Month and Year, and Country	Patient Age (Years), Gender, and Presentation	History of Epilepsy	Pertinent Medical History	Presentation of Seizure/Status Epilepticus	COVID-19 Diagnosis	Workup (Imaging, CSF)	EEG Findings	Outcome
Balloy et al., August 2020; France[13]	59, M, fever, dyspnea, and cough prompting intubated for respiratory failure	No	Atrial fibrillation	Impaired level of consciousness and behavioral disturbance following weaning of midazolam	Initial NP (−), repeat TA (+)	MRI and CSF PCR negative, including CSF SARS-CoV-2 RNA	Predominantly frontal runs of rhythmic delta discharges with superimposed spikes x 5–6 min	Improved on levetiracetam and clobazam
Moriguchi et al., May 2020; Japan[14]	24, M, fever, URI x 9 days	No	None	GTC sz x 1 min	NP(−), CSF(+)	MRI: DWI hyperintensity-R lateral ventricle wall, R MTL CSF: SARS-CoV-2 RNA (+), 12 WBCs (mononuclear predominant), OP-320 mm H_2O	N/A	Treated with levetiracetam, ceftriaxone, vancomycin, acyclovir, steroids, and favipravir
Kadono et al., June 2020; Japan[15]	44, M, anosmia, left hand and face numbness.	Yes	Cerebral venous sinus thrombosis complicated by hemorrhagic infarct and epilepsy, status post-R Fr-T decompression 6 months prior	Intermittent L hand and face twitching that secondarily generalized	NP(+)	CTH with worsening R temporal lobe edema. MRI with no new stroke. CSF deferred	N/A	Episodes resolved with levetiracetam. Treated with hydroxychloroquine and azithromycin

Reference	Presentation		Past medical history	Seizure description	NP PCR	MRI/CSF	EEG after discharge	Treatment
Lyons et al., June 2020; Ireland[16]	20, M, myalgias and lethargy x 3 days, then GTC sz at home	No	None	GTC sz	NP(−), repeat after 2 days NP(+)	MRI unremarkable. CSF with lymphocytic pleocytosis (21 cells/mm, 99% mononuclear cells), CSF SARS-CoV-2 PCR(−)	EEG after discharge-normal	Treated with levetiracetam, ceftriaxone, vancomycin, and acyclovir
Haddad et al., May 2020, USA[17]	41, M, dry cough, fever, and confusion x 6 days	No	Well-controlled HIV on dolutegravir-lamivudine and recurrent HSV on chronic suppressive therapy	Worsening mentation followed by GTC sz	NP(+)	MRI unremarkable. CSF with no WBCs	Diffuse slowing, no epileptiform activity	Clinically improved with hydroxychloroquine and azithromycin
Karimi et al., March 2020; Iran[18]	30, F, dry cough fever x 5 days	No	None	GTC sz in sleep 2 days prior to presentation, followed by recurrent (5) szs every 8 h	NP(+)	MRI and CSF studies normal. CSF SARS-CoV-2 PCR negative	N/A	Treated with phenytoin, levetiracetam, chloroquine, and lopinavir-ritonivir

(−), negative; (+), positive; b/l, bilateral; C, central; CKD, chronic kidney disease; CTH, computed tomography of head; COPD, chronic obstructive pulmonary disease; COVID-19, coronavirus disease 2019; CSF, cerebrospinal fluid; DWI, diffusion weighted images; EEG, electroencephalogram; ESRD, end-stage renal disease; F, female; Fr, frontal; GTC, generalized tonic clonic; HSV, herpes simplex virus; L, left; M, male; MRI, magnetic resonance imaging; MTL, mesial temporal lobe; N/A, not available; NC, nonconvulsive; NP, nasopharyngeal swab PCR; OP, opening pressure; R, right; P, parietal; PCR, polymerase chain reaction; PD, periodic discharges; SARS-CoV-2, severe acute respiratory syndrome coronavirus 2; SE, status epilepticus; sz, seizure; T, temporal; TA, tracheal aspirate PCR; TBI, traumatic brain injury; URI, upper respiratory infection; x = lasting for; WBC, white blood cells.

Encephalopathy is one of the most common neurologic manifestations of COVID-19 infection.[20] However, some studies did not reveal any seizure activity on EEG.[20, 22] In addition to encephalopathy, a few cases of suspected SARS-CoV-2 associated encephalitis have been reported.[14, 23, 24] In one case series of encephalopathy with encephalitis diagnosed by increased CSF levels of anti-S1 IgM and abnormal CSF cytokines, consistent with direct central nervous system involvement by SARS-CoV-2, though with undetectable CSF RNA, two of the three patients exhibited multifocal myoclonus.[24] Overall, this promotes the possibility that mechanisms including peri-infectious inflammation mediated by antibodies, complement, vasculopathy, or altered neurotransmission, other than direct brain infection, might account for the cause.

Even with an increasing amount of data regarding seizures and COVID-19 infection, the question of whether or not concurrent SARS-CoV-2 infection further increases the risk of seizures in patients with a known history of epilepsy remains. Overall, evidence at this point demonstrates that the risk of seizures is not significantly increased in patients with epilepsy. The majority of cases of seizure associated with COVID-19 infection were in patients with no previously known history of epilepsy.

Certain epilepsy syndromes where seizures may be triggered by fever, such as Dravet syndrome, may theoretically have worsening of their seizure frequency during COVID-19 infection. However, in a study from Spain that assessed the impact of national lockdown on patients in developmental and epileptic encephalopathies from the caregiver's perspective, epilepsy remained stable in 86% of cases, and of the 14.1% of patients with increased seizure frequency, one had status epilepticus.[25] Patients with epileptic encephalopathies may be at higher risk of seizures in the setting of COVID-19 infection due to factors that include triggers, antiseizure medications,[25] and additional comorbid medical conditions, including respiratory disease.

A multicenter retrospective study in China performed during the early COVID-19 pandemic (January to February 2020) demonstrated no cases of new onset seizure or status epilepticus in 304 patients diagnosed with COVID-19 infection, even though patients had multiple risk factors including prior stroke, traumatic brain injury, central nervous system infection, and severe metabolic disturbances. None of these patients had a history of epilepsy.[26] This suggests that even in the presence of underlying risk factors, infection with SARS-CoV-2 did not increase the risk of seizure occurrence. However, no routine or long-term EEG was recorded in that cohort due to risk of virus exposure, so the presence of subclinical seizures could have gone unnoticed. Several reports of ischemic stroke associated with a suspected hypercoagulable state have been documented in COVID-19 infection.[19] Although it is reasonable to believe that this would result in an associated risk of poststroke epilepsy, there have been no reports of this at the time of publication.

Since the publication of whole genome sequence analysis on January 5, 2020, the SARS-COV2 genome has remained largely unchanged in some regions while others have shown diversity, and 198 filtered recurrent mutations in the SARS-CoV-2 genome have been revealed until the date of this publication.[27] Genomic mutations are sometimes known to be associated with variable clinical features. There are no studies published thus far, relating neurological manifestations to this, let alone occurrence of seizures in those who are infected.

SEIZURES IN COVID-19 INFECTION

Although reports of seizures in COVID-19 positive patients are relatively rare as compared to other neurologic manifestations, it is reasonable to expect seizures as a presenting or complicating feature of the illness given the possibly associated systemic disturbances including hypoxia, metabolic derangements, and multiorgan failure. Seizure semiology has included both generalized and focal seizures in various stages of COVID-19 infection. Patients have also been reported to be in status epilepticus, more so with focal status epilepticus presenting as focal myoclonus or twitching with consistent EEG findings (Table 5.1). There is a single report of a COVID-19 positive patient presenting with nonepileptic spells, suspected to be due to convulsive syncope in the setting of autonomic dysfunction due to abnormal sympathetic skin response.[28] Furthermore, postinfection inflammation was suggested in one case report 6 weeks after initial COVID-19 diagnosis who had refractory status epilepticus.[29]

EPILEPSY IN COVID-19 INFECTION

The current pandemic has also raised the question whether or not patients with epilepsy are at a higher risk of becoming infected with the SARS-CoV-2 virus as compared to the general population. Limited information from regions significantly affected by the virus early in the pandemic suggested that patients with epilepsy are not at higher risk for being infected with the SARS-CoV-2 virus. We should not forget, however, that patients with epilepsy may also have additional comorbid conditions that put them at risk of infection, including diabetes, hypertension, heart disease, and old age. To further support these findings, most patients with epilepsy do not appear to be at risk of more severe COVID-19 symptoms simply due to their history of epilepsy alone.[30] Nevertheless, patients undergoing treatment with corticosteroids or immune modulating therapies such as everolimus for syndromes such as West Syndrome or Tuberous Sclerosis may be at higher risk from infection due to effects of their medication regimen.[28]

Conversely, Cabezudo-Garcia et al. conducted a cross-sectional observational study in Spain that found that the cumulative incidence of COVID-19 infection in epilepsy patients was higher than in patients without epilepsy (1.2% vs 0.5%).[31] The case fatality rate was found to be higher in patients with active epilepsy; however, it was not statistically different when accounting for only patients who were real-time polymerase chain reaction positive. Hypertension was found to be independently associated with fatality. The majority of these patients were dependent on others for care and one-third of them were institutionalized, suggesting that these patients may have poor reserve at baseline and significant comorbidities that may put them at higher risk. Among deceased patients, there was a particularly higher incidence of hypertension and diabetes. In addition, these patients had a higher mean age (57.8 years).[31] Of note, focal epilepsy was the most common epilepsy type in these patients with structural causes being the most common etiology, including vascular malformations, meningiomas, and malignancy.[31]

Medical comorbidities such as hypertension, diabetes, and obesity are more frequent in patients with epilepsy, providing a possible explanation as to why patients with epilepsy appear to have a higher incidence of COVID-19 infection when compared to the general population.[32] Hypertension has been indicated as the most common comorbid condition associated with COVID-19 infection.[33] In addition, patients with epilepsy have a threefold increased risk of developing pneumonia compared to the general population, and this risk is associated with higher mortality rates, especially in the pediatric population.[34] This may also contribute to the previously mentioned higher fatality rates in these patients. Although some data suggests that the incidence of COVID-19 infection is higher in patients with epilepsy, it is unclear if this may also be in part due to increased testing in this vulnerable population. It is possible that due to the increased number of multiple medical comorbidities in patients with epilepsy, as well as their higher risk for decompensation, they are more likely to be hospitalized and tested than the general population.[31]

DIAGNOSIS
EEG Procedure
Electroencephalography can be an efficient and safe method to evaluate for seizures in the setting of COVID-19 infection if used with appropriate precautions and personal protective equipment. Given the risks of exposure to health-care personnel, it is important to weigh the risks and benefits of obtaining EEG recordings in attempts to characterize clinical spells or guide management. Multiple variables should be taken into account when ordering neurodiagnostic testing in suspected COVID-19 positive patients, including the urgency of the procedure, how the results will guide management, the level of exposure to staff performing the procedure, and the availability of appropriate personal protective equipment.[35] During the early months of the pandemic, there were no clear guidelines regarding specific precautions needed and changes to the process of obtaining neurodiagnostic evaluation in order to decrease infection risk while adequately using and preserving resources. Since then, multiple different organizations including the American Epilepsy Society,[36] American Clinical Neurophysiology Society,[37] and American Academy of Neurology[38] have released resources and statements with general recommendations regarding workflow, safety, and resource optimization during the COVID-19 pandemic.

It is now generally agreed upon that in COVID-19 positive patients, EEG should be limited to cases where the findings would change clinical management in order to minimize the risk of exposure to the EEG technologist. This has been demonstrated by a survey conducted in Italy by Assenza et al., who noted that the average weekly number of EEGs decreased from a baseline of 46.1 per week to 11 per week during the COVID-19 pandemic.[39] Nonurgent EEGs should be deferred to a later date if there is significant concern of COVID-19 infection.[40]

It is also reasonable for protocol changes to be made in favor of decreasing the amount of time that EEG technologists spend at the bedside of a COVID-19 positive patient in order to decrease the risk of exposure. One retrospective time analysis in a Texas hospital looked at time of exposure in EEG technologists prior to and after COVID-19 protocol revisions and found that their exposure time decreased from 99 to 51 min.[35] The decrease in time was primarily noted during EEG setup, which decreased from 60 to 33 min, and was felt to be due to the use of a reduced electrode array as well as use of paste or tape as an adhesive as opposed to collodion, which requires an air gun to dry, which bears a potential for aerosolization. Alterations to the standard procedure, such as single-use subdermal needle electrodes and the use of reduced montages, may be implemented to reduce the risk of exposure to the EEG technologist.[41] Prioritizing the deployment of experienced EEG technologists in order to minimize exposure time while troubleshooting and remote EEG monitoring outside of the patient's room are additional methods to help reduce exposure to the care team. Additional measures include the omission of hyperventilation and photic stimulation, extended equipment quarantine following use, and the use of specific "COVID-19 rule-out" machines. It is also reasonable to avoid the initiation of EEG monitoring shortly after use of a nebulizer in order to decrease possible contact with aerosolized viral particles.[35] At times hospitals favored long-term EEG monitoring over routine EEG to limit repeated exposure, especially in comatose patients with suspected nonconvulsive seizures.[41]

When interpreting the EEG, it is important to note the position of the patient during these recordings, especially if the patient is prone in the setting of acute respiratory distress syndrome.[42] Respiratory artifacts are common in mechanically ventilated patients. However, it is of utmost importance to avoid overinterpretation of both respiratory and head movement artifacts, which will be more frontally predominant in prone positioning as opposed to the usual occipitally dominant artifacts due to movement of the back of the head against the occipital leads. In addition, the electroencephalographer ought to be comfortable with EEG patterns commonly seen in critically ill patients, including that in the setting of metabolic encephalopathy, hypoxia, anoxia, and sepsis.[42]

EEG Findings in COVID-19

Initial reported EEG recordings in COVID-19 positive patients demonstrated generalized slowing and nonspecific patterns similar to those seen in metabolic encephalopathy.[43, 44] There is limited data regarding specific electrographic ictal patterns that have been encountered in SARS-CoV-2 infected patients presenting with clinical features suggestive of seizures.[20] One retrospective study performed in New York using eight-channel headband EEGs (Ceribell, Inc., Mountain View, CA, United States) found that in patients who were COVID-19 positive, there was a higher clinical suspicion for seizures compared to COVID-19 negative patients. This led EEG orders to be increased by 63.6% in COVID-19 positive patients in contrast to 33.3% in COVID-19 negative patients.[20] The authors of this study found that 40.9% of COVID-19 positive patients who underwent EEG due to concern for either clinical or subclinical seizures had

epileptiform discharges captured on recording. On the other hand, only one COVID-19 negative patient had epileptiform discharges. No seizures were recorded in COVID-19 positive patients. The most common epileptiform discharges were frontal sharp waves (typically bifrontal and asymmetric), encompassing 88.9% of the recordings. Conversely, a study from Italy reported fewer EEGs being performed on COVID-19 positive patients as compared to COVID-19 negative patients.[39] It is possible that the concern for infection and exposure to medical personnel played an important factor and limited the number of studies being performed in COVID-19 positive patients.

Similar EEG patterns have been reported in other studies. In March 2020, Vespignani et al. investigated 26 COVID-19 positive patients who underwent EEG monitoring for further evaluation of altered mental status and loss of consciousness during hospitalization. Five patients were found to have generalized periodic discharges (GPDs) consisting of high amplitude, frontally predominant delta waves. Three patients had myoclonic jerks due to seizure activity. Frontally predominant lateralized periodic discharges (LPDs) were additionally seen on EEG, with no associated clinical manifestations. EEGs on 19 patients demonstrated nonspecific, generalized theta and alpha activity with intermixed delta activity with no focality or periodicity.[45]

Another retrospective, systematic analysis of EEGs performed in SARS-CoV-2 positive patients was performed in France between March 2020 and June 2020 and investigated a total of 40 EEGs in 36 COVID-19 positive patients.[46] The majority of these EEGs were obtained to evaluate fluctuating mental status (57.5%) and poor responsiveness of sedation in the intensive care unit (15%). Abnormal EEG or an EEG that demonstrated mild background slowing was noted in 23 of these patients (57.5%). The remaining patients had an abnormal EEG, ranging from a moderately abnormal, theta range background to critically abnormal with continuous periodic or rhythmic activity or absent reactivity. The most common abnormal patterns were generalized periodic discharges, multifocal periodic discharges, and rhythmic delta activity, with the latter seen in 32.5% of patients and being the most common. No seizures were recorded on EEG in any of these patients.

An additional case series of eight COVID-19 positive patients performed by Pilato et al. also demonstrated generalized background slowing as the most common finding in all the patients.[10] Five of the studied patients had a history of epilepsy. Two seizures were captured, one focal seizure in a patient with a history of focal epilepsy, and new onset focal status epilepticus in a patient with no prior history of epilepsy. Focal findings, such as focal slowing and sharp waves, were similarly seen in patients with known focal pathologies. It was suggested that COVID-19 positive patients who are more likely to develop neurologic symptoms and have EEG include those with risk factors for epilepsy, underlying neurologic diagnoses, prior head trauma, or craniotomies.

As commonly encountered in the intensive care unit setting, background slowing and theta activity on EEG are likely due to toxic-metabolic encephalopathy, sedation, and hypoxia.[45] In the setting of clinical events, the findings of frontally predominant LPDs raise the possibility of focal brain injury, either from the virus itself or associated hypoxia and anoxia. However, as the studied patients had CSF negative for SARS-CoV-2, it appears less likely that these may be a result of direct injury from the virus itself.[45]

Considering the previously mentioned studies, there has not been a particular EEG pattern that has consistently been demonstrated in COVID-19 positive patients. Many of the EEG abnormalities recorded in these studies, such as rhythmic delta activity, triphasic waves, and generalized periodic discharges, are nonspecific and may be associated with ongoing medical comorbidities at the time of COVID-19 infection, including those of metabolic, hypoxic, and toxic etiologies. These findings are commonly encountered in the inpatient setting and are often seen outside of the coronavirus infection.[46] At this time, there remains minimal evidence regarding EEG patterns associated with COVID-19 infection.

Some studies have evaluated the use of EEG in the characterization of central nervous system involvement and outcome severity in the setting of COVID-19 infection. A study performed by Cechetti et al. evaluating 18 COVID-19 positive patients suggested that EEG may be a useful tool to assess central nervous system involvement due to SARS-CoV-2 infection. Out of 18 patients, 16 (88.9%) had generalized slowing on EEG with an anterior predominance observed in 10/18 (55.6%) patients. The authors found an association between oxygen saturation on presentation and the degree of EEG abnormalities, as well as a linear relationship between the severity of EEG derangements and alteration of laboratory markers such as white blood cell count, sodium level, and coagulation function.[47] These findings support the idea that patients presenting with a delay in oxygenation or significant hypoxia may have more severe cerebral dysfunction.

In an additional retrospective cohort study evaluating 10 critically ill, mechanically ventilated patients,

Pati et al. found that quantitative EEG can be used to predict neurologic outcome in patients with SARS-CoV-2 infection.[48] EEG epochs, including baseline activity and reactivity in response to verbal and tactile stimulation, were assessed in patients with both good and poor neurologic outcomes. Patients with good outcomes were noted to have greater temporal variance in activity than those with poor outcomes. The most significant predictor of good outcomes was found to be an increase in theta power and temporal variance during reactivity.[48] Additional findings by Louis et al. at Cleveland Clinic suggested that there was no relationship between the presence of epileptiform activity on EEG and in-hospital patient mortality.[49]

MANAGEMENT

As epilepsy is one of the most common neurologic disorders worldwide, it is likely that millions of patients have had their care altered by the COVID-19 pandemic. Since the rise of COVID-19 cases, multiple organizations have released consensus statements with recommendations regarding how to best care for epilepsy patients during the COVID-19 pandemic. The main focus of these recommendations is to provide safe epilepsy management from the patient's home in order to prevent infection exposure in the health-care setting.[30]

Recommendations include increasing the accessibility of telemedicine visits, as well as prescribing adequate amounts of antiseizure drugs, initiating a rescue therapy plan if indicated, and ensuring easy access to refills.[50] As the goal is to keep patients out of the emergency department and clinic, physicians may have a lower threshold to prescribe rescue therapy for fast medication availability at home. Patient and caregiver counseling becomes even more important in this setting in order to increase medication adherence and to ensure a proper maintenance treatment regimen and rescue therapy plan. Caregivers should be educated regarding the natural history of seizures and informed about any concerning features that would warrant evaluation in the hospital, including seizures lasting longer than 5 min and a prolonged postictal state. General counseling regarding the importance of abstaining from alcohol and drug use, as well as maintaining a regular sleep schedule, should be reinforced.[30] It is important for physicians to provide safe and effective care to their patients, while also prioritizing patient safety. It may be appropriate to delay changes to an ongoing treatment plan, including medication weaning and neuromodulation setting changes in order to decrease exposure and avoid possible increase in seizure frequency at the time of these changes. In the setting of new onset seizures, further outpatient workup such as neuroimaging and laboratory evaluation may be delayed unless these studies will result in urgent therapeutic changes.[50] Urgent magnetic resonance imaging for evaluation of the first-time seizure may be limited to those with a high suspicion for serious underlying pathology depending on local infection patterns. This includes patients who present with focal signs or symptoms, as well as those with acute onset, frequent seizures.[50] There are multiple different treatment aspects that should be taken into account when treating epilepsy patients who have become infected with COVID-19. One of the primary areas of concern is the safety of antiviral medications in patients with epilepsy. Seizures have rarely been reported with the use of antimalarial agents such as hydroxychloroquine and chloroquine, as well as azithromycin.[51] A recent systematic review found that there is no significant class I evidence supporting the concern that chloroquine and hydroxychloroquine increase the risk of seizures, and two clinical trials demonstrated that there was no increased risk of seizure with these medications.[51] Prior clinical trials have not been able to support the claim of increased seizure risk listed on the package insert of these medications, and data regarding occurrence of seizures in the setting of chloroquine or hydroxychloroquine use is limited to case reports. These reports should be taken into consideration when managing epilepsy patients with SARS-CoV-2 infection; however, these medications are not contraindicated in patients with a history of epilepsy.[30]

When initiating either antiviral or antiseizure medication in COVID-19 positive patients, clinicians should consider the possibility of drug–drug interactions between COVID-19 therapies and antiseizure medications, specifically those metabolized by the CYP 450 system[51] (Table 5.2). Many different agents used for the treatment of COVID-19 infection have been found to alter the metabolism of antiseizure medications. Chloroquine and hydroxychloroquine, as well as tocilizumab, may also decrease the efficacy of medications such as phenytoin, carbamazepine, oxcarbazepine, lamotrigine, and phenobarbital. Close clinical and drug level monitoring may be required in patients taking these medications concurrently. Lopinavir/ritonavir can induce glucuronidation of lamotrigine, and may additionally increase the metabolism of phenytoin and valproate. This may require an increase in lamotrigine dose up to 200% in order to achieve adequate concentrations, whereas CYP3A and CYP2D6 are inhibited by ritonavir, which may lead to increased levels of antiseizure medications including

lacosamide, zonisamide, carbamazepine, cannabidiol, parampanel, and ethosuximide.[52]

Alternatively, antiseizure medications may alter the metabolism of many medications used as treatment for COVID-19 infection. Antiseizure medications that induce cytochrome P450 enzymes, such as carbamazepine, phenytoin, and phenobarbital, may decrease the effectiveness of antiviral medications also metabolized by these enzymes, such as hydroxychloroquine and chloroquine, in addition to lopinavir and sofosbuvir. These COVID-19 targeting medications may need to undergo increases in dosage in order to reach therapeutic levels; however, these doses have not been formally investigated. Cannabidiol, a significant enzyme inhibitor, may increase plasma levels of hydroxychloroquine when used simultaneously.[53]

Despite these interactions, it is not recommended to change a patient's established antiseizure medication regimen if seizures are well controlled, and the patient is to be started on antiviral treatment. However, close monitoring of drug levels may be required in these situations to ensure adequate dosing as well as closer clinical monitoring to evaluate for signs of medication toxicity.

In addition to the significant cardiac manifestations of the SARS-CoV-2 virus, including myocarditis and heart failure, clinicians must be aware of the cardiac effects that may be encountered in the setting of co-administration of antiseizure medications and antiviral therapies, and even antiseizure medication use alone. Steps to minimize the risk of cardiac side effects include baseline electrocardiogram monitoring with repeat monitoring following initiation of QTc prolonging agents, avoidance of additional QTc prolonging agents such as antiemetics, as well as strict electrolyte monitoring and replacement. Lacosamide should be avoided if possible in patients with cardiac manifestations or those with conduction abnormalities.[54] In addition, when considering treatment of seizure-like activity in COVID-19 positive patients with severe respiratory symptoms, the use of benzodiazepines should be used cautiously in nonintubated patients given the risk of respiratory compromise.

It is important to consider the patient's overall clinical status including renal and hepatic function when choosing an antiseizure medication in COVID-19 positive patients given the significant adverse effects that may be encountered. Liver and renal function should be monitored closely, and dose adjustments should be made accordingly in those with known or suspected impairment. Multiple antiseizure medications may require dose adjustments in the setting of associated

TABLE 5.2
Clinically Relevant Drug–Drug Interaction Between AEDs and Medications Used in the Treatment of COVID-19 Patients.

Drugs reported (constantly updated): ATV, atazanavir; DRV/c, darunavir/cobicistat; LPV/r, lopinavir/ritonavir; RDV, remdesivir/GS-5734; FAVI, favipiravir; CLQ, chloroquine; HCLQ, hydroxychloroquine; NITA, nitazoxanide; RBV, ribavirin; TCZ, tocilizumab; IFN-β-1a; interferon β-1a; OSV, oseltamivir.

	ATV	*DRV/c[1]	*LPV/r	RDV[2]	FAVI	CLQ	HCLQ	NITA	RBV	TCZ[2]	IFN-β-1a[4]	OSV
Brivaracetam	↔	↔	↓	↔	↔	↑	↑	↔	↑	↔	↔	↔
Carbamazepine	⇓↑	⇓↑	⇓↑	⇓	↔	⇓	⇓	↔	↔	↓	↔	↔
Cannabidiol	↔	↑	↑	↔	↔	↑	↑	↔	↔	↔	↔	↔
Cenobamate	⇓	⇓	⇓	↔	↔	⇓	⇓	↔	↔	↔	↔	↔
Clonazepam	↑	↑	↑	↔	↔	↔	↔	↔	↔	↔	↔	↔
Clobazam	↑	↑	↑	↔	↔	↔	↔	↔	↔	↔	↔	↔
Diazepam	↑	↑	↑	↔	↔	↔	↔	↔	↔	↔	↔	↔
Eslicarbazepine	⇓♥	⇓	⇓♥	⇓	↔	⇓	⇓	↔	↔	↔	↔	↔
Ethosuximide	↑	↑	↑	↔	↔	↔	↔	↔	↔	↔	↔	↔
Felbamate	↓	⇓	↓	↔	↔	♥↓	♥↓	↔	↔	↔	↔	↔
Gabapentin	↔	↔	↔	↔	↔	↔	↔	↔	↔	↔	↔	↔
Lacosamide	♥↔	⇑	♥↔	↔	↔	↔	↔	↔	↔	↔	↔	↔
Lamotrigine	↔	↑	↓	↔	↔	↔	↔	↔	↔	↔	↔	↔
Levetiracetam	↔	↔	↔	↔	↔	↔	↔	↔	↔	↔	↔	↔
Lorazepam	↔	↔	↔	↔	↔	↔	↔	↔	↔	↔	↔	↔
Oxcarbazepine	⇓	⇓↓	⇓	⇓	↔	⇓	⇓	↔	↔	↔	↔	↔
Perampanel	↑	⇓	↑	↔	↔	↔	↔	↔	↔	↔	↔	↔
Phenytoin	⇓	⇓	⇓	⇓	↔	⇓	⇓	↑	↔	↓	↔	↔
Phenobarbital	⇓	⇓↓	⇓	⇓	↔	⇓	⇓	↔	↔	↓	↔	↔
Pregabalin	↔	↔	↔	↔	↔	↔	↔	↔	↔	↔	↔	↔
Primidone	⇓	⇓	⇓↓	⇓	↔	⇓	⇓	↔	↔	↓	↔	↔
Retigabine	↔	↔	↔	↔	↔	↔	↔	↔	↔	↔	↔	↔
Rufinamide	⇓	⇓	⇓	⇓	↔	⇓	⇓	↔	↔	↔	↔	↔
Sulthiame	↑	↑	↑	↔	↔	↔	↔	↔	↔	↔	↔	↔
Tiagabine	↑	↑	↑	↔	↔	↔	↔	↔	↔	↔	↔	↔
Topiramate	↔	⇓	↔	↔	↔	↔	↔	↔	↔	↔	↔	↔
Valproic acid	↔	⇓	⇑	↔	↔	↔	↔	↔	↔	↔	↔	↔
Vigabatrin	↔	↔	↔	↔	↔	↔	↔	↔	↔	↔	↔	↔
Zonisamide	↔	↑	↔	↔	↔	↔	↔	↔	↔	↔	↔	↔

*Should not be administered without booster drug (ritonavir or cobicistat).

↑   Potential increased exposure of the co-medication;
↓   Potential decreased exposure of the co-medication;
⇑   Potential increased exposure of COVID drug;
⇓   Potential decreased exposure of COVID drug;
↔   No significant effect;
♥   One or both drugs may cause QT and/or PR prolongation

	Drugs should not be co-administered
	Potential interaction which may require a dose adjustment or close monitoring
	Potential interaction likely to be of weak intensity. Additional acts monitoring or dosage adjustment unlikely to be required.
	No clinically significant interaction expected.

[1] Currently, the *Johnson & Johnson*, holder of *Jansson Pharmaceutica* owner of the drug **Darunavir**, highlighted the lack of evidence to support use of Darunavir-based treatments for SARS-CoV-2 (https://www.jnj.com/lack-of-evidence-to support-darunavir-based-hiv-treatments-for-coronavirus).

[2] Some data on drug interactions of Remdesivir are not available yet.

[3] An increase in IL-6, as well as other cytokines, can improve plasmatic concentration of administered drugs reducing hepatic metabolism (CYP-mediated), a treatment with **Tocilizumab** (anti-IL 6R) could reduce plasmatic concentrations of other previous co-treatments duo to hepatic metabolism normalization[2].

[4] No studies have been performed yet in humans to assess drugs-interactions.

Notes:
- Ritonavir is a strong inhibitor of CYP 3A and 2D6 *per se*, independently to co-administered antiviral.
- Atazanavir can increase midazolam plasmatic concentration until 4-fold.
- Also refer to SmPC for further information.

1. Aitken, A. E. Richardson, T. A. & Morgan, E. T. Regulation of drug-metabolizing enzymes and transporters in inflamation *Annu. Rev. Pharmacol. Toxicol.* 46, 123–149 (2006).
2. Kim, S., Oster, A. J. K. & Nisar, M. K. Interleukin-6 and cytochrome-P450, reason for concern? *Rheumatology International* 32, 2601–2604 (2012).

By E. Russo and L. Iannone (School of Pharmacology, University of Catanzaro, Mater Domini University Hospital, Catanzaro, Italy)

(Adapted from ILAE website[52]).

severe hepatic failure, including phenytoin, valproate, carbamazepine, lamotrigine, phenobarbital, topiramate, brivaracetam, and cannabidiol. In the setting of renal failure, medications such as levetiracetam, gabapentin, pregabalin, topiramate, zonisamide, and perampanel may require dose adjustments. Intermittent hemodialysis can remove a significant amount of majorly water-soluble antiseizure medications such as levetiracetam and lacosamide and supplementary dosage after dialysis could be considered along with therapeutic drug monitoring to ensure adequate blood levels. In addition, extracorporeal membrane oxygenation (ECMO) required in the setting of severe respiratory failure can alter the pharmacokinetics of multiple antiseizure drugs, especially those that are highly protein bound, such as phenytoin, valproic acid, clobazam, and perampanel. This usually occurs as the medications are sequestered in the ECMO circuits for an unpredictable amount of time prior to being released, causing variable blood levels.[55]

As status epilepticus is one of the most common serious neurologic conditions managed in the intensive care unit, it is likely that the management of status epilepticus in COVID-19 negative patients will also be affected due to various reasons, including limitations in staffing and ventilator availability. Prompt management of suspected convulsive and nonconvulsive seizures and status epilepticus is recommended in order to avoid sedation and intubation.

Given the uncertainty regarding nonsteroidal antiinflammatory drug use in the setting of active COVID-19 infection, many patients have been instructed to avoid these medications. In patients with epilepsy syndromes such as Dravet syndrome where fever control may be more important, acetaminophen can be used.[30] Medications often found in over-the-counter cough and cold formulations, such as pseudoephedrine and diphenhydramine, should be avoided in patients with a known history of seizures as these may lower the seizure threshold.[30]

COVID-19 VACCINE AND EPILEPSY

A variety of COVID-19 vaccines on different generic platforms are being developed, and given the proven general safety and expected efficacy in the initial clinical trials, some vaccines were authorized for emergency use in the United States, starting mid-December 2020, and across the world. Multiple epilepsy organizations including the American Epilepsy Society, International League Against Epilepsy, and other organizations formulated statements supporting the use of COVID-19

vaccine in epilepsy patients. The risk of acquiring COVID-19 infection is greater than the potential risk of the vaccine itself. Given the occurrence of fever in some cases after the vaccine, administering antipyretics is suggested during that period for patients with a history of febrile seizures, fever-sensitive epilepsies such as Dravet syndrome, or in patients with a history of fever exacerbating their seizures. It is advised to have a seizure action plan including rescue treatment in case the vaccine or the fever triggers a seizure.[56]

IMPACT OF COVID-19 ON PATIENTS AND THEIR CARE

Comorbid psychiatric diagnoses, such as depression and anxiety, are commonly seen in epilepsy patients and may be worsened in the setting of the pandemic. Patients and their caregivers should be reassured and given appropriate referrals and adequate resources for management.[30] Symptoms of depression may be seen in up to 20%–30% of patients with epilepsy, and patients with epilepsy have a 40%–50% increased risk of suicide compared to the general population.[55] It is believed that the impact of symptoms of depression may be as impairing as the seizures themselves in epilepsy patients. This may be due in part to the stress of managing a chronic illness, hopelessness regarding lack of seizure control, limitations in daily activities such as inability to drive, as well as socioeconomic concerns. The additional impact of the COVID-19 pandemic on the mental health of patients with epilepsy was assessed in China by Kuroda. Patients with epilepsy reported increased levels of psychological distress during the early months of the COVID-19 pandemic and spent more time following media reports regarding the pandemic as compared to the general population.[55] Behavioral deterioration was reported by 30.3% of caregivers during lockdowns, with anxiety and depression being the most common features. No studies have investigated the risk of sudden unexpected death in epilepsy (SUDEP) in patients with COVID-19 infection.

In addition, patients with epilepsy often have complex psychosocial factors that may limit them from receiving necessary care in the time of a pandemic, leading to worse outcomes.[55] As a number of patients with epilepsy rely on caregivers, the care of these patients may be significantly affected in the setting of either self-isolation or isolation of caregivers due to infection.[57]

In an effort to alleviate the challenges of healthcare delivery, the American Epilepsy Society released a statement suggesting that the prescriptions be refilled for 90 days in advance.[58] The Center for Medicare and Medicaid Services has supported increased access to telehealth services, flexible health-care plan coverage, and allowing mail delivery of medications.[59] Telemedicine is evidently appreciated by patients with seizures who cannot drive or need a caregiver to drive for their appointments and allows consultations with their physician without risk of exposure, preventing infection spread among patients, their care providers, and other health-care workers.

Overall, the COVID-19 pandemic has changed how the care is delivered for patients with seizures and epilepsy. Health-care systems across the world are in the process of reconfiguring services and clinical practices, responding in the most effective way for better patient care during the pandemic. It is possible that after this pandemic, some of the transformational changes will continue to some extent for convenient, efficient, and enhanced care for patients with epilepsy.

REFERENCES

1. de Wit E, van Doremalen N, Falzarano D, Munster VJ. SARS and MERS: recent insights into emerging coronaviruses. *Nat Rev Microbiol.* 2016;14(8):523–534.
2. Bohmwald K, Gálvez NMS, Ríos M, Kalergis AM. Neurologic alterations due to respiratory virus infections. *Front Cell Neurosci.* 2018;12:386.
3. Hung EC, Chim SS, Chan PK, et al. Detection of SARS coronavirus RNA in the cerebrospinal fluid of a patient with severe acute respiratory syndrome. *Clin Chem.* 2003;49(12):2108–2109.
4. Lau KK, Yu WC, Chu CM, Lau ST, Sheng B, Yuen KY. Possible central nervous system infection by SARS coronavirus. *Emerg Infect Dis.* 2004;10(2):342–344.
5. Li Y, Li H, Fan R, et al. Coronavirus infections in the central nervous system and respiratory tract show distinct features in hospitalized children. *Intervirology.* 2016;59(3):163–169.
6. Saad M, Omrani AS, Baig K, et al. Clinical aspects and outcomes of 70 patients with Middle East respiratory syndrome coronavirus infection: a single-center experience in Saudi Arabia. *Int J Infect Dis.* 2014;29:301–306.
7. Vollono C, Rollo E, Romozzi M, et al. Focal status epilepticus as unique clinical feature of COVID-19: a case report. *Seizure.* 2020;78:109–112.
8. Somani S, Pati S, Gaston T, Chitlangia A, Agnihotri S. De novo status epilepticus in patients with COVID-19. *Ann Clin Transl Neurol.* 2020;7:1240–1244.
9. Hepburn M, Mullaguri N, George P, et al. Acute symptomatic seizures in critically ill patients with COVID-19: is there an association? *Neurocrit Care.* 2020;1–5.
10. Pilato MS, Urban A, Alkawadri R, et al. EEG findings in coronavirus disease. *J Clin Neurophysiol.* 2020. https://doi.org/10.1097/WNP.0000000000000752.
11. Sohal S, Mossammat M. COVID-19 presenting with seizures. *IDCases.* 2020;20, e00782.
12. Flamand M, Perron A, Buron Y, Szurhaj W. Pay more attention to EEG in COVID-19 pandemic. *Clin Neurophysiol.* 2020;131:2062–2064.
13. Balloy G, Leclair-Visonneau L, Péréon Y, et al. Non-lesional status epilepticus in a patient with coronavirus disease 2019. *Clin Neurophysiol.* 2020;131(8):2059–2061.
14. Moriguchi T, Harii N, Goto J, et al. A first case of meningitis/encephalitis associated with SARS-Coronavirus-2. *Int J Infect Dis.* 2020;94:55–58.
15. Kadono Y, Nakamura Y, Ogawa Y, et al. A case of COVID-19 infection presenting with a seizure following severe brain edema. *Seizure.* 2020;80:53–55.
16. Lyons S, O'Kelly B, Woods S, et al. Seizure with CSF lymphocytosis as a presenting feature of COVID-19 in an otherwise healthy young man. *Seizure.* 2020;80:113–114.
17. Haddad S, Tayyar R, Risch L, et al. Encephalopathy and seizure activity in a COVID-19 well controlled HIV patient. *IDCases.* 2020;21, e00814.
18. Karimi N, Razavi AS, Rouhani N. Frequent convulsive seizures in an adult patient with COVID-19: a case report. *Iran Red Crescent Med J.* 2020;22(3), e102828.
19. Mao L, Jin H, Wang M, et al. Neurologic manifestations of hospitalized patients with coronavirus disease 2019 in Wuhan, China. *JAMA Neurol.* 2020;77(6):1–9.
20. Galanopoulou AS, Ferastraoaru V, Correa DJ, et al. EEG findings in acutely ill patients investigated for SARS-CoV-2/COVID-19: a small case series preliminary report. *Epilepsia Open.* 2020;5(2):314–324.
21. Li YC, Bai WZ, Hashikawa T. The neuroinvasive potential of SARS-CoV2 may play a role in the respiratory failure of COVID-19 patients. *J Med Virol.* 2020;92(6):552–555.
22. Pastor J, Vega-Zelaya L, Martín Abad E. Specific EEG encephalopathy pattern in SARS-CoV-2 patients. *J Clin Med.* 2020;9(5):1545.
23. Poyiadji N, Shahin G, Noujaim D, Stone M, Patel S, Griffith B. COVID-19-associated acute hemorrhagic necrotizing encephalopathy: imaging features. *Radiology.* 2020;296(2):E119–E120.
24. Benameur K, Agarwal A, Auld SC, et al. Encephalopathy and encephalitis associated with cerebrospinal fluid cytokine alterations and coronavirus disease, Atlanta, Georgia, USA, 2020. *Emerg Infect Dis.* 2020;26(9):2016–2021.
25. Aledo-Serrano A, Mingorance A, Jiménez-Huete A, et al. Genetic epilepsies and COVID-19 pandemic: lessons from the caregiver perspective. *Epilepsia.* 2020;61(6):1312–1314.
26. Lu L, Xiong W, Liu D, et al. New-onset acute symptomatic seizure and risk factors in coronavirus disease 2019: a retrospective multicenter study. *Epilepsia.* 2020;61(6):e49–e53.
27. van Dorp L, Acman M, Richard D, et al. Emergence of genomic diversity and recurrent mutations in SARS-CoV-2. *Infect Genet Evol.* 2020;83:104351.
28. Logmin K, Karam M, Schichel T, Harmel J, Wojtecki L. Non-epileptic seizures in autonomic dysfunction as the initial symptom of COVID-19. *J Neurol.* 2020;1–2.

29. French JA, Brodie MJ, Caraballo R, et al. Keeping people with epilepsy safe during the COVID-19 pandemic. *Neurology.* 2020;94(23):1032–1037.

30. Cabezudo-Garcia P, Ciano-Petersen NL, Mena-Vasquez N, Pons-Pons G, Castro-Sanchez MV, Serrano-Castro PJ. Incidence and case fatality rate of COVID-19 in patients with active epilepsy. *Neurology.* 2020;95(10):e1417–e1425.

31. Keezer MR, Sisodiya SM, Sander JW. Comorbidities of epilepsy: current concepts and future perspectives. *Lancet Neurol.* 2016;15(1):106–115.

32. Zhou F, Yu T, Du R, et al. Clinical course and risk factors for mortality of adult inpatients with COVID-19 in Wuhan, China: a retrospective cohort study. *Lancet.* 2020;395(10229):1054–1062.

33. Gaitatzis A, Carroll K, Majeed A, Sander JW. The epidemiology of the comorbidity of epilepsy in the general population. *Epilepsia.* 2004;45(12):1613–1622.

34. Haines S, Caccamo A, Chan F, Galaso G, Catinchi A, Gupta PK. Practical considerations when performing neurodiagnostic studies on patients with COVID-19 and other highly virulent diseases. *Neurodiagn J.* 2020;60(2):78–95.

35. American Epilepsy Society. n.d.COVID-19 Delivery of Care. https://www.aesnet.org/about_aes/position_statements/covid-19/delivery-of-care. Accessed July 29, 2020.

36. American Clinical Neurophysiology Society. n.d. Guidelines and Consensus Statements. https://www.acns.org/practice/guidelines. Accessed 29 July 2020.

37. American Academy of Neurology. n.d. COVID-19 Neurology Resource Center. https://www.aan.com/tools-and-resources/covid-19-neurology-resource-center. Accessed 29 July 2020.

38. Assenza G, Lanzone J, Ricci L, et al. Electroencephalography at the time of Covid-19 pandemic in Italy. *Neurol Sci.* 2020;41(8):1999–2004.

39. Centers for Medicare and Medicaid Services. n.d. Non-Emergent, Elective Medical Services, and Treatment Recommendations. https://www.cms.gov/files/document/cms-non-emergent-elective-medical-recommendations.pdf. Accessed 29 July 2020.

40. Gélisse P, Rossetti AO, Genton P, Crespel A, Kaplan PW. How to carry out and interpret EEG recordings in COVID-19 patients in ICU? *Clin Neurophysiol.* 2020;131(8):2023–2031.

41. Ramadan AR, Alsrouji OK, Cerghet M, et al. Tales of a department: how the COVID-19 pandemic transformed Detroit's Henry Ford Hospital, Department of Neurology—part I: the surge. *BMJ Neurol Open.* 2020;2(1), e000070.

42. Helms J, Kremer S, Merdji H, et al. Neurologic features in severe SARS-CoV-2 infection. *N Engl J Med.* 2020;382(23):2268–2270.

43. Filatov A, Sharma P, Hindi F, Espinosa PS. Neurological complications of coronavirus disease (COVID-19): encephalopathy. *Cureus.* 2020;12(3), e7352.

44. Vespignani H, Colas D, Lavin BS, et al. Report on electroencephalographic findings in critically ill patients with COVID-19. *Ann Neurol.* 2020;88(3):626–630.

45. Petrescu AM, Taussig D, Bouilleret V. Electroencephalogram (EEG) in COVID-19: a systematic retrospective study. *Neurophysiol Clin.* 2020;50(3):155–165.

46. Cecchetti G, Vabanesi M, Chieffo R, et al. Cerebral involvement in COVID-19 is associated with metabolic and coagulation derangements: an EEG study. *J Neurol.* 2020;267(11):3130–3134.

47. Pati S, Toth E, Chaitanya G. Quantitative EEG markers to prognosticate critically ill patients with COVID-19: a retrospective cohort study. *Clin Neurophysiol.* 2020;131(8):1824–1826.

48. Louis S, Dhawan A, Newey C, et al. Continuous electroencephalography (cEEG) characteristics and acute symptomatic seizures in COVID-19 patients. *Clin Neurophysiol.* 2020;131(11):2651–2656.

49. Adan GH, Mitchell JW, Marson T. Epilepsy care in the COVID-19 era. *Clin Med (Lond).* 2020;20(4):e104–e106.

50. Pati S, Houston T. Assessing the risk of seizures with chloroquine or hydroxychloroquine therapy for COVID-19 in persons with epilepsy. *Epilepsy Res.* 2020;165:106399.

51. Russo E, Iannone L. n.d.Clinically Relevant Drug-Drug Interaction Between AEDs and Medications used in the Treatment of COVID-19 Patients. https://www.ilae.org/files/dmfile/Antiepileptic-drugs-interactions_in_COVID-19.pdf. Accessed 29 July 2020.

52. Asadi-Pooya A, Attar A, Moghadami M, Karimzadeh I. Management of COVID-19 in people with epilepsy: drug considerations. *Neurol Sci.* 2020;41(8):2005–2011.

53. Farrokh S, Tahsili-Fahadan P, Ritzl EK, Lewin 3rd JJ, Mirski MA. Antiepileptic drugs in critically ill patients. *Crit Care.* 2018;22(1):153.

54. Kuroda N. Mental health considerations for patients with epilepsy during COVID-19 crisis. *Epilepsy Behav.* 2020;111:107198.

55. International League against Epilepsy. COVID-19 Vaccines and People with Epilepsy. https://www.ilae.org/patient-care/covid-19-and-epilepsy/covid-19-vaccines-and-people-with-epilepsy. Accessed 04/05/2021, 2021.

56. Kuroda N. Epilepsy and COVID-19: associations and important considerations. *Epilepsy Behav.* 2020;108:107122.

57. American Epilepsy Society. n.d. AES Statement on COVID-19. https://www.aesnet.org/about_aes/position_statements/covid-19. Accessed 29 July 2020.

58. Centers for Medicare and Medicaid Services. n.d., CMS Issues Guidance to Help Medicare Advantage and Part D plans respond to COVID-19. https://www.cms.gov/newsroom/press-releases/cms-issues-guidance-help-medicare-advantage-and-part-d-plans-respond-covid-19. Accessed 24 March 2020.

CHAPTER 6

COVID-19 and Autoimmune Demyelinating Diseases

ANZA B. MEMON[a,b] • NATALIE STEC[a] • HELENA BULKA[a] • MIRELA CERGHET[a,b]
[a]Department of Neurology, Henry Ford Hospital, Detroit, MI, United States, [b]Wayne State University, School of Medicine, Detroit, MI, United States

ABBREVIATIONS

AQP4	aquaporin 4
CNS	central nervous system
CSF	cerebrospinal fluid
FDA	US food and drug administration
IgG	immunoglobulin G
IVIG	human immunoglobulin
IVMP	intravenous methylprednisolone
MOG	myelin oligodendrocyte glycoprotein
MS	multiple sclerosis
NMO	neuromyelitis optica
NMOSD	neuromyelitis optica spectrum disorder
PLEX	plasmapheresis
SARS-CoV-2	severe acute respiratory syndrome coronavirus 2

DEMYELINATING CONDITIONS ASSOCIATED WITH HUMAN CORONAVIRUS INFECTION BEFORE COVID-19

Viral infections can unsettle the body's immune mechanism in several ways and can lead to immunosuppression in animals and humans.[1] Several mechanisms are involved in viral-induced immunopathogenesis, such as impairment of T cell-mediated immunity, upregulation of MHC antigen expression, and molecular mimicry, resulting in overstimulation of B cells and/or T cells.[2] The interaction of viruses with the host immune system is diverse and complex and has not been entirely elucidated. For example, studies have shown that mice infected with a neurotropic murine coronavirus [JHM mouse hepatitis virus (MHV-4)] show central nervous system (CNS) effects, such as acute encephalitis, chronic demyelination, and subacute paralysis.[3–6]

SARS-CoV, HCoV-OC43, and HCoV-229E are human coronaviruses (HCoVs) with neurotropic and neuroinvasive properties and the potential to be neurovirulent. Association of HCoV infection with MS has been described, and coronavirus-like particles have been detected in autopsied brain tissue from MS patients and in mice infected with murine neurotropic CoV.[7,8] Moreover, HCoV viral RNA and intrathecal production of anti-HCoV antibodies have been detected in autopsied brain tissues from patients with MS.[9,10]

A study that assessed a large panel of human brain autopsy samples from donors who had various neurological diseases (25 nondiseased, 39 MS, and 26 other neurological disorders) reported a significantly higher detection of HCoV-OC43 RNA in MS patients (35.9%; 14 of 39) than in nondiseased donors (13.7%; 7 of 51).[11] However, the presence of viral particles in the brain does not always mean that the virus has caused neurological pathology.

HCoV could induce CNS demyelination through several mechanisms, as has been shown in mouse studies, such as oligodendrocyte destruction,[12] overexpression of cytotoxic antigens by glial cells, and overexpression of inflammatory markers (e.g., interleukin-1b, tumor necrosis factor, interleukin-6 [IL-6], and type 2 nitric oxide synthase).[13] Other studies in rodents have shown the loss of myelin in the CNS during the acute phase of infection with murine coronavirus, with myelin degeneration occurring 2–3 weeks after infection.[14]

In humans, a case of acute disseminated encephalomyelitis (ADEM) was reported in a 15-year-old patient who had upper respiratory symptoms secondary to HCoV-OC43 infection, where the virus was detected in cerebrospinal fluid (CSF) and nasopharyngeal samples.[15] Also, a case of MERS-CoV infection-induced CNS demyelination was reported in a 71-year-old patient who developed inflammatory lesions in the periventricular deep white matter, corpus callosum, bilateral pons, midbrain, left cerebellum, and upper cervical cord that were detected on the 24th day of the disease.[16]

Neurological Care and the COVID-19 Pandemic. https://doi.org/10.1016/B978-0-323-82691-4.00010-8

The compelling evidence from studies in mice and observations in humans on the potential for coronavirus CNS involvement underlines the importance of assessing the potential for SARS-CoV-2 in not only causing CNS pathology but also exacerbating preexisting neurological disease during infection. Here, we present the effects of SARS-CoV-2 infection in patients with CNS autoimmune demyelinating disorders, and important considerations surrounding disease-modifying therapies (DMT) and their effects on the course of COVID-19. The main focus will be on multiple sclerosis and neuromyelitis optica spectrum disorder, the two most prevalent CNS demyelinating disorders, with brief discussions of other less common demyelinating diseases.

MULTIPLE SCLEROSIS AND SARS-COV-2 INFECTION

Multiple Sclerosis

Multiple sclerosis (MS) is a chronic inflammatory, demyelinating disease of the CNS. Like other chronic autoimmune disorders, etiopathogenesis is complicated because of the interplay between genetic and environmental factors.[17] In MS, the blood-brain barrier breaks down,[18] and access to autoreactive lymphocytes to the CNS promotes a local neuroinflammatory process.[19] Both B cells and T cells play a role in neuroinflammation during MS and contribute to the development of neuronal and axonal injury, astrocyte scar formation, and loss of oligodendrocytes and the myelin sheath, which may ultimately result in the presence of demyelinating plaques in the white and gray matter.[20–23]

At the onset of MS, approximately 80%–85% of patients have a relapsing course of disease consisting of an acute demyelination event (with or without axonal injury) followed by a recovery or remission phase, where incomplete restoration of myelin and improvement of axonal injury are seen.[24] Ultimately, about 80% of patients with MS evolve to a progressive phase.[25] Incomplete repair after relapses, oxidative damage, abnormal energy metabolism, activation of microglia, and exhaustion of compensatory mechanisms are some of the proposed mechanisms that lead to an insidious and irreversible worsening of neurological function.[26–29]

DMTs, the treatments of choice for MS, are used to prevent relapses and delay disease progression; thus choosing the proper DMT for patients with MS requires an individualized approach. All DMTs alleviate disease activity and may slow the accumulation of disability by reducing the relapse rate and preventing the expansion of new T2 lesions in the CNS. Options for DMTs have

significantly increased in the past decade, with more than 18 FDA-approved therapies currently available and several in clinical trials. Newer DMTs offer improved effectiveness and convenience, but they can also cause serious adverse effects,[30] including increased risk for infections.

Multiple Sclerosis and Infectious Disease

People with MS have an increased risk of infection, which leads to increased hospital admissions and a higher mortality rate.[31,32] Reported risk factors associated with severe infections are age, significant disability (e.g., patients who require wheelchair assistance or are bedbound), presence of comorbidities,[32] sex (higher risk in men), and MS phenotype.[31]

DMTs, with the exception of first-generation glatiramer acetate and interferon beta, may increase the risk of infection.[33] DMTs that suppress leukocyte trafficking (e.g., natalizumab and fingolimod) are associated with higher rates of respiratory infection, herpes zoster virus infection, and progressive multifocal leukoencephalopathy. DMTs that deplete lymphocytes (ocrelizumab, rituximab, alemtuzumab, and cladribine) have also been associated with increased susceptibility to a variety of infections.[34,35]

Multiple Sclerosis and SARS-CoV-2 Infection

The COVID-19 pandemic has created fear and concern in MS patients and their physicians.[36] Patients who are not receiving DMT have a higher risk of recurrence of clinical and radiographic disease and a lower risk for acquiring new infections due to the absence of the immunosuppressive state induced by DMTs. Notably, for MS patients who are not on DMT, the risk of being infected with the SARS-CoV-2 virus and contracting COVID-19 was shown to be similar to that for the general population.[37] Over the past year, the National MS Society in the United States (NMSS) has regularly updated its information related to COVID-19 in MS patients. Some patients with MS are more susceptible to acquiring a severe case of COVID-19, and risk factors for a more severe disease course include primary progressive MS phenotype, age over 60 years, male sex, Black and South Asian ethnicity, presence of certain disabilities (e.g., MS patients who need assistance for walking/expanded disability status scale score ≥ 6), associated comorbidities (e.g., obesity, diabetes, heart or lung disease), and use of specific disease-modifying therapies.[38,39]

Interestingly, despite the logical concern that DMTs may increase infectious disease risk because of immunosuppression, it has been shown that DMTs may be beneficial for controlling the overly activated immune system triggered by SARS-CoV-2 infection, the main cause of serious illness.[37] Several case series pertinent to the safety of DMT in MS patients with COVID-19 have been published and are outlined in Table 6.1.[40–55]

Infection with SARS-CoV-2 induces an innate immune response that is followed by an adaptive immune response. Because many cases of COVID-19 are asymptomatic, it is postulated that the innate immune system (monocytes and macrophages) followed by an adaptive CD8 + cytotoxic T cell response is the dominant mechanism responsible for SARS-CoV-2 containment and clearance.[56] Supporting this idea, in vitro experiments and autopsy samples from a COVID-19 patient have shown a predominance of macrophages and monocytes in infected tissues.[57] After the innate and T cell responses, B cell-mediated immunoglobulin production occurs and confers an undetermined level of protection against SARS-CoV-2 reinfection. Interruption of either innate or adaptive immunity interferes with the immune system's ability to fight and eradicate SARS-CoV-2 effectively. One study suggested that low peripheral CD8 + T cell levels in patients with severe COVID-19 symptoms portend a poor prognosis.[58] Macrophages produce cytokines, such as IL-6 and IL-1, which are thought to instigate a cytokine storm, resulting in acute respiratory distress syndrome (ARDS) and rapid respiratory decline.

Relative lymphopenia associated with COVID-19 may be multifactorial and linked with disease severity and viral load. Potential causative factors for lymphopenia in COVID-19 include lymphocyte sequestration during the antiviral response, CD8 T cell exhaustion (as in advanced age), direct macrophage activity, and atrophy of lymphoid tissues.[56,58]

Mechanisms and Potential Effects of DMTs in COVID-19 Infection

COVID-19 has created many challenges for MS specialists in managing immunomodulatory/immunosuppressive therapies. Most of the newer DMTs can cause lymphopenia, which raises concern for increased risk of infection while patients are on treatments. A recent review by Amor et al.[59] elaborates on the role of DMTs in the setting of COVID-19, and an overview of these therapies is outlined below.

But to understand the role of DMTs and their potential impact on COVID-19 in MS patients, a review of some basic immunological principles may be helpful. Two primary immunological responses occur within the context of infection: the innate and the adaptive immune responses. The innate immune response is the first line of defense, and its purpose is to immediately halt the spread of pathogens (viral or bacterial). Multiple host cells generate type 1 interferons that inhibit viral replication during viral infections, and natural killer (NK) innate immune cells eradicate infected cells. Macrophages, neutrophils, and dendritic cells are also part of the innate response, and they activate the adaptive immune system by presenting pathogenic antigens to adaptive immune cells.

The adaptive immune response has two key players: T cells and B cells. Specifically, cytotoxic CD8 T cells directly kill virus-infected cells, and B cells generate protective antibodies. Pathogen-specific antibodies create long-lasting immunity against many but not all viral pathogens and are essential for preventing future infections.

Most DMTs target the adaptive immune system, although some DMTs may affect innate immunity to some degree.[37] DMTs with immunomodulatory effects, such as interferons and glatiramer acetate, are considered low risk for MS patients infected with SARS-CoV-2 as they have no harmful effects on the innate immune system=.[59] B cell-depleting DMTs affect mature B cells and not the immature B cells responsible for producing antibodies to fight infections. Additionally, very few DMTs have a significant effect on CD8 T cells, which, if they did, would limit protection against COVID-19.[59]

Studies of two other coronaviruses, SARS-CoV and the Middle East respiratory syndrome (MERS) virus, have shown that these viruses inhibit innate immunity and interferon production[37,60]; thus interferon-based therapies could potentially have a protective role and may assist with the initial innate response during SARS-CoV-2 infection.[37,60–64]

Glatiramer acetate is presumed to induce T helper cells and macrophages, promoting an antiinflammatory response with no suppressive effects on NK cells and CD4 or CD8 T cells. Therefore glatiramer acetate therapy is expected to encourage an immune landscape sufficient for defense against infections.[60–65]

Teriflunomide selectively and reversibly inhibits de novo pyrimidine biosynthesis by blocking the mitochondrial enzyme dihydroorotate dehydrogenase, resulting in reduced proliferation of activated T and B cells. Persistent lymphopenia with this therapy is found in 2.3% of patients.[37,66] Although upper respiratory infections such as influenza have been described within the context of teriflunomide therapy, no serious infections or increased morbidity/mortality have been associated with this drug .[37,67] These results may indicate that teriflunomide has a limited effect on the innate and adaptive immune response and is safe in the setting of COVID-19. Also, increased levels of IL-6 have been

TABLE 6.1
Published Case Series on the Safety of DMT in Multiple Sclerosis Patients with COVID-19 Infection.

	MS Type	DMT	Comorbidities	COVID-19 Symptoms	COVID-19 Treatment	DMT Modification	Outcomes
Chaudhury et al.[40] n = 40 F:M = 24:16	PPMS: 3 RRMS: 30 SPMS: 6 Unspecified: 1	ALZ: 1 DMF: 6 FNG: 2 GA: 3 INF: 2 IV steroids: 1 NTZ: 2 OCZ: 12 TFL: 3 None: 8	DM, HTN, HLD, asthma/COPD	Fever, cough, myalgia, shortness of breath, diarrhea, sore throat, headache, altered mental status	HXQ: 14 ABX: 13 Steroid: 10	Held	Hospitalized: 20 ICU: 5 Death: 4
Crescenzo et al.[41] n = 29 F:M = 15:14	PPMS: 6 RRMS: 23	AZA:1 DMF: 12 FNG: 4 NTZ: 2 OCZ: 7 TFL: 2 None: 1	CVD, lung disease, malignancy, smoking	Fever, hypoxia	HXQ or lopinavir/ritonavir: 2	N/A	Hospitalized: 2 ICU: 0 Death: 0
Hughes et al.[42] n = 307 F:M = 171:94 Unreported sex: 42	PPMS: 47 RRMS: 128 Not reported: 132	OCZ: 307	DM, cancer, CAD, CKD, obesity, HTN, COPD	N/A	N/A	N/A	Hospitalized: 100 Death: 17 Not reported/missing: 60
Hughes et al.[43] n = 51 F:M = 34:17	PPMS: 13 RRMS: 38	OCZ: 51	N/A	N/A	N/A	N/A	Hospitalized: 16 Death: 3 Not reported/missing: 3
Kataria et al.[44] n = 3 F:M = 1:2	RRMS: 3	DMF: 1 GA: 1 OCZ: 1	HTN, HLD, DM	Severe; hypoxia Fever, hypoxia	HXQ ABX Ritonavir	Held: 2 Discontinued: 1	Recovered: 3
Loonstra et al.[45] n = 43 F:M = 28:15	PPMS: 4 RRMS: 30 SPMS: 7 Missing: 2	DMF: 8 FNG: 7 GA: 1 IFN: 2 IVIg: 1 NTZ: 3 OCZ: 8 Stem cells: 1 None: 9	Asthma/COPD, obesity, CVD, DM, cancer, rheumatic disease, hypothyroidism, chronic liver disease	N/A	N/A	N/A	Hospitalized: 22 ICU: 3 Death: 4

Study	MS type	DMT	Comorbidities	Symptoms	Treatment	DMT management	Outcomes
Louapre et al.[46] n = 347 F:M = 249:98	CIS: 6 PPMS: 17 RRMS: 276 SPMS: 48	ALZ: 1 CLB: 3 DMF: 35 FNG: 42 GA: 33 IFN: 20 NTZ: 57 OCZ: 38 RTX: 17 TFN: 33 Other: 5 None: 63	CVD, lung disease, DM, obesity, smoking	Asthenia, fever, cough, anosmia, ageusia, headache	N/A	N/A	Unable to obtain this information (graph in study does not provide numbers)
Mallucci et al.[47] n = 14 F:M = 12:2	N/A	FNG: 6 NTZ: 8	Hashimoto's disease, psoriatic arthritis, tetralogy of Fallot	Dyspnea, fever, cough	Paracetamol	Held: 6 No modification: 2 N/A: 6	Hospitalized: 6 ICU: 1 N/A: 2 Not reported: 3 Death: 1
Meca-Lallana et al.[48] n = 7	SAP: 1 PPMS: 1 RRMS: 4 SPMS: 1	OCZ: 6 RTX: 1	Smoking, HTN, HLD	Fever, cough, dyspnea, headache, hyposmia	HXQ: 2 Lopinavir/ritonavir: 2 ABX: 1	Held: 2	Hospitalized: 3 Deaths: 0
Montero-Escribano et al.[49] n = 9 F:M = 7:2	NMO: 1 PPMS: 3 RRMS: 4 SPMS: 1	OCZ: 2 RTX: 7	N/A	Fever, cough, anosmia, ageusia, GI disturbance, odynophagia, fatigue, dyspnea, pneumonia	N/A	N/A	Hospitalized: 1 Death: 0
Parotta et al.[50] n = 37 F:M = 23:14	PPMS: 0 RRMS: 25 SPMS: 10 Other: 2	Anti-CD20: 14 DMF: 2 GA: 4 IFN: 1 IVIg: 1 LFN: 1 NTZ: 3 S1P inhibitor: 4 None: 7	HTN, obesity, DM, VTE, CAD, cancer	N/A	N/A	N/A	Ongoing treatment: 7 Recovered: 25 Death: 5

Continued

TABLE 6.1
Published Case Series on the Safety of DMT in Multiple Sclerosis Patients with COVID-19 Infection—cont'd

	MS Type	DMT	Comorbidities	COVID-19 Symptoms	COVID-19 Treatment	DMT Modification	Outcomes
Reder et al.[51] n = 344 F:M = 267:77	N/A	Anti-CD20: 123 Anti-CD52: 3 Anti-VLA4: 28 DHO-DH inhibitor: 13 Fumarate: 45 GA: 35 IFN: 40 S1P modulator: 29 Other: 28	CKD, COPD, DM, CVD. cancer, HTN	N/A	N/A	N/A	Hospitalized: 74 Death: 12
Safavi et al.[52] n = 34 F:M = 27:7	PPMS: 7 RRMS: 27	DMF: 2 FNG: 5 IFN: 3 TFL: 1 RTX: 21 None: 2	DM, HLD, HTN, asthma/COPD	Fever, cough, shortness of breath, diarrhea, sore throat, sneezing, rhinorrhea, GI distress	N/A	N/A	Hospitalized: 2 ICU: 0 Death: 0
Salter et al.[53] n = 1626 F:M = 1202:421	PMS: 280 RRMS/CIS: 1275	ALZ: 9 CLB: 14 DMF: 208 DRF: 3 FNG: 106 GA: 84 IFN: 53 IVIG: 6 MTX: 2 MP: 2 NTZ: 170 OCZ: 484 OFM: 3 OZD: 1 RTZ: 77 SP: 17 TFL: 82 Other: 10 None: 237	Cancer, CVD, CKD, chronic liver disease, lung disease, neurological disease, DM, HTN, immunodeficiency, obesity	Fever, fatigue, cough, shortness of breath, anosmia, headache, myalgia, ageusia, sore throat, chills, GI disturbance, neurological	N/A	N/A	Not hospitalized: 1293 Hospitalized: 200 ICU: 79 Death: 54

Sormani et al.[54] n=844 F:M=593:251	PPMS: 44 RRMS: 676 SPMS: 91 Missing: 33	ALZ: 14 AZA: 10 CLB:11 CX: 70 DMF: 174 FNG: 94 IFN: 73 MX: 1 MTX: 1 NTZ: 85 OCZ: 89 RTX: 5 TFL: 64 Other: 2 None: 151	DM, CVD, HTN, HLD, hepatitis B	N/A	N/A	Hospitalized: 96 ICU: 38 Death: 13
Zabalza et al.[55] n=93 F:M=62:31	CIS: 5 PPMS: 5 RRMS: 66 SPMS: 17	COVID-confirmed (n=48): ALZ: 2CX: 2 DMF: 5 FNG: 4 IFN: 12 NTZ: 2 OCZ: 3 RTX: 7 TFL: 5 Other: 1	Smoking, lung disease, DM, obesity, HTN, liver disease, cancer	Fever, cough, dyspnea, hyposmia, anosmia, dyspepsia, fatigue, conjunctivitis, rhinorrhea	N/A	Hospitalized: 19 Recovered: 72 Improving: 18 Worsening: 1 Death: 2

ABX, antibiotics; *ALZ*, alemtuzumab; *AZA*, azathioprine; *CAD*, coronary artery disease; *CIS*, clinically isolated syndrome; *CKD*, chronic kidney disease; *CLB*, cladribine; *COPD*, chronic obstructive pulmonary disease; *CX*, copaxone; *CVD*, cardiovascular disease; *DHODH*, dihydroorotate dehydrogenase; *DM*, diabetes mellitus.; *DMF*, dimethyl fumarate; *DRF*, diroximel fumarate; *F*, female; *FNG*, fingolimod; *GA*, glatiramer acetate; *HLD*, hyperlipidemia; *HTN*, hypertension; *HXQ*, hydroxychloroquine; *IFN*, interferon; *IG*, immunoglobulin; *IV*, intravenous; *LFN*, leflunomide; *M*, male; *MP*, mycophenolate; *MTX*, methotrexate; *MX*, mitoxantrone; *N/A*, not available; *NMO*, neuromyelitis optica; *NTZ*, natalizumab; *OCZ*, ocrelizumab; *OFM*, ofatumumab; *OZD*, ozanimod; *PPMS*, primary progressive multiple sclerosis; *RRMS*, relapsing remitting multiple sclerosis; *RTX*, rituximab; *S1P*, sphingosine 1-phosphate; *SAP*, single attack progressive; *SP*, siponimod; *SPMS*, secondary progressive multiple sclerosis; *TFL*, teriflunomide; *VTE*, venous thromboembolism.

detected in patients with severe COVID-19, and since teriflunomide may decrease the release of proinflammatory cytokines such as IL-6 and IL-8, this agent could potentially have positive effects during COVID-19 by increasing viral clearance and helping reduce runaway inflammation.[59,60] A case series has described 5 teriflunomide-treated MS patients who continued their therapy during COVID-19 and had favorable outcomes.[68] Other case reports have described MS patients who remained on teriflunomide therapy during active SARS-CoV-2 infection and had good clinical recovery.[69] Therefore the authors speculate that teriflunomide therapy should be continued in patients with COVID-19, since it may play a protective role against pathogenic inflammatory mechanisms triggered by infection.[68,69]

Dimethyl fumarate (DMF) has a mechanism of action that is not well understood; however, through one of its mechanisms, DMF affects erythroid-derived 2-related factor (Nrf2) and causes loss of lymphocytes of the adaptive immune system. Phase 3 trials and other studies have shown little difference in the overall risk of infection between DMF and placebo. DMF blocks proinflammatory cytokine production and can inhibit macrophage function in vitro, thus suppressing inflammation and possibly providing some benefits during COVID-19, such as inhibition of the "cytokine storm".[37,67,70]

Modulators of sphingosine-1-phosphate (S1P) (fingolimod, siponimod, ozanimod, ponesimod) limit the egress of B cells and T cells from secondary lymphoid organs. However, the actual degree of lymphopenia that these drugs elicit is not associated with their efficacy or increased risk of severe infection, and opportunistic infections in patients receiving this therapy are rare.[71] Also, patients on fingolimod appear to have no additional complications during infection with exotic viruses such as the dengue virus.[72] Therefore the use of S1P modulators may have a relatively low risk for complications during COVID-19. It is hypothesized that sequestering lymphocytes may assist with blunting the immune response during severe COVID-19, and fingolimod is currently being studied in a clinical trial in a COVID-19 cohort [NCT04280588]. Fingolimod, however, does blunt vaccine responses, indicating that both innate and adaptive immune responses are affected by this therapy.[71] Therefore, if possible, patients should be vaccinated at least 2–4 weeks before starting an S1P modulator. If a patient is already taking an S1P modulator, the COVID-19 vaccine is still recommended, with no adjustments.[38]

Cladribine inhibits DNA synthesis and repair and causes apoptosis of lymphocytes,[37] but it has minor effects on innate immune cells. Cladribine treatment depletes 50% of T lymphocytes (mostly CD4 cells and fewer CD8 cells),[73] and lymphocyte depletion has been implicated in a poor COVID-19 prognosis. In clinical trials, varicella-zoster virus infections were more frequent in patients taking cladribine than in the placebo group. Importantly, when viral infections did occur, they were mild to moderate in severity.[71,74] Given the substantial and sustained decrease of lymphocytes resulting from cladribine therapy, a theoretical concern exists for increased susceptibility to SARS-CoV-2 in patients who are receiving this drug; however, this does not necessarily suggest the promotion of worst outcomes.

Natalizumab prevents the transmigration of T lymphocytes across the blood-brain barrier by blocking the alpha 4 subunit of the integrin vascular cell adhesion molecule (VCAM). One cohort study found no significant increase in the general risk of infection during natalizumab therapy than during platform therapies,[37] and patients on natalizumab have been shown to clear dengue virus infections without complications, which is reassuring.[71,72] Given its central acting effects, natalizumab may not pose a significant risk for COVID-19, with a few exceptions. For example, natalizumab blocks the immune surveillance in the CNS; therefore patients with COVID-19-related encephalitis could be in danger of a significant complication during natalizumab treatment. Another consideration is that natalizumab decreases lymphocyte migration in the gastrointestinal tract, and SARS-CoV-2 has been shown to cause gastrointestinal tract infections in 3%–4% of people with COVID-19. Caution within both settings is necessary, and withholding natalizumab treatment is recommended to decrease chances of viral replication.[37,72,75] However, withholding natalizumab treatment for more than 6 weeks may increase the risk of an MS relapse, and this should be taken into consideration. Different outcomes for COVID-19 patients who are on natalizumab have been reported, and in one reported case fatality, the patient's comorbidities may have played a role in disease severity.[48,76] The COViMS registry (COVID-19 Infections in MS and related diseases) currently includes 262 COVID-19 patients who were on natalizumab during their illness, and three of them have died.[77]

Rituximab, ocrelizumab, and ofatumumab are anti-CD20 monoclonal antibodies that reduce levels of memory and mature B cells by binding to the B cell surface CD20 molecule and targeting cells for apoptosis. Thus these therapies reduce proinflammatory B cell effects and cytokine levels. Rituximab, ocrelizumab, and ofatumumab selectively deplete circulating CD20

B cells, but not hematopoietic stem cells and immature antibody-producing B cells.[78] CD20 therapies also have a minor effect on T cell levels and no effect on the innate immune system, further emphasizing that these therapies are unlikely to increase the risk of severe viral infection.[37] B cells are not necessary for viral elimination, and in the setting of a mild infection, the innate immune system and antiviral T cells may provide sufficient protection.[59,79] As only 2% of the body's total B cell population is in the peripheral blood, resistance of tissue-residing B cells might account for the relative safety of anti-CD20 therapies.[80]

Additionally, the observation that people with X-linked agammaglobulinemia, who lack B cell lymphocytes, can recover from COVID-19 without needing ICU admission or oxygen ventilation further supports the idea that B cells do not have a direct role in virus clearance.[81] Interestingly, several cases of patients who recovered from COVID-19 after having received anti-CD20 therapies have been reported, suggesting that selective immunosuppression before infection with SARS-CoV-2 could protect patients from the potentially fatal hyperinflammatory phase of the disease, perhaps through lowering the release of proinflammatory cytokines such as IL-6.[59,71,77] In a study that assessed ocrelizumab-treated MS patients who developed COVID-19, analysis of internal clinical trial data showed no association between duration of exposure to ocrelizumab and development of COVID-19, and analysis of external real-world data showed similar rates of hospitalization, need for ventilation, and death in MS patients regardless of ocrelizumab therapy.[42] However, a preliminary large analysis of data from a global data-sharing initiative, which analyzed MS patients with COVID-19, found an association of rituximab and ocrelizumab use with an increased risk of ICU admission and hospitalization from COVID-19 compared to dimethyl fumarate use.[82] However, the study found no association of rituximab or ocrelizumab use with the risk of death in this population.

While CD8 T cells help eliminate SARS-CoV-2, virus-specific antibodies produced by B cells are essential for generating long-lasting immunity and preventing reinfection. More studies and case observations are needed to verify the effects of anti-CD20 monoclonal antibody therapies on COVID-19, but the lack of an increased risk for influenza with these therapies is heartening. Because B cell precursors are continuously repopulated, immunologic recovery is possible when treatment is interrupted.[78]

Alemtuzumab is a monoclonal antibody therapy directed against the CD52 protein on the surface of T and B cell lymphocytes, inducing antibody depletion and cytokine-dependent cellular cytotoxicity.[83] Alemtuzumab treatment results in prolonged lymphopenia for up to 12–13 months and B cell depletion for approximately 7 months, which increase the risk of serious infection, especially with viruses such as herpes simplex virus or varicella-zoster virus.[37] Because of the known infectious risks with alemtuzumab, this therapy may pose a higher risk of severe COVID-19 following treatment,[37,59] and more research is needed. Several case reports of MS patients on alemtuzumab therapy have reported that these patients had mild symptoms during COVID-19, and the authors hypothesize that lymphocyte reconstitution induced by alemtuzumab may offer protection from cytokine storm.[84–86] However, the NMSS cautions that more data are needed to assess the safety of using alemtuzumab and cladribine during the COVID-19 pandemic.[38]

Caring for Patients With MS During the COVID-19 Pandemic

At the onset of the COVID-19 pandemic, initial expert recommendation (Societa Italiana di Neurologia [SIN] and the Association of British Neurologists [ABN]) advised discontinuing DMTs for MS patients with COVID-19,[56] even therapies with a lower efficacy. Subsequently, numerous suggested revisions have been published by expert communities in response to emerging findings on COVID-19 immunopathophysiology. Overall, when considering the distinct pathways driving MS and COVID-19, DMTs are unlikely to appreciably interrupt the physiological immune response during COVID-19.[56]

The direct effects of immunomodulatory and immunosuppressive MS therapies on COVID-19 are currently under study in several trials, including investigations of interferons and the S1P modulator fingolimod.[71] Further analysis of MS patients on DMT who develop COVID-19 will reveal whether the moderate immunosuppression induced by DMTs protects against severe COVID-19 pathology.[59] In addition to mechanistic principles, the revisions proposed below are further supported by a large volume of case reports showing favorable outcomes in MS patients who continued their DMTs despite SARS-CoV-2 infection. For example, a multicenter cohort study of 274 patients with MS in France identified risk factors for severe COVID-19, including neurologic disability, age, and obesity; however, no association between DMTs (all agents as mentioned above included) and COVID-19 severity was found, and DMT use was associated with a lower risk of hospitalization.[87] A cohort study from New York University of 76 patients concluded that most patients with MS and COVID-19 did not require hospitalization, despite being on DMTs. Also, no DMT class was associated with an increased risk of hospitalization or fatal outcome, and DMT use was not a predictor of poor COVID-19 outcome.[71] Thus these cumulative findings serve as a rationale for supporting proposed revisions to the initial expert recommendation.[50,53,67] Table 6.2 summarizes the expert recommendations for DMT use in MS patients during the COVID-19 pandemic.[38,56,71,88-90]

Another concern for patients with MS who are receiving certain DMTs is whether they will have an effective response to a SARS-CoV-2 vaccine. Most DMTs prescribed for MS do not have significant long-term effects on the CD8 T cells necessary for protection from and clearance of SARS-CoV-2 and do not generally affect B cell development, thus allowing antibody production for prevention of reinfection and an adequate vaccine response. The NMSS has published guidelines for COVID-19 vaccination in MS patients and updates it periodically. Their overall view (as of April 2021) is that the COVID-19 vaccines approved for emergency use in the United States are safe for people with MS (mRNA vaccines from Pfizer-BioNtech and Moderna and the vector vaccine from Johnson & Johnson).[38] But one possible exception that may be of concern for vaccine effectiveness could be anti-CD20 DMTs, which may blunt initial vaccine responses; however, antibodies to SARS-CoV-2 have been found in COVID-19 patients who had taken anti-CD20 therapies,[79] and preexisting adaptive immunity is mainly unaffected by short-term treatment with anti-CD20 therapies.[78] A study of responses to several non-COVID-19 vaccines in patients with relapsing MS found that patients with peripheral B cell depletion (from ocrelizumab) were able to mount a humoral response, although the response to non-live vaccines was somewhat attenuated.[91]

Coordination of vaccine timing for patients undergoing anti-CD20 therapy may be essential.[37,59] Current recommendations from the NMSS suggest starting ocrelizumab, rituximab, ofatumumab, or cladribine at least 4 weeks after complete COVID-19 vaccination, if possible. For patients already on ocrelizumab or rituximab, an ideal time for COVID-19 vaccination is 12 weeks from the last infusion. For alemtuzumab, the ideal time for COVID-19 vaccination is 24 weeks or more after the last infusion, and infusions can be resumed 4 weeks or more after complete vaccination. However, the NMSS recognizes that their scheduling recommendations may not be possible, and that getting a vaccination against COVID-19 once the vaccine becomes available to a patient may be the most important consideration.[38]

Neuromyelitis Optica Spectrum Disorders (NMOSD, MOG)

Neuromyelitis optica spectrum disorder (NMOSD) is an inflammatory CNS syndrome that includes at least three defined phenotypes: aquaporin 4-IgG-associated disease (AQP4-IgG), myelin oligodendrocyte glycoprotein IgG-associated disease (MOG-IgG), and AQP4 negative IgG-associated disease.[92] Neuromyelitis optica (NMO) was first described by Eugen Devic in 1804[93] and was considered a form of MS affecting the optic nerve and spinal cord only. Although Devic disease was clinically and radiologically different from MS, the discovery of AQP4-IgG[94] led to the recognition that NMO is a separate disorder from MS, with different pathology. Moreover, the availability of the NMO-IgG test helped to clarify our understanding of the variability in clinical presentation and to define diagnostic criteria for NMOSD.[95]

Currently, serum markers are used to diagnose two autoimmune disorders under the umbrella of NMOSD: AQP4-IgG and MOG-IgG. AQP4-IgG-associated NMOSD is considered an immune astrocytopathy.[96] Approximately 25% of patients with negative test results for AQP4-IgG have the anti-MOG-IgG antibody, which targets myelin, not astrocytes.[97,98] Clinically, these two disorders can appear similar, although they vary in terms of age of onset and sex distribution.[92,99]

Compared to MS and other autoimmune neurological disorders (e.g., myasthenia gravis), NMOSD occurs in a relapsing pattern,[100] and early treatment during the acute relapsing phase can improve patient outcomes.[101] The acute phase of NMOSD can be treated with intravenous methylprednisolone (IVMP) as first-line therapy. Plasmapheresis (PLEX) can be used to treat severe relapses and in patients where high-dose steroids are not effective. Immunosuppressive treatment is initiated to prevent future relapses, particularly in seropositive patients.[102]

Neuromyelitis Optica Spectrum Disorder and COVID-19

Several risk factors for severe infection with SARS-CoV-2, such as older age, comorbidities (pulmonary disorders, heart disease, obesity, diabetes), and chronic disabling neurological diseases that affect the pulmonary function or require long-term treatment with immunosuppressive drugs, have become evident from the abundant studies performed since the pandemic began.[39] Episodes of NMOSD can affect the functions of spinal cord and brain stem function, increasing the risk for infections and pneumonia and potentially resulting in significant disability, such as limited mobility.

TABLE 6.2
Various Expert Recommendations on DMT Management During COVID-19.

At Risk Category[a]	DMT	BHATIA ET AL.[88]			BROWNLEE ET AL.[89]			BAKER ET AL.,[56] GIOVANNONI ET AL.,[71] ZHENG ET AL.[90]			NATIONAL MS SOCIETY[38]		
		Initiate	Continue	COVID19 Infection	Initiate	Continue	COVID19 Infection	Initiate	Continue	COVID19 Infection	Initiate	Continue	COVID19 Infection
Very low	Interferon-beta	Yes	Yes	–	Yes	Yes	–	Yes	Yes	Continue	Yes	Yes	–
Very low	Glatiramer acetate	Yes	Yes	–	Yes	Yes	–	Yes	Yes	Continue	Yes	Yes	–
Very low	Teriflunomide	Yes (with caution)	Yes	–	Yes	Yes, ensure neutrophils >1000 mm³	–	Yes	Yes	Continue	Yes	Yes	–
Low	Dimethyl fumarate	Yes	Yes	–	Yes	Yes, ensure lymphocytes >500–800 mm³	–	Probable safe	Yes, but switched if lymphopenic	Continue	Yes	Yes	–
Low (EID) Intermediate (SID)	Natalizumab	Yes	Yes	–	Yes	Yes, consider EID	–	Yes	Continue	Continue or temporary suspension	Yes	Yes	–
Intermediate	S1P receptor modulators (Fingolimod, siponimod, ozanimod, ponesimod)	No	Yes	–	Consider delaying	Yes, ensure lymphocytes >200–300 mm³	–	Probable safe	Continue	Continue or temporary suspension	Yes	Yes	–
Intermediate	Anti-CD20 (ocrelizumab, rituximab, ofatumumab)	No	Withhold/ delay	–	Consider delaying	Consider EID and CD19, lymphocytes counts	–	Probable safe	Continue or suspend based on risk	Temporary suspension	Can be considered	Possible, but discuss with physician	–
Intermediate	Cladribine	–	–	–	No	Delay	–	Probable safe	Continue or suspend based on risk	Temporary suspension	More data needed	Possible, but discuss with physician	–
High	Alemtuzumab	No	Withhold/ delay	–	No	Delay	–	No	Suspend	Suspend	More data needed	Possible, but discuss with physician	–
High	Mitoxantrone	–	–	–	–	–	–	No	Suspend	Suspend	–	–	–
High	HSCT	–	–	–	No	Suspend	Suspend	No	Suspend	Suspend	–	–	–

Abbreviations: *EID*, extended-interval dosing; *SID*, standard interval dosing; *HSCT*, hematopoietic stem cell transplantation.
[a]Refers to risk of acquiring infection during immunodepleting phase.

Also, long-term treatment with immunosuppressive therapies increases the risk of disease in patients with NMOSD.

Little is known about how SARS-CoV-2 infection affects patients with NMOSD, and very few case reports have been published so far. Creed et al. described a patient with AQP4-IgG NMOSD who was on long-term treatment with rituximab. This patient had presented with fever, myalgia, and headache and had a positive SARS-CoV-2 RNA PCR test result. The patient also had mild COVID-19 respiratory symptoms despite having been treated with B cell depletion therapy.[103] In a telephone survey study of 130 patients with NMOSD in Iran, five patients on rituximab treatment reported infection with SARS-CoV-2, of these three of these patients required hospitalization and subsequently recovered.[104] However, this small study demonstrated that the rate of infection in patients treated with targeted B cell therapy was the same as that in the general population despite the therapy's immunosuppressive effects.[105]

Neuromyelitis Optica Spectrum Disorder Treatment and COVID-19

Treatment of NMOSD requires immunosuppression, which can potentially increase the risk of infection with SARS-CoV-2 and promote potential complications from COVID-19.[106] However, a survey conducted in China reported no increased risk of COVID-19 in a cohort of 2129 patients with NMOSD, irrespective of receiving DMT, although stringent preventive measures to reduce SARS-CoV-2 infection were used.[107]

Also, the requirement of intravenous delivery of NMOSD therapies at infusion centers or hospitals is concerning for a possibly increased risk of SARS-CoV-2 exposure and infection.[37] NMOSD acute episodes are usually severe and require prompt treatment with corticosteroids, hospitalization for PLEX, or PLEX combined with corticosteroids.[108,109] But the general view is that treatment of acute episodes of NMOSD should not be withheld because of COVID-19, since withholding treatment can lead to long-term disability.[110,111]

Long-term corticosteroid treatment for NMOSD may increase the risk of infection[97,98]; however, short-term use is less likely to increase infection risk[99] and is recommended when necessary.[110] The use of glucocorticoids in patients infected with SARS-CoV-2 is debatable because of conflicting evidence. A recent report showed the benefits of dexamethasone treatment in COVID-19 patients who required respiratory support in a hospital setting; however, no differences were seen in hospitalized patients who did not require respiratory support.[112]

Reports on the effects of PLEX and intravenous human immunoglobulin (IVIG) in the context of COVID-19 are limited, but these treatments are viewed as being a mild risk for infection or severe COVID-19.[110] Moreover, IVIG may be a preferred option during COVID-19 because of its antiviral and immune-boosting effects.[106] Therefore options for treatment of acute NMOSD relapses in patients with COVID-19 may include oral corticosteroids for mild relapses, PLEX or IVIG for severe relapses, and avoidance of high-dose IVMP in a hospital setting, specifically for older patients who may have comorbidities that increase the risk of severe COVID-19.[106]

Maintenance treatments used for NMOSD vary. Classically, azathioprine, mycophenolate mofetil, methotrexate, and rituximab have been used as off-label therapies for patients with NMOSD[92]; however, eculizumab, inebilizumab, and satralizumab are FDA-approved drugs specific for the treatment of NMOSD.

Azathioprine, mycophenolate mofetil, and drugs that deplete lymphocytes increase the risk of infections, which could include SARS-CoV-2.[113,114] Eculizumab, a humanized monoclonal antibody that inhibits the terminal complement protein C5, is approved by the FDA as an add-on therapy or monotherapy for NMOSD.[115] Eculizumab increases the risk of infection with encapsulated bacteria but does not seem to increase the risk for viral infection. Leukopenia and lymphopenia due to eculizumab are extremely rare, and treatment has not been associated with hypogammaglobulinemia.[106,115] Also, eculizumab treatment does not affect vaccinations.[106] As such, eculizumab is viewed as not posing an increased risk of severe COVID-19.[110] As a proof-of-concept study to explore complement inhibition within the context of COVID-19, 80 patients with severe COVID-19 were enrolled, and 35 were treated with eculizumab. Estimated survival at 15 days was higher in patients treated with eculizumab than in patients treated with standard of care.[116] Small case series describing patients with various disorders for which they were taking eculizumab have reported mixed results,[117] and several clinical trials investigating complement inhibition treatment in patients with COVID-19 are ongoing (NCT04346797, NCT04288713, NCT 04369469, NCT04390464).

Inebilizumab is an anti-CD19 antibody that depletes CD19-expressing B cells and has been approved by the FDA to treat NMOSD.[118] However, inebilizumab can increase the risk of infection and cause hypogammaglobulinemia.[119] International and national recommendations on treatment with DMTs and one Italian study suggest that B cell-depleting therapies may increase the risk of severe COVID-19[120]; however, clear evidence is lacking. The increased risk may depend on the duration of inebilizumab treatment since immunoglobulin deficiency occurs more frequently after 2–3 years of treatment.[121] Also, the period of immunoglobulin depletion from inebilizumab may decrease over time, with a reduction in peripheral B cells lasting 5–6 months after the patient's last dose.[122] Studies have shown that treatment with B cell-depleting therapies (rituximab, ocrelizumab, and ofatumumab) for neuroinflammatory disorders in individual patients can be initiated during COVID-19, especially for younger patients with no comorbidities known to increase the risk of severe COVID-19.[37,105,109]

Satralizumab is an FDA-approved humanized anti-IL-6 monoclonal antibody for the treatment of AQP4-positive and -negative NMOSD. In clinical trials, satralizumab has been shown to be highly effective for treating NMOSD.[123] However, satralizumab was reported to increase the risk of upper respiratory infections compared to placebo. Satralizumab as a self-subcutaneous injection may be preferable during the COVID-19 pandemic, as this strategy does not require administration at an infusion center and exposure to health-care personnel.

Currently, more than 160 vaccines against SARS-CoV-2 are being investigated.[124] In general, live-attenuated vaccines are contraindicated for patients with NMOSD who are on immunosuppressive agents. While nonlive vaccines should be considered, patients on B cell-depleting therapies are more likely to have an attenuated humoral response, possibly reducing the vaccine's effectiveness.[90] In the race for finding a vaccine against SARS-CoV-2, new vaccine strategies have emerged, including mRNA vaccines. However, no data showing how these new vaccines may be influenced by immunosuppressive therapies or how they may affect patients with neuroinflammatory disorders exist.[125] Currently, seven inactive COVID-19 vaccines are available worldwide: BNT162b2 (Pfizer-BioNTech) and mRNA1273 (Moderna) are mRNA vaccines; AdV26.CoV2·S (Johnson & Johnson), AZD1222/ChAdOx1 nCoV-19 (AstraZeneca, Oxford), and Sputnik V (Gamaleya Research Institute Russia) are nonreplicating viral vector vaccines; CoronaVac (Sinovac) is an inactivated virus vaccine; and NVX-CoV2373 (Novovax) is a protein subunit vaccine. At the time of writing, the first three vaccines have been approved in the United States for emergency use.

The COViMS registry has been gathering information on patients with COVID-19 and includes patients with MS, NMOSD, and MOG antibody disorder. At present, 66 patients with NMOSD and 15 patients with MOG antibody disorder who developed COVID-19 are included in the registry, and the mortality is reported at 10.4% for NMOSD patients and 0% for patients with MOG antibody disorder. The registry also currently includes five patients on eculizumab with no reported deaths.[77]

In conclusion, some therapies for NMOSD may increase the risk of SARS-CoV-2 infection or development of severe COVID-19; however, NMOSD patients should be started on preventive therapies and should continue treatments because of the risk for severe relapse and the potential for disability due to relapse.[105,109] Guidance and recommendations for the treatment of NMOSD during the COVID-19 pandemic are still emerging. Patients and health-care providers face multiple uncertainties regarding SARS-CoV-2 in the context of NMOSD, including the potential of NMOSD therapies to increase the risk of infection and severity of the disease, the possibility of viral exposure during monitoring of NMOSD and administration of therapies, and the unknown impact that NMOSD therapies might have on future vaccinations against SARS-CoV-2.[126,127]

OTHER AUTOIMMUNE INFLAMMATORY AND DEMYELINATING CNS DISEASES

Immune-mediated CNS manifestations of SARS-CoV-2 infection, including acute necrotizing encephalitis, myelitis, meningoencephalitis, and acute disseminated encephalomyelitis, have been reported[128–139] (Table 6.3). Such complications underscore the neurotropic and micro-invasive potential of the SARS-CoV-2 virus. These complications could result from neuronal retrograde dissemination of the virus, innate or adaptive immune responses, or the immune-mediated neurotoxicity initiated by the cytokine storm secondary to immune system perturbance by the viral infection (see Chapter 2 for a possible mechanism of SARS-CoV-2 entering and affecting CNS). Secondary effects on the nervous system could also occur from hypoxic metabolic derangements secondary to pulmonary, renal, and cardiac complications of SARS-CoV-2 infection.

Acute Necrotizing Encephalitis

Several acute necrotizing encephalitis (ANE) cases in patients with confirmed COVID-19, many of them women, have been reported in various international geographic locations,[128–131] and patients often manifested neurological symptoms 3–10 days after COVID-19 symptoms had appeared. MRI and CT assessment of patients with COVID-19-associated ANE

TABLE 6.3

Selected Case Report Summaries of COVID-19 Associated Other Autoimmune Inflammatory and Demyelinating CNS Diseases.

Study	Geographic Location	Age	Gender	Comorbidities	Symptom Onset/Onset of Neurologic Syndrome (Days)	CNS/PNS Symptomatology	Nasopharyngeal SARS-CoV 2 RT-PCR	CSF SARS-CoV 2 RT-PCR	MRI	Treatment	Outcome
Poyiadji et al.[128] Case report ANE	Detroit, MI, USA	58	F	HTN	4 days after cough, fever and myalgia	AMS	Positive	Negative	BL thalamic and medial temporal lobe hemorrhages	IVIG + IVMP + HCQ + AZI	Recovered
Dixon et al.[129] Case report ANE	London, UK	59	F	Transfusion dependent aplastic anemia	10 days after fever, cough, sorethroat, myalgia, dyspnea and headache	AMS, Seizures	Positive	Negative	Symmetrical hemorrhagic lesions in the amygdalae, putamen, brain stem, and thalamic nuclei	levetiracetam, ceftriaxone, aciclovir, amoxicillin, clarithromycin, steroids	Died
Elkady et al.[130] Case report ANE	Egypt	33	F	None	4 days after fatigue, fever, headache, nasal congestion	Status epilepticus, coma,	Positive	Not tested	BL hemorrhagic thalamic and cerebellar lesions	IVMP + IV midazolam + valproic acid	Died
Virhammar et al.[131] Case report ANE	Sweden	55	F	None	7 days after Fever, myalgia, pneumonia	Lethargy, unresponsiveness, stupor, multifocal myoclonus	Positive	Negative × 3 (N gene was positive)	BL thalamic, hypocampal, medial temporal lobes, cerebral peducnle and pontine lesions	IVIG + acyclovir + PLEX + Convalescent plasma	Recovered
Piloto et al.[132] Case report SRE	Italy	60	M	None	2 days after fever and cough	Irritability, confusion, asthenia, akinetic mutism	Positive	Negative × 2	Normal	IVMP 1 g × 5 days	Recovered
Moriguchi et al.[133] Case report ME	Japan	24	M	NR	9 days after headache, generalized fatigue, fever, sorethroat	AMS, seizure	Negative	Positive	Right mesial temporal lobe, hippocampus, dural enhancement	Laninamivir + AP + Flavipravir + ceftriaxone + vancomycin + acyclovir + LVT	Not reported
Duong et al.[134] Case report ME	CA, USA	41	F	Diabetes, obesity	NR	Fever, Headache, seizure, disorientation, hallucination	Positive	Not tested	Not done	Ceftrixone, vancomycin, acyclovir, HCQ	Recovered
Sotoca et al.[135] Case report ANM	Spain	69	F	None	8 days after fever and dry cough	Cervical pain, imbalance, motor weakness, left hand numbness	Positive	Negative	LETM from medulla to C7 level with diffuse patchy enhancement.	IVMP 1 g × 5 days × 2, PLEX and presdnisone taper	Recovered

Study	Location	Age	Sex	Past medical history	Onset	Symptoms			MRI findings	Treatment	Outcome
Maideniuc et al.[136] Case report ANM	Michigan, USA	61	F	HTN, HLD, Hypothyroidism, Nasopharyngeal and uterine cancer	7 days after runny nose and chills	Paresthesias, quadreparesis, bowel and bladder dysnfunction	Positive	Negative	LETM from C2 to cervico-thoracic junction level with patchy enhancement.	IVMP 1 g×5 days×2 and PLEX	Recovered
Parsons et al.[137] Case report ADEM	CT, USA	51	F	NR	18 days after dyspnea, fever, vomiting, pneumonia	Coma and an impaired oculocephalic response	Positive	Negative	BL cortical, juxtacortical and DWM lesions	IVMP 1 g×5 days, IVIG 0.4 g/kg×5 days	Recovered
Novi et al.[138] Case report ADEM		64	F	HTN, Vitiligo, MGUS	21 days after influenza like syndrome, anosmia, ageusia	BL vision loss, right leg sensory deficits	PRC Negative but IgG antibody positive	Positive	Multiple T1 post-Gd enhancing lesions of the brain, T8 cord lesion, BL optic nerve enhancement	IVMP 1 g×5 days, IVIG 0.4 g/kg×5 days, oral prednisone	Recovered
Zenin et al.[139] Case report ADEM?	Brescia, Italy	54	F	(AComA) aneurysm treated surgically 20 years ago	Several days of anosmia, ageusia, pneumonia	AMS, seizures	Positive	Positive	DWM brain, bulbomedullary junction and multiple cervical cord lesions	Lacosamide, levetiracetam, phenytoin, dexamethasone 20 mg/die×10 days and 10 mg/die×10 days	Recovered

Abbreviations: AMS, altered mental status; ANE, acute necrotizing encephalopathy; ANM, acute necrotizing myelitis; AZI, azithromycin; DM, diabetes mellitus; HTN, hypertension; HCQ, hydroxychloroquine; IV, Intravenous; I.G, immunoglobulin; MP, methylprednisolone; NR, nor reported; PLEX, plasmapheresis; Rx, treatment.

generally showed hemorrhagic lesions[128–130] and/or diffuse brain stem swelling.[129,130] In one report, a woman with ANE had positive test results for SARS-CoV-2 from an initial nasopharyngeal swab; however, two CSF samples had shown negative SARS-CoV-2 test results before a third CSF sample taken 19 days after symptom onset showed positive results.[131] Although seemingly rare, ANE is a severe and potentially fatal possible complication in patients with COVID-19.[128–131]

Steroid Responsive Encephalitis

One case of steroid-responsive encephalitis was reported in a 60-year-old man who had positive test results for COVID-19 from a nasopharyngeal swab. He had presented with acute encephalopathy and akinetic mutism 7 days after having had a mild respiratory illness. The patient had normal brain MRI results, an EEG showed generalized theta slowing, and CSF had negative SARS-CoV-2 test results. The patient was treated with IV methylprednisolone for 5 days, and increased IL-8 and tumor necrosis factor-α levels were detected in CSF. Other infectious, limbic, and autoimmune test results were negative, and the patient showed clinical improvement after steroid treatment.[132]

Meningoencephalitis

Cases of meningoencephalitis in the presence of COVID-19 have also been reported. A 24-year-old man in Japan, for instance, presented with altered consciousness and a new-onset seizure 8 days after having had a fever, malaise, and sore throat. Results from RT-PCR for SARS-CoV-2 were positive from CSF but negative from a nasopharyngeal swab. Results from brain MRI with various imaging strategies were interpreted as hippocampal sclerosis with postconvulsive encephalopathy. The patient did not receive immunotherapy, and the outcome was not reported.[133]

Another case of meningoencephalitis was reported in a 41-year-old California woman who had positive SARS-CoV-2 test results from a nasopharyngeal swab.[134] She had presented with seizures, headache, neck stiffness, and fever, but she had no respiratory symptoms. The patient's CSF was analyzed for white and red blood cells, but the health-care team could not obtain SARS-CoV-2 testing for the CSF. The patient had normal CT results, a clear chest X-ray, and an MRI of brain was not done. Throughout her illness, the encephalopathy worsened; she became disoriented and lethargic and experienced hallucinations. This patient did not receive any immunotherapy and eventually recovered.[134] This case highlights that SARS-CoV-2 may be involved in CNS disease in the absence of respiratory illness.

Acute Necrotizing Myelitis

Several cases of acute necrotizing myelitis (ANM) have been reported to date. There are two initial case reports published in the literature from different geographic locations (Spain and the United States), which are worth describing here. The mean age of the patients was 65 (both women). These patients presented with longitudinally extensive transverse myelitis (LETM). Both patients received IVMP and plasmapheresis, and subsequently recovered.[135,136]

Acute Disseminated Encephalomyelitis

Several cases of acute disseminated encephalomyelitis (ADEM) have been reported. In one case, a 51-year-old woman who had positive COVID-19 test results from a nasopharyngeal swab developed an altered level of consciousness and coma, and she required intubation 18 days after COVID-19 pneumonia. A brain MRI showed demyelinating lesions indicating ADEM. Her CSF was negative for viral pathogens, including for SARS-CoV-2. The patient received treatment with IVMP and IVIG and made a recovery over several weeks.[137]

In another case of ADEM, a 64-year-old woman presented with a right lower extremity sensory loss and bilateral vision loss 18 days after COVID-19 symptoms. MRI of the brain revealed optic nerve, brain, and spine involvement. Nasopharyngeal swab test results were negative for SARS-CoV-2 but positive for immunoglobulin G. CSF was negative for infectious and other autoimmune conditions (AQP4 and MOG antibodies). The patient received treatment with IVMP and IVIG and made clinical improvement.[138]

Another case report described a 54-year-old woman who presented with an altered level of consciousness and clinical and subclinical seizures. Test results for SARS-CoV-2 were positive, and multiple demyelinating lesions were reported in the brain and cervical spinal cord. This patient required ICU admission and mechanical ventilation. An electroencephalogram showed epileptiform activity, and she was given antiepileptic drugs. CSF analysis was negative for infections, including for SARS-CoV-2. This patient was treated with dexamethasone and showed reduced pneumonia with subsequent neurological recovery. The patient was successfully weaned off ventilation 15 days later and was discharged to a rehabilitation facility where she experienced no neurological deficits.[139]

SUMMARY

While the COVID-19 pandemic is still raging across the globe, many questions remain about how SARS-CoV-2 affects the CNS and what impact the virus might have on patients with neurological disorders. Many neurological manifestations of COVID-19 have been reported; however, the pandemic has also affected the health of patients who have preexisting chronic neuroimmunological diseases. At present, the strategy of using immunomodulatory and immunosuppressive drugs to treat patients who have a preexisting demyelinating disease and COVID-19 is not entirely clear, and we do not yet have a full understanding of the ramifications of this approach. Most DMTs, with the exception of a few, appear to be generally safe to use in patients with COVID-19 and some may even confer some protection against the systemic inflammatory response syndrome and cytokine storm seen in severe infections. Keeping up-to-date with the current guidelines regarding the care of patients with MS and other demyelinating conditions will prove essential as more is learned about the pathogenesis of neurological disease in COVID-19.

CONFLICT OF INTEREST

All authors declare they have no known conflicts of interest.

ACKNOWLEDGMENTS

The authors thank Karla D Passalacqua, PhD, at Henry Ford Hospital for editorial assistance.

The authors thank Stephanie Stebens, MLIS, and AHIP librarian at Henry Ford Hospital for reference assistance.

REFERENCES

1. McChesney MB, Oldstone MBA. Viruses perturb lymphocyte function: selected principles characterizing virus-induced immunosuppression. *Annu Rev Immunol.* 1987;5(1):279–304.
2. Mims CA. Interaction of viruses with the immune system. *Clin Exp Immunol.* 1986;66(1):1–16.
3. Suzumura A, Levi E, Weiss SR, Silberberg DH. Coronavirus infection induces H-2 antigen expression on oligodendrocytes and astrocytes. *Science.* 1986;232(4753):991–993.
4. Watanabe R, Wege H, ter Meulen V. Adoptive transfer of EAE-like lesions from rats with coronavirus-induced demyelinating encephalomyelitis. *Nature.* 1983;305(5930):150–153.
5. Wege H, Siddell S, ter Meulen V. The biology and pathogenesis of coronavirus. *Curr Top Microbiol Immunol.* 1982;99:165–200.
6. Bender SJ, Weiss SR. Pathogenesis of murine coronavirus in the central nervous system. *J Neuroimmune Pharmacol.* 2010;5(3):336–354.
7. Tanaka R, Iwasaki Y, Koprowski H. Intracisternal virus-like particles in brain of a multiple sclerosis patient. *J Neurol Sci.* 1976;28(1):121–126.
8. Burks JS, DeVald BL, Jankovsky LD, Gerdes JC. Two coronaviruses isolated from central nervous system tissue of two multiple sclerosis patients. *Science.* 1980;209(4459):933–934.
9. Salmi A, Ziola B, Hovi T, Reunanen M. Antibodies to coronaviruses OC43 and 229E in multiple sclerosis patients. *Neurology.* 1982;32(3):292–295.
10. Stewart JN, Mounir S, Talbot PJ. Human coronavirus gene expression in the brains of multiple sclerosis patients. *Virology.* 1992;191(1):502–505.
11. Arbour N, Day R, Newcombe J, Talbot P. Neuroinvasion by human respiratory coronaviruses. *J Virol.* 2000;74(19):8913–8921.
12. Weber T, Major EO. Progressive multifocal leukoencephalopathy: molecular biology, pathogenesis and clinical impact. *Intervirology.* 1997;40(2–3):98–111.
13. Lane TE, Asensio VC, Yu N, Paoletti AD, Campbell IL, Buchmeier MJ. Dynamic regulation of alpha- and beta-chemokine expression in the central nervous system during mouse hepatitis virus-induced demyelinating disease. *J Immunol.* 1998;160(2):970–978.
14. Wu GF, Perlman S. Macrophage infiltration, but not apoptosis, is correlated with immune-mediated demyelination following murine infection with a neurotropic coronavirus. *J Virol.* 1999;73(10):8771–8780.
15. Yeh EA, Collins A, Cohen ME, Duffner PK, Faden H. Detection of coronavirus in the central nervous system of a child with acute disseminated encephalomyelitis. *Pediatrics.* 2004;113(1 Pt 1):e73–e76.
16. Algahtani H, Subahi A, Shirah B. Neurological complications of Middle East respiratory syndrome coronavirus: a report of two cases and review of the literature. *Case Rep Neurol Med.* 2016;2016:3502683.
17. Nourbakhsh B, Mowry EM. Multiple sclerosis risk factors and pathogenesis. *Continuum (Minneap Minn).* 2019;25(3):596–610.
18. Sormani MP, Bruzzi P. MRI lesions as a surrogate for relapses in multiple sclerosis: a meta-analysis of randomized trials. *Lancet Neurol.* 2013;12(7):669–676.
19. Frohman EM, Racke MK, Raine CS. Multiple sclerosis-the plaque and its pathogenesis. *N Engl J Med.* 2006;354(9):942–955.
20. Pettinelli CB, McFarlin DE. Adoptive transfer of experimental allergic encephalomyelitis in SJL/J mice after in vitro activation of lymph node cells by myelin basic protein: requirement for Lyt1+2-T lymphocytes. *J Immunol.* 1981;127(4):1420–1423.
21. Krumbholz M, Derfuss T, Hohlfeld R, Meinl E. B cells and antibodies in multiple sclerosis pathogenesis and therapy. *Nat Rev Neurol.* 2012;8(11):613–623.

22. Hohlfeld R, Dornmair K, Meinl E, Wekerle H. The search for the target antigens in multiple sclerosis, part 2: CD8+T cells, B cells and antibodies in the focus of reverse-transletional research. *Lancet Neurol.* 2016;15(3):317–331.

23. Peterson JW, Bo L, Mork S, Chang A, Trapp BD. Transected neurites, apoptotic neurons, and reduced inflammation in cortical multiple sclerosis lesions. *Ann Neurol.* 2001;50(3):389–400.

24. Confavreux C, Vukusic S. Natural history of multiple sclerosis: a unifying concept. *Brain.* 2006;129(Pt 3):606–616.

25. Tutuncu M, Tang J, Zeid NA, et al. Onset of progressive phase is an age-dependent clinical milestone in multiple sclerosis. *Mult Scler.* 2013;19(2):188–198.

26. Mahad DH, Trapp BD, Lassmann H. Pathological mechanisms in progressive multiple sclerosis. *Lancet Neurol.* 2015;14(2):183–193.

27. Pitt D, Werner P, Raine CS. Glutamate excitotoxicity in a model of multiple sclerosis. *Nat Med.* 2000;6(1):67–70.

28. Gilgun-Sherki Y, Melamed E, Offen D. The role of oxidative stress in the pathogenesis of multiple sclerosis: the need for effective antioxidant therapy. *J Neurol.* 2004;251(3):261–268.

29. Lassman H. Hypoxia-like tissue injury as a component of multiple sclerosis lesions. *J Neurol Sci.* 2003;206(2):187–191.

30. Bowen JD. Highly aggressive multiple sclerosis. *Continuum (Minneap Minn).* 2019;25(3):689–714.

31. Montgomery S, Hillert J, Bahmanyar S. Hospital admission due to infections in multiple sclerosis patients. *Eur J Neurol.* 2013;20(8):1153–1160.

32. Nelson RE, Xie Y, DuVall SL, et al. Multiple sclerosis and risk of infection-related hospitalization and death in US veterans. *Int J MS Care.* 2015;17(5):221–230.

33. Lalmohamed A, Bazelier MT, van Staa TP, et al. Causes of death in patients with multiple sclerosis and matched referent subjects: a population-based cohort study. *Eur J Neurol.* 2012;19(7):1007–1014.

34. Wijnands JMA, Zhu F, Kingwell E, et al. Disease-modifying drugs for multiple sclerosis and infection risk: a cohort study. *J Neurol Neurosurg Psychiatry.* 2018;89(10):1050–1056.

35. Kordzadeh-Kermani E, Khalili H, Karimzadeh I, Salehi M. Prevention strategies to minimize the infection risk associated with biologic and targeted immunomodulators. *Infect Drug Resist.* 2020;13:513–532.

36. Berger J, Brandstadter R, Bar-Or A. COVID-19, and MS disease-modifying therapies. *Neurol Neuroimmunol Neuroinflamm.* 2020;7, e761.

37. Mateen FJ, Rezaei S, Alakel A, Gazdag B, Kumar AR, Vogel A. Impact of COVID-19 on U.S. and Canadian neurologists' therapeutic approach to multiple sclerosis: a survey of knowledge, attitudes, and practices. *J Neurol.* 2020;1–9. https://doi.org/10.1007/s00415-020-10045-9.

38. https://www.nationalmssociety.org/coronavirus-covid-19-information/multiple-sclerosis-and-coronavirus.

39. Centers for Disease Control and Prevention. *Coronavirus disease 2019 (COVID-19): people with certain medical conditions;* 2020. https://www.cdc.gov/coronavirus/2019-ncov/need-extra-precautions/people-with-medical-conditions.html?CDC_AA_refVal=https%3A%2F%2Fwww.cdc.gov%2Fcoronavirus%2F2019-ncov%2Fneed-extra-precautions%2Fgroups-at-higher-risk.html. Accessed 17 September 2020.

40. Chaudhry F, Bulka H, Rathnam AS, et al. COVID-19 in multiple sclerosis patients and risk factors for severe infection. *J Neurol Sci.* 2020;418:117147. https://doi.org/10.1016/j.jns.2020.117147.

41. Crescenzo F, Marastoni D, Bovo C, Calabrese M. Frequency and severity of COVID-19 in multiple sclerosis: a short single-site report from northern Italy. *Mult Scler Relat Disord.* 2020;44. https://doi.org/10.1016/j.msard.2020.102372, 102372.

42. Hughes R, Whitley L, Fitovski K, et al. COVID-19 in ocrelizumab-treated people with multiple sclerosis. *Mult Scler Relat Disord.* 2021;49:102725.

43. Hughes R, Whitley L, Fitovski K, et al. COVID-19 in ocrelizumab-treated people with multiple sclerosis. *Mult Scler Relat Disord.* 2020;49:102725. https://doi.org/10.1016/j.msard.2020.102725.

44. Kataria S, Tandon M, Melnic V, Sriwastava S. A case series and literature review of multiple sclerosis and COVID-19: Clinical characteristics, outcomes and a brief review of immunotherapies. *eNeurological Sci.* 2020;21:100287. https://doi.org/10.1016/j.ensci.2020.100287.

45. Loonstra FC, Hoitsma E, Le van Kempen Z, Killestein J, Mostert JP. COVID-19 in multiple sclerosis: the Dutch experience. *Mult Scler.* 2020;26(10):1256–1260. https://doi.org/10.1177/1352458520942198.

46. Louapre C, Collongues N, Stankoff B, et al. Clinical characteristics and outcomes in patients with coronavirus disease 2019 and multiple sclerosis. *JAMA Neurol.* 2020;77(9):1079–1088.

47. Mallucci G, Zito A, Baldanti F, et al. Safety of disease-modifying treatments in SARS-CoV-2 antibody-positive multiple sclerosis patients. *Mult Scler Relat Disord.* 2021;49:102754.

48. Meca-Lallana V, Aguirre C, Río B, Cardeñoso L, Alarcon T, Vivancos J. COVID-19 in 7 multiple sclerosis patients in treatment with ANTI-CD20 therapies. *Mult Scler Relat Disord.* 2020;44:102306.

49. Montero-Escribano P, Matías-Guiu J, Gómez-Iglesias P, Porta-Etessam J, Pytel V, Matias-Guiu JA. Anti-CD20 and COVID-19 in multiple sclerosis and related disorders: a case series of 60 patients from Madrid. *Spain Mult Scler Relat Disord.* 2020;42:102185.

50. Parrotta E, Kister I, Charvet L, et al. COVID-19 outcomes in MS: observational study of early experience from NYU Multiple Sclerosis Comprehensive Care Center. *Neurol Neuroimmunol Neuroinflamm.* 2020;7(5):e835. https://doi.org/10.1212/NXI.0000000000000835.

51. Reder AT, Centonze D, Naylor ML, et al. COVID-19 in patients with multiple sclerosis: associations

with disease-modifying therapies. *CNS Drugs.* 2021 Mar;35(3):317–330. https://doi.org/10.1007/s40263-021-00804-1.

52. Safavi F, Nourbakhsh B, Azimi AR. B-cell depleting therapies may affect susceptibility to acute respiratory illness among patients with multiple sclerosis during the early COVID-19 epidemic in Iran. *Mult Scler Relat Disord.* 2020 Aug;43:102195. https://doi.org/10.1016/j.msrad.2020.102195.

53. Salter A, Fox RJ, Newsome SD, et al. Outcomes and risk factors associated with SARS-CoV-2 infection in a north American registry of patients with multiple sclerosis. *JAMA Neurol.* 2021;19. https://doi.org/10.1001/jamaneurol.2021.0688, e210688.

54. Sormani MP, De Rossi N, Schiavetti I. Disease-modifying therapies and coronavirus disease 2019 severity in multiple sclerosis. *Ann Neurol.* 2021;89(6):780–789.

55. Zabalza A, Cárdenas-Robledo S, Tagliani P, Arrambide G, Otero-Romero S. Carbonell-Mirabent et al. COVID-19 in multiple sclerosis patients: susceptibility, severity risk factors and serological response. *Eur J Neurol.* 2020;19. https://doi.org/10.1111/ene.14690.

56. Baker D, Amor S, Kang AS, Schmierer K, Giovannoni G. The underpinning biology relating to multiple sclerosis disease modifying treatments during the COVID-19 pandemic. *Mult Scler Relat Disord.* 2020;43:102174.

57. Xu Z, Shi L, Wang Y, et al. Pathological findings of COVID-19 associated with acute respiratory distress syndrome. *Lancet Respir Med.* 2020;8(4):420–422.

58. Du RH, Liang LR, Yang CQ, et al. Predictors of mortality for patients with COVID-19 pneumonia caused by SARS-CoV-2: a prospective cohort study. *Eur Respir J.* 2020;55(5):2000524.

59. Amor S, Baker D, Khoury SJ, Schmierer K, Giovannoni G. SARS-CoV-2 and multiple sclerosis: not all immune depleting DMTs are equal or bad. *Ann Neurol.* 2020;87(6):794–797.

60. Mohn N, Pul R, Kleinschnitz C, et al. Implications of COVID-19 outbreak on immune therapies in multiple sclerosis patients-lessons learned from SARS and MERS. *Front Immunol.* 2020;11:1059.

61. de Wilde AH, Raj VS, Oudshoorn D, et al. MERS-coronavirus replication induces severe in vitro cytopathology and is strongly inhibited by cyclosporine A or interferon-alpha treatment. *J Gen Virol.* 2013;94(Pt 8):1749–1760.

62. Hart BJ, Dyall J, Postnikova E, et al. Interferon-betal and mycophenolic acid are potent inhibitors of Middle East respiratory syndrome coronavirus in cell-based assays. *J Gen Virol.* 2014;95(Pt 3):571–577.

63. Hensley LE, Fritz LE, Jahrling PB, Karp CL, Huggins JW, Geisbert TW. Interferon-beta 1a and SARS coronavirus replication. *Emerg Infect Dis.* 2004;10(2):317–319.

64. Spiegel M, Pichlmair A, Muhlberger E, Haller O, Weber F. The antiviral effect of interferon-beta against SARS-coronavirus is not mediated by MxA protein. *J Clin Virol.* 2004;30(3):211–213.

65. Ruggieri M, Avolio C, Livrea P, Trojano M. Glatiramer acetate in multiple sclerosis: a review. *CNS Drug Rev.* 2007;13(2):178–191.

66. Wallin MT, Culpepper WJ, Campbell JD, et al. The prevalence of MS in the United States: a population-based estimate using health claims data. *Neurology.* 2019;92(10):e1029–e1040.

67. Grenbenciucova E, Pruitt A. Infections in patients receiving multiple sclerosis disease modifying therapies. *Curr Neurol Neurosci Rep.* 2017;17(11):88.

68. Maghzi AH, Houtchens MK, Preziosa P, et al. COVID-19 in teriflunomide-treated patients with multiple sclerosis. *J Neurol.* 2020;267(10):2790–2796. https://doi.org/10.1007/s00415-020-09944-8.

69. Capone F, Motolese F, Luce T, Rossi M, Magliozzi A, Di Lazzaro V. COVID-19 in teriflunomide-treated patients with multiple sclerosis: a case report and literature review. *Mult Scler Relat Disord.* 2021 Feb;48:102734. https://doi.org/10.1016/j.msard.2020.102734.

70. Albrecht P, Bouchachia I, Goebels N, et al. Effects of dimethyl fumarate on neuroprotection and immunomodulation. *J Neuroinflammation.* 2012;9:163.

71. Giovannoni G, Hawkes C, Lechner-Scott J, Levy M, Waubant E, Gold J. The COVID-19 pandemic and the use of MS disease-modifying therapies. *Mult Scler Relat Disord.* 2020;39:102073.

72. Fragoso YD, Gama PDD, Gomes S, et al. Dengue fever in patients with multiple sclerosis taking fingolimod or natilizumab. *Mult Scler Relat Disord.* 2016;6:64–65.

73. Pawlitzki M, Zett UK, Ruck T, Rolfes L, Hartung HP, Meuth SG. Merits and culprits of immunotherapies for neurological diseases in times of COVID-19. *EBioMedicine.* 2020;56:102822.

74. Cook S, Vermersch P, Comi G, et al. Safety and tolerability of cladribine tablets in multiple sclerosis: the CLARITY (CLAdRIbine Tablets treating multiple sclerosis orallY) study. *Mult Scler.* 2011;17(5):578–593.

75. Ghosh S, Goldin E, Gordon FH, et al. Natalizumab for active Crohn's disease. *N Engl J Med.* 2003;348(1):24–32.

76. Rimmer K, Farber R, Thakur K, et al. Fatal COVID-19 in an MS patient on natalizumab: a case report. *MSJ-Exp Transl Clin.* 2020;6(3). https://doi.org/10.1177/2055217320942931, 2055217320942931.

77. www.COViMS.Org. Accessed 4 May 2021.

78. Barry B, Shin RK. AntiCD20+ agents. *Pract Neurol (Fort Wash Pa).* 2020;19(2):33–36.

79. Baker D, Pryce G, Amor S, Giovannoni G, Schmierer K. Learning from other autoimmunities to understand targeting of B cells to control multiple sclerosis. *Brain.* 2018;141(10):2834–2847. https://doi.org/10.1093/brain/awy239.

80. Gelfand JM, Cree BAC, Hauser SL. Ocrelizumab and other CD20(+) B-cell-depleting therapies in multiple sclerosis. *Neurotherapeutics.* 2017;14(4):835–841.

81. Soresina A, Moratto D, Chiarini M, et al. Two X-linked agammaglobulinemia patients develop pneumonia as COVID-19 manifestation but recover. *Pediatr Allergy Immunol.* 2020;31(5):565–569.

82. Simpson-Yap S, De Brouwer E, Kalincik T, et al. Associations of DMT therapies with COVID-19 severity in multiple sclerosis. *MedRxiv.* 2021. https://doi.org/10.1101/2021.02.08.21251316, 21251316.

83. Matias-Guiu J, Montero-Escribano P, Pytel V, Porta-Etessam J, Matias-Guiu JA. Potential COVID-19 infection in patients with severe multiple sclerosis treated with alemtuzumab. *Mult Scler Relat Disord.* 2020;44:102297.

84. Matias-Guiu J, Montero-Escribano P, Pytel V, et al. Potential COVID-19 infection in patients with severe multiple sclerosis treated with alemtuzumab. *Mult Scler Relat Disord.* 2020;40:102297.

85. Fiorella C, Galleguillos L. COVID-19 in multiple sclerosis patient treated with alemtuzumab: insight to the immune response after COVID. *Mult Scler Relat Disord.* 2020;46:102447.

86. Carandini T, Pietobani AM, Sacchi L, et al. Alemtuzumab in multiple sclerosis during the COVID19 pandemic: a mild uncomplicated infection despite intense immunosupression. *Mult Scler J.* 2020;26:1268–1269.

87. Louapre C, Collongues N, Stankoff B, et al. Clinical characterisitcs and outcomes in patients with coronavirus disease 2019 and multiple sclerosis. *JAMA Neurol.* 2020;77(9):1–10.

88. Bhatia R, Srivastava MVP, Khurana D, et al. Consensus statement on immune modulation in multiple sclerosis and related disorders during the COVID-19 pandemic: expert group on behalf of the Indian Academy of Neurology. *Ann Indian Acad Neurol.* 2020;23(Suppl 1):S5–14.

89. Brownlee W, Bourdette D, Broadley S, Killestein J, Ciccarelli O. Treating multiple sclerosis and neuromyelitis optica spectrum disorder during the COVID-19 pandemic. *Neurology.* 2020;94(22):949–952.

90. Zheng C, et al. Multiple sclerosis disease-modifying therapy and the COVID-19 pandemic: implications on the risk of infection and future vaccination. *CNS Drugs.* 2020;34(9):879–896.

91. Bar-Or A, Calkwood JC, Chognot C, et al. Effect of ocrelizumab on vaccine and responses in patients with multiple sclerosis: the Veloce study. *Neurology.* 2020;95(14):e1999–e2008. https://doi.org/10.1212/WNL.0000000000010380.

92. Weinshenker BG, Wingerchuk DM. Beuromyelitis spectrum disorders. *Mayo Clin Proc.* 2017;92(4):663–679.

93. Jarius S, Wildemann B. The case of the Marquis de Causan (1804): an early account of visual loss associated with spinal cord inflammation. *J Neurol.* 2012;259(7):1354–1357.

94. Lennon VA, Wingerchuk DM, Kryzer TJ, et al. A serum autoantibody marker for neuromyelitis optica: distinction from multiple sclerosis. *Lancet.* 2004;364(9451):2106–2112.

95. Wingerchuck DM, Banwell B, Bennett JL, et al. International consensus diagnostic criteria for neuromyelitis optica spectrum disorders. *Neurology.* 2015;85(2):177–189.

96. Marignier R, Nicolle A, Watrin C, et al. Oligodendrocytes are damaged by neuromyelitis optica immunoglobulin G via astrocyte injury. *Brain.* 2010;133(9):2578–2591.

97. Ikeda K, Kiyota N, Kuroda H, et al. Severe demyelination but no astrocytopathy in clinically definite neuromyelitis optica with anti-myelin-oligodendrocyte glycoprotein antibody. *Mult Scler.* 2015;21(5):656–659.

98. Peschl P, Bradl M, Hoftberger R, Berger T, Reindl M. Myelin oligodendrocyte glycoprotein: deciphering a target in inflammatory demyelinating diseases. *Front Immunol.* 2017;8:529.

99. Weber MS, Derfuss T, Metz I, Bruck W. Defining distinct features of anti-MOG antibody associated central nervous system demyelination. *Ther Adv Neurol Disord.* 2018;11, 1756286418762083.

100. Palace J, Lin DY, Zeng D, et al. Outcome prediction models in AQP4-IgG positive neuromyelitis optica spectrum disorders. *Brain.* 2019;142(5):1310–1323.

101. Kleiter I, Gahlen A, Borisow N, et al. Apheresis therapies for NMOSD attacks: a retrospective study of 207 therapeutic interventions. *Neurol Neuroimmunol Neuroinflamm.* 2018;5(6), e504.

102. Wu Y, Zhong L, Geng J. Neuromyelitis optica spectrum disorder: pathogenesis, treatment and experimental models. *Mult Scler Relat Disord.* 2019;27:412–418.

103. Creed MA, Ballesteros E, Greenfield Jr LJ, Imitola J. Mild COVID-19 infection despite chronic B cell depletion in a patient with aquaporin-4-positive neuromyelitis optica spectrum disorder. *Mult Scler Relat Disord.* 2020;44:102199.

104. Sahraian MA, Azimi A, Navardi S, Rezaeimanesh N, Naser MA. Evaluation of COVID-19 infection in patients with neuromyelitis optica spectrum disorder (NMOSD): a report from Iran. *Mult Scler Relat Disord.* 2020;44:102245.

105. Signorelli C, Scognamiglio T, Odone A. COVID-19 in Italy: impact of containment measures and prevalence estimates of infection in the general population. *Acta Biomed.* 2020;91(3–S):175–179.

106. Abboud H, Zheng C, Kar I, Chen CK, Sau C, Serra A. Current and emerging therapeutics for neuromyelitis optica spectrum disorder: relevance to the COVID-19 pandemic. *Mult Scler Relat Disord.* 2020;44:102249.

107. Fan M, Qui W, Bu B, et al. Risk of COVID-19 infection in MS and neuromyelitis optica spectrum disorders. *Neurol Neuroimmunol Neuroinflamm.* 2020;7(5), e787.

108. Wingerchuck DM, Hogancamp WF, O'Brien PC, Weinshenker BG. The clinical course of neuromyelitis optica (Devic's syndrome). *Neurology.* 1999;53(5):1107–1114.

109. Abboud H, Petrak A, Mealy M, Sasidharan S, Siddique L, Levy M. Treatment of acute relapses in neuromyelitis optica: steroids alone versus steroids plus plasma exchange. *Mult Scler.* 2016;22(2):185–192.

110. Korsukewitz C, Reddel SW, Bar-Or A, Wiendl H. Neurological immunotherapy in the era of COVID-19 - looking for consensus in the literature. *Nat Rev Neurol.* 2020;16(9):493–505.

111. Carnero Contenti E, Correa J. Immunossupression during the COVID-19 pandemic in neuromyelitis optica spectrum disorders patients: a new challenge. *Mult Scler Relat Disord*. 2020;41:102097.

112. Horby P, Lim WS, Emberson JR, et al. Dexamethasone in hospitalized patients with Covid-19 – preliminary report. *N Engl J Med*. 2020;384(8):693–704. https://doi.org/10.1056/NEJMoa2021436.

113. Nikoo Z, Badihian S, Shaygannejad V, Asgari N, Ashtari F. Comparison of the efficacy of azathioprine and rituximab in neuromyelitis optica spectrum disorder: a randomized clinical trial. *J Neurol*. 2017;264(9):2003–2009.

114. Russell B, Moss C, George G, et al. Associations between immune-suppressive and stimulating drugs and novel COVID-19-a systemic review of current evidence. *Ecancermedicalscience*. 2020;14:1022.

115. Pittock SJ, Berthele A, Fujihara K, et al. Eculizumab in aquaporin-4 positive neuromyelitis optica spectrum disorder. *N Engl J Med*. 2019;381(7):614–625.

116. Annane D, Heming N, Grimaldi-Bendouda L, et al. Eculizumab as an emergency treatment for adult patients with severe COVID-19 in the intensive care unit: a proof-of-concept study. *EClinicalMedicine*. 2020;28:100590.

117. Pike A, Muus P, Munir T, et al. COVID-19 infection in patients on anti-complement therapy: the Leeds national paroxysmal nocturnal Haemoglobinuria service experience. *Br J Haematol*. 2020;191:e1–e4.

118. Cree BAC, Bennett JL, Kim HJ, et al. Inebilizumab for the treatment of neuromyelitis optica spectrum disorder (N-MOmentum): a double-blind, randomised placebo-controlled phase 2/3 trial. *Lancet*. 2019;394(10206):1352–1363.

119. US Food and Drug Administration. *FDA approves new therapy for rare disease affecting optic nerve, spinal cord: second FDA approved therapy for neuromyelitis optica spectrum disorder offers patients additional treatment option*; 2020. https://www.fda.gov/news-events/press-announcements/fda-approves-new-therapy-rare-disease-affecting-optic-nerve-spinal-cord. Accessed 18 September 2020.

120. Parrotta E, Kister I, Chravet L, et al. COVID-19 outcomes in MS: observational study of early experience from NYU multiple sclerosis comprehensive care center. *Neurol Neuroimmunol Neuroinflamm*. 2020;7(5), e835.

121. Tallantyre EC, Whittman DH, Jolles S, et al. Secondary antibody deficiency: a complication of anti-CD20 therapy for neuroinflammation. *J Neurol*. 2018;265(5):1115–1122.

122. Cohen SB, Emery P, Greenwald MW, et al. Rituximab for rheumatoid arthritis refractory to anti-tumor necrosis factor therapy: results of a multicenter, randomized, double-blind, placebo-controlled, phase III trial evaluating primary efficacy and safety at twenty-four weeks. *Arthritis Rheum*. 2006;54(9):2793–2806.

123. Traboulsee A, Greenberg BM, Bennett JL, et al. Safety and efficacy of satralizumab monotherapy in neuromyelitis optica spectrum disorder: a randomised, double-blind, multicentre, placebo-controlled, phase 3 trial. *Lancet Neurol*. 2020;19(5):402–412.

124. World Health Organization. *Draft landscape of COVID-19 candidate vaccines*; 2020. https://www.who.int/publications/m/item/draft-landscape-of-covid-19-candidate-vaccines. Accessed 18 September 2020.

125. Ciotti JR, Valtcheva MV, Cross AH. Effects of MS disease modifying therapies on response to vaccination: a review. *Mult Scler Relat Disord*. 2020;45:102439.

126. Razaei SJ, Vogel AC, Gazdag B, Alakel N, Kumar AR, Mateen FJ. Neuromyelitis optica practice and prescribing changes in the setting of Covid19: a survey of neurologists. *J Neuroimmunol*. 2020;346:577320.

127. Salama S, Giovannoni G, Hawkes CH, Lechner-Scott J, Waubant E, Levy M. Changes in patient and physician attitudes resulting from COVID-19 in neuromyelitis optica spectrum disorder and multiple sclerosis. *Mult Scler Relat Disord*. 2020;42:102259.

128. Poyiadji N, Shahin G, Noujaim D, Stone M, Patel S, Griffith B. COVID-19-associated acute hemorrhagic necrotizing encephalopathy: imaging features. *Radiology*. 2020;296(2):E119–E120.

129. Dixon L, Varley J, Gontsarova A, et al. COVID-19-related acute necrotizing encephalopathy with brainstem involvement in a patient with aplastic anemia. *Neurol Neuroimmunol Neuroinflamm*. 2020;7, e789.

130. Elkady A, Rabinstein AA. Acute necrotizing encephalopathy and myocarditis in a young patient with COVID-19. *Neurol Neuroimmunol Neuroinflamm*. 2020;7(5), e801.

131. Virhammar J, Kumlien E, Fällmar D, Frithiof R. Jackmanns, Skold MK, et al. acute necrotizing encephalopathy with SARS-CoV-2 RNA confirmed in cerebrospinal fluid. *Neurology*. 2020;95(10):445–449.

132. Pilotto A, Odolini S, Masciocchi S, et al. Steroid-responsive encephalitis in coronavirus disease 2019. *Ann Neurol*. 2020;88(2):423–427.

133. Moriguchi T, Harii N, Goto J, et al. A first case of meningitis/encephalitis associated with SARS-Coronavirus-2. *Int J Infect Dis*. 2020;94:55–58.

134. Duong L, Xu P, Liu A. Meningoencephalitis without respiratory failure in a young female patient with COVID-19 infection in Downtown Los Angeles, early April 2020. *Brain Behav Immun*. 2020;87:33.

135. Sotoca J, Rodrıguez-Alvarez Y. COVID-19-associated acute necrotizing myelitis. *Neurol Neuroimmunol Neuroinflamm*. 2020;7(5), e803.

136. Maideniuc C, Memon AB. Retracted article: acute necrotizing myelitis and acute motor axonal neuropathy in a COVID-19 patient. *J Neurol*. 2021 Feb;268(2):739. https://doi.org/10.1007/s00415-020-10145-6.

137. Parsons T, Banks S, Bae C, Gelber J, Alahmadi H, Tichauer M. COVID-19-associated acute disseminated encephalomyelitis (ADEM). *J Neurol*. 2020;267:2799–2802.

138. Novi G, Rossi T, Pedemonte E, et al. Acute disseminated encephalomyelitis after SARS-CoV-2 infection. *Neurol Neuroimmunol Neuroinflamm*. 2020;7(5), e797.

139. Zanin L, Saraceno G, Panciani PP, et al. SARS-CoV-2 can induce brain and spine demyelinating lesions. *Acta Neurochirurgica (Wein)*. 2020;162(7):1491–1494.

CHAPTER 7

COVID-19 and Neuromuscular Disorders

NAGANAND SRIPATHI • DANIEL NEWMAN • KAVITA M. GROVER
Wayne State University, Henry Ford Hospital, Detroit, MI, United States

SARS-CoV-1 caused severe acute respiratory syndrome in 2002–03 and this epidemic affected close to 8000 patients worldwide. Aggressive public health efforts to contain the virus along with relative lack of easy transmissibility limited the original outbreak.[1] Very few neurologic complications were reported during this epidemic limited to large vessel strokes, axonal peripheral neuropathy, myopathy, and one case of olfactory neuropathy. Neurologic complications with SARS developed 2–3 weeks after the initial symptoms. COVID-19 infection, with higher infectivity and possibly reduced lethality compared to SARS, became a global pandemic very quickly. There are more than 25 million cases worldwide with 843,586 deaths as of August 31, 2020. Neurologic manifestations during the current COVID-19 (SARS-CoV-2) have been reported to be as high as 57.4% of the patients.[2] Another notable difference compared to SARS is the occurrence of neurologic complications earlier in the course of COVID-19 infection and seen in patients with more severe disease.

CRANIAL NEUROPATHY

The proposed mechanisms of central and peripheral nervous system involvement in SARS-CoV-2 are direct neuroinvasion, neurotropism leading to neurovirulence, and finally host's adaptive immune response to infection.[3] Neurologic complications seen in SARS-CoV and MERS-CoV are presumed to be from either hematogenous spread or retrograde neuronal dissemination.[4] It has been documented that entry of COVID-19 spike protein into respiratory cells is mediated by ACE-2 receptors and also by binding to sialic acid moiety attached to cell surface glycoproteins and gangliosides.[5] Costello and Dalakas favor an autoimmune mechanism for the neuropathies seen in COVID-19 infections.[3, 6] Cross reactivity between COVID-19 S-protein gangliosides and peripheral nerve glycolipids could also trigger an autoimmune reaction.

The most plausible route of CNS infection by the virus is through the olfactory route, as olfactory bulb is not protected by the dura.

In a retrospective case series, taste and smell impairment were reported in 5.6% and 5.1%, respectively, in 214 patients admitted with Covid-19.[7] In one large study of 204 mildly symptomatic patients, 64% reported olfactory dysfunction.[8] A case-control study of confirmed COVID-19 infection showed smell dysfunction in 98% of patients, 35% being aware of their deficit, and the other 58% being either anosmic or microsmic.[9] Sudden olfactory dysfunction (OD) has been recognized as a marker for COVID-19 infection. Anosmia and dysgeusia often happen in mild or asymptomatic cases. Olfactory receptor cells lack both ACE-2 receptors and cell surface protease TMPRSS2 gene that are necessary for direct invasion of viral particle.[10] Olfactory ensheathing glial cells surround olfactory receptor cell axons and fila, and it appears that these cells may be responsible for ACE-2-independent viral transfer by the way of exosomes. Abnormal taste in the patients may also be attributable to the olfactory dysfunction rather than damage to the taste buds, as detecting flavor depends on retro-nasal olfaction. In a multicenter European study including 417 patients with confirmed COVID-19 infection of mild to moderate severity, 85.6% and 88% reported olfactory and gustatory dysfunction respectively.[11] In 18.2% of the patients without nasal obstruction and rhinorrhea, almost 80% of them were either hyposmic or anosmic. An early olfactory recovery was reported in 44% of the patients. A proposed approach for the assessment and management of COVID-19-related olfactory dysfunction (OD) recommends a full otolaryngologic examination, which includes a three-pass naso-endoscopy when appropriate personal protective equipment is available, followed by CT to assess the paranasal sinuses, and MRI brain to examine brain and olfactory tracts if needed.[12] MRI brain has been reported to demonstrate

Neurological Care and the COVID-19 Pandemic. https://doi.org/10.1016/B978-0-323-82691-4.00011-X

transient edema in the olfactory cleft,[13] changes in the gyrus rectus, edema of olfactory cleft as well as olfactory atrophy.[14, 15] A psychophysical assessment using validated tests of odorants and tastants should complement the subjective assessment. Treatment may be needed if symptoms persist for more than 2 weeks. This includes olfactory training by sniffing specific odorants such as rose, lemon, cloves, and eucalyptus for 20 s each, at least twice daily for 3 months or longer. Other therapies which work in other postinfectious OD include intranasal vitamin A and systemic Omega-3 but these have not been tested in post-COVID-19 OD specifically. Whitcroft did not recommend corticosteroids, whether oral or intranasal, due to lacking evidence of benefit and potential harm.[12] However, a small percentage of patients received nasal corticosteroids (8%) and oral corticosteroids (3%) as reported in the study by Lechien et al.[11]

Isolated cases involving other cranial nerves have also been reported. In a large case series, one case of late optic neuritis was reported suggesting an immune-mediated etiology.[2] Another patient has been described with unilateral ocular neuritis with optic disc edema along with panuveitis in the setting of COVID-19 infection.[16]

Dinkin reported two patients with cranial neuropathies.[17] One patient presented with cough, fever, and diplopia due to right abducens palsy with MRI evidence of enhancement of optic nerve sheaths and posterior Tenon capsules. Treatment included hydroxychloroquine for COVID-19 infection and oxygen after the nasal swab RT-PCR came back positive. The diplopia gradually improved over 2 weeks. The second case presented with unilateral ptosis, diplopia, and leg paresthesia, preceded by cough and fever. MRI brain showed left oculomotor nerve enhancement and enlargement. Intravenous immunoglobulins (IVIg) were given for presumed Miller-Fisher syndrome along with hydroxychloroquine, resulting in partial resolution of the deficits.

A case of isolated facial nerve palsy in a previously healthy 27-year-old male was reported by Goh et al.[18] Soon after returning from Spain, the patient was admitted to a hospital, with flu-like symptoms and unilateral throbbing headache for 4 days without clinical evidence of meningitis. Left facial weakness was noted on day 6. Nasopharyngeal swab PCR was positive for SARS-CoV-2. Cerebrospinal fluid was noninflammatory and PCR for SARS-CoV-2 and other viruses was negative. MRI showed contrast enhancement of the left facial nerve. He was treated with prednisone, valacyclovir, and lopinavir/ritonavir.

Pellitero reported a case of acute vestibular dysfunction in a 30-year-old woman presenting with nausea, vomiting, and disequilibrium 3 weeks after developing anosmia and ageusia. Her RT-PCR for COVID-19 was positive on admission. Her MRI of the brain was normal, and she improved with vestibular suppressants and antiemetics.[19]

ANTERIOR HORN CELL/MOTOR NEURON DISEASE

There are no reports of acute presentation of anterior horn cell dysfunction similar to West Nile poliomyelitis. A case series from Scotland did not report any change in the new diagnosis of motor neuron disease (MND) during the COVID-19 pandemic and reported two cases with MND with confirmed or suspected COVID-19 infection, who died.[20] Another case report described two patients with MND on noninvasive ventilatory support at baseline, with multifocal pneumonia. One patient with confirmed COVID-19 recovered after treatment with remdesivir and solumedrol and the other patient with suspected for COVID-19 infection recovered after treatment with antibiotics and increased respiratory support.[21]

BRACHIAL AND LUMBOSACRAL PLEXUS

Brachial plexopathy has been reported in association with COVID-19 infection. Two case series described brachial plexus involvement along with isolated upper limb neuropathies, which were felt to be due to compression or stretch injury secondary to prone positioning while being artificially ventilated.[22, 23] A patient with hypoxic respiratory failure due to COVID-19 infection, not treated with proning was reported to have brachial plexitis. There was purpuric rash consistent with COVID-19-induced microangiopathy. MRI brachial plexus showed T2 hyperintensity and thickening of the entire brachial plexus. Fascicular involvement on electrodiagnostic testing was consistent with COVID-19-induced hypercoagulability causing thrombosis of the vasa nervorum and microvascular infarction.[24]

Compressive lumbar plexopathy has been described in four patients with COVID-19 infection, on anticoagulation, secondary to the development of a retroperitoneal hematoma.[25] There have been no reported cases of lumbosacral plexitis or plexopathy directly related to COVID-19 infection, so far.

PERIPHERAL NERVE

Guillain-Barre syndrome or its variants were reported in 19 patients with COVID-19 so far.[25] Two of these patients developed a febrile illness 7 days after the symptoms of GBS, and in the other 17, neuropathy developed between 7 and 24 days (median 7 days) after respiratory or systemic symptoms. Tetraparesis was seen in 11 patients, with or without sensory loss, and eight of them developed respiratory failure. Autonomic dysfunction including sphincter dysfunction and hypertension was seen in three patients. Electrodiagnostic studies showed demyelinating neuropathy in eight and axonal loss in four patients. Miller Fischer variant was seen in two patients. SARS-CoV-2 was detected through respiratory swab in 16 and in two the sample was not specified. One patient also had rhinovirus infection. One of the patients had antibody titers to COVID-19. Albumino-cytological dissociation was seen in 11 of the 13 patients who underwent lumbar puncture. RT-PCR for SARS-CoV-2 was negative in all the CSF samples. Two of the eight patients needing ventilatory support died. A total of 15 patients were treated with IVIg. In all, 12 patients improved and an additional five patients were discharged with disability.

First patient of Guillain-Barre syndrome with COVID-19 was reported from Wuhan province.[26] A 61-year-old female from Wuhan presented with ascending bilateral lower extremity weakness without initial fever, respiratory, or GI symptoms. CSF showed elevated protein with normal cell count. Absent F-waves were seen on EMG, consistent with early findings of GBS. Patient received a course of IVIg. Eight days later, she developed a fever and a dry cough, and tested positive for SARS-CoV-2. She was treated with arbidol, lopinavir, and ritonavir. She completely recovered by day 30 with full strength and return of reflexes.

Gutierrez reported two cases of Miller-Fisher syndrome (MFS) and polyneuritis cranialis.[27] The first patient, a 50-year-old man developed the cardinal features of Miller-Fisher syndrome (ataxia, areflexia, and ophthalmoparesis) 5 days after the onset of flu-like illness. He was found to have positive GD1b antibodies and albumin-cytologic dissociation. He was treated with IVIg for 5 days and made a complete recovery, except for residual anosmia and ageusia. The second patient, a 39-year-old man presented with bilateral abducens palsies 3 days after diarrhea and fever. He was areflexic but had a normal appendicular strength and sensation with no dysmetria or ataxia. While albumin-cytological dissociation was present, antiganglioside antibodies testing was not performed. Patient received treatment with

acetaminophen and made a complete recovery. RT-PCR assay of oropharyngeal swab test for SARS-Cov-2 was positive in both patients and the test was negative in the cerebrospinal fluid.

Three hospitals in Northern Italy reported a series of five COVID-19 cases who presented with GBS symptoms 5–10 days after onset of respiratory symptoms.[28] Four had paraparesis progressing to tetraparesis/tetraplegia and one had facial diplegia. Antiganglioside antibodies were tested in three patients and were negative. Albumino-cytological dissociation was demonstrated in 3/5 patients. CSF was negative for SARS-CoV-2 PCR in all patients. Three had electrodiagnostic findings consistent with an axonal variant of GBS, whereas two had demyelinating features. All received IVIg and one had plasmapheresis in addition. At 4 weeks, two patients were still mechanically ventilated, one was discharged, and two were undergoing physical rehabilitation.

Arnaud et al. reported a 64-year-old man who presented to a hospital outside of Paris, France with a severe case of COVID-19.[29] He was treated with cefotaxime, azithromycin, and hydroxychloroquine and discharged. Seven days after discharge, he returned to the hospital with rapidly progressive lower extremity weakness. His exam showed flaccid paraparesis, areflexia, and a length-dependent neuropathy in the lower extremities. CSF showed an albumino-cytologic dissociation with no pleocytosis. Otherwise, an extensive laboratory workup was negative. EMG showed classic demyelinating features including conduction block meeting criteria for GBS. He received IVIg and responded well.

NEUROMUSCULAR JUNCTION

Patients with myasthenia gravis (MG) face several challenges. Majority of the patients are maintained on immunosuppressive treatments, which put them at risk for infection, while serious infection in these patients may precipitate myasthenic crises. Furthermore, several antibiotics used for the treatment of severe sepsis as well as hydroxychloroquine which is widely used as a prophylactic and therapeutic agent in patients with COVID-19 infection can worsen myasthenic control.

Ramaswamy reported a patient with refractory myasthenia gravis on immunosuppressive therapy, who recovered without modifying the therapy after undergoing quarantine for 14 days.[30]

Delly et al. reported a patient with myasthenia gravis and connective tissue disorder presenting with fever and respiratory distress requiring intubation.

Her maintenance regimen included pyridostigmine, prednisone 20 mg a day and biweekly 650 mg/kg of IVIg for 2 days, as well as, hydroxychloroquine 200 mg twice a day for her mixed connective tissue disorder. She had never experienced severe respiratory problems needing intubation. She was initially started on a combination of vancomycin, cefepime, and azithromycin. Her PCR for COVID-19 came back positive on day 2 when her antibiotics were stopped, and hydroxychloroquine was restarted. Her prednisone was increased to 40 mg a day and IVIg to 400 mg/kg for 5 days. She was successfully extubated on day 13. Her maintenance dose of IVIg was given as her proximal weakness worsened on day 19. She was able to walk by day 25. Authors postulated cytokine dysregulation from COVID-19 along with the combination of azithromycin and hydroxychloroquine might have contributed to developing myasthenic crisis.[31]

Anand et al. reviewed five MG patients admitted with COVID-19 over 1 month. Four of them were AChR receptor antibody positive, and one had MuSK antibody. Two patients required intubation and one required supplemental oxygen. These three patients received hydroxychloroquine and azithromycin as part of the COVID-19 treatment. One of the intubated patients received tocilizumab and was successfully extubated and the other remained on mechanical ventilation. Two patients received intravenous immunoglobulin therapy (one was continued on the home IVIg regimen) without developing thromboembolic complications.[32]

International MG/COVID-19 working group consisting of experts on MG and LEMS published guidance for management of MG and LEMS patients.[33] According to the guidelines, maintenance treatment with pyridostigmine and 3,4-diaminopyridine carries no increased risk for infection. Patients already established on immunosuppressive treatments (corticosteroids, azathioprine, mycophenolate) should be continued on their medications. Targeted C5 complement inhibition with eculizumab has not been reported to increase susceptibility to COVID-19 and can be continued. Initiation of B-cell depleting treatment with rituximab should be delayed if possible, and individual risk and benefits may need to keep in mind when considering such treatment. Consideration of continuing routine surveillance of immunotherapy with blood work should also be based on local COVID-19 incidence and need for monitoring. MG patients with active COVID-19 infection may need an increase in corticosteroid dosage similar to other infections/stress steroid protocols. Standard immunosuppressive medications

(azathioprine, mycophenolate) may be continued as drug wash-out time is quite long and there is delay in building the medication effect if medication is stopped and then restarted at a later time. Immune-depleting therapies, however, should be withheld. As there is no approved treatment for COVID-19, treatment protocols must be individualized keeping in mind the potential for medication-induced MG worsening.

SKELETAL MUSCLE INJURY

Myalgia, rhabdomyolysis, and myositis have all been reported with COVID-19 infection. Generalized muscle aching, pain, and fatigue are known to be a part of a viral symptom complex. Myalgia was reported in 11%–50% of the patients in various studies.[34–36]

Mao et al. reported evidence of skeletal muscle injury with elevated CK in 10.7% of their patients.[7] COVID-19 patients with muscle injury had higher neutrophil counts, lower lymphocyte counts, higher C-reactive protein, and higher D-dimer levels regardless of the severity of the infection. The elevated D-dimer and C-reactive protein most likely indicate increased inflammatory response and coagulopathy. Multiorgan failure was also more common in patients with muscle injury. These abnormalities may be due to pro-inflammatory cytokine damage to the muscle, or from a direct invasion of skeletal muscle by COVID-19. Postmortem studies in SARS-CoV-1 infection, however, did not detect SARS-CoV-1 N-protein and RNA polymerase gene fragments in the skeletal muscle.[37]

Guan reported rhabdomyolysis in two patients and elevated CK levels in 13.7% of their series.[38] Rhabdomyolysis can be an initial presentation or a late manifestation. Suwanwongse reported an 88-year-old presenting with acute onset of bilateral lower extremity pain and weakness, with a CK of 13,581 U/L.[39] He was subsequently diagnosed with COVID-19 infection. Even though, he was treated with intravenous fluids, he developed acute renal failure on day 7 of hospitalization. CK trended down to 368 u/L with hydration over 8 days. He had been taking simvastatin for years and the report did not indicate whether simvastatin was stopped during the hospitalization.

A 38-year-old male presented with few days' history of fever, cough, and myalgias after being exposed to a coworker with COVID infection. His CK on presentation was >42,670 U/L. He felt symptomatically better with hydration despite CK remaining high and CK levels started to drop by day 7 preceded by the reduction of other inflammatory markers such as ferritin, CRP, and LDH.[40]

Jin and Tong reported a case who developed rhabdomyolysis during the course of Covid-19 infection. The patient presented with fever and respiratory symptoms initially with normal CK levels. Nine days into hospitalization, he developed lower extremity weakness and pain and was found to have markedly elevated CK, myoglobin, and LDH. Over the next few days, with treatment, his muscle pain and fatigue improved.[41]

Rhabdomyolysis associated with viral infection is more common in children but rather rare in elderly. Apart for influenza, human immunodeficiency virus (HIV), enteroviruses, Epstein-Barr virus (EBV), cytomegalovirus (CMV), adenovirus, herpes simplex virus (HSV), and varicella viruses are implicated as rare cause of viral-induced rhabdomyolysis. Immune-mediated mechanism such as cytokine storm may be contributing to rhabdomyolysis as opposed to direct viral invasion.[40–42]

Beydon reported a patient presenting with acute onset of proximal lower extremity weakness and pain and was found to have elevated CK (> 24,000 U/L).[42] Patient developed fever on day 4 and desaturated on day 7. Patient had two negative PCR for Covid-19 by nasopharyngeal swabs twice and finally tested positive on bronchial lavage on day 11 of the hospital admission. MRI showed evidence of muscle edema in external obturators and vastus medialis consistent with myositis.

SUMMARY

COVID-19 infection has been reported to be associated with neuromuscular involvement, predominantly cranial neuropathies, Guillain-Barre syndrome, and muscle involvement, which may at times, be the presenting symptom. This is similar to what has been reported with other acute viral illnesses. A few patients with known diagnosis of myasthenia gravis with COVID-19 have been reported, all of whom had variable course and outcome, and the use of hydroxychloroquine and azithromycin was not conclusively reported to be either beneficial or harmful. There have been no reports of any other preexisting neuromuscular disorder with COVID-19 infection. There is no consensus on viral-specific treatment in COVID-19 patients with neuromuscular complications. Treatment should be individualized per the neuromuscular disease-specific guidelines along with supportive care and virus-specific treatment guided by institutional recommendations.

REFERENCES

1. Peiris JSM, Yuen KY, Osterhaus ADME, Stohr K. The severe acute respiratory syndrome. *N Engl J Med.* 2003;349(25):2431–2441.
2. Romero-Sánchez CM, Díaz-Maroto I, Fernández-Díaz E, et al. Neurologic manifestations in hospitalized patients with COVID-19: the ALBACOVID registry. *Neurology.* 2020. Epub June 1.
3. Costello F, Dalakas M. Cranial neuropathies and COVID-19: neurotropism and autoimmunity. *Neurology.* 2020. https://doi.org/10.1212/WNL.0000000000009921. June 2.
4. Desforges M, Le Coupanec A, Stodola JK, Meessen-Pinard M, Talbot PJ. Human coronaviruses: viral and cellular factors involved in neuroinvasiveness and neuropathogenesis. *Virus Res.* 2014;194:145–158.
5. Fantini J, Di Scala C, Chahinian H, Yahi N. Structural and molecular modelling studies reveal a new mechanism of action of chloroquine and hydroxychloroquine against SARS-CoV-2 infection. *Int J Antimicrob Agents.* 2020;55(5):105960. https://doi.org/10.1016/j.ijantimicag.2020.105960.
6. Dalakas MC. Pathogenesis of immune-mediated neuropathies. *Biochim Biophys Acta.* 2015;1852(4):658–666.
7. Mao L, Jin H, Wang M, et al. Neurologic manifestations of hospitalized patients with coronavirus disease 2019 in Wuhan, China. *JAMA Neurol.* 2020;77(6):683–690. https://doi.org/10.1001/jamaneurol.2020.1127.
8. Spinato G, Fabbris C, Polesel J, et al. Alterations in smell or taste in mildly symptomatic outpatients with SARS-CoV-2 infection. *JAMA.* 2020. https://doi.org/10.1001/jama.2020.6771 [Published online April 22].
9. Moein ST, et al. Smell dysfunction: a biomarker for COVID19. *Int Forum Allergy Rhinol.* 2020. https://doi.org/10.1002/alr.22587 [Published online April 17].
10. Brann DH, Tsukahara T, Weinreb C, et al. Non-neural expression of SARS-CIV-2 entry genes in the olfactory epithelium suggests mechanisms underlying anosmia in COVD-19 patients. *bioRxiv.* 2020. https://doi.org/10.1101/2020.03.25.009084. Epub 09 April 2020.
11. Lechien JR, Chiesa-Estomba CM, De Siati DR, et al. Olfactory and gustatory dysfunctions as a clinical presentation of mild-to-moderate forms of the coronavirus disease (COVID-19): a multicenter European study. *Eur Arch Otorhinolaryngol.* 2020;277(8):2251–2261. https://doi.org/10.1007/s00405-020-05965-1.
12. Whitcroft KL, Hummel T. Olfactory dysfunction in COVID-19: diagnosis and management. *JAMA.* 2020;323(24):2512–2514. https://doi.org/10.1001/jama.2020.8391.
13. Eliezer M, Hamel A, Houdart E, Herman P, Housset J, et al. Loss of smell in patients with COVID-19: MRI data reveal a transient edema of the olfactory clefts. *Neurology.* 2020;95(23):e3145–e3152. https://doi.org/10.1212/WNL.0000000000010806.
14. Politi LS, Salsano E, Grimaldi M. Magnetic resonance imaging alteration of the brain in a patient with coronavirus

disease 2019 (COVID-19) and anosmia. JAMA Neurol. 2020;77(8):1028–1029. https://doi.org/10.1001/jamaneurol.2020.2125.

15. Chiu A, Fischbein N, Wintermark M, et al. COVID-19-induced anosmia associated with olfactory bulb atrophy. *Neuroradiology*. 2021;63:147–148. https://doi.org/10.1007/s00234-020-02554.

16. François J, Collery AS, Hayek G, et al. Coronavirus disease 2019–associated ocular neuropathy with panuveitis: a case report. *JAMA Ophthalmol*. 2021;139(2):247–249. https://doi.org/10.1001/jamaophthalmol.2020.5695.

17. Dinkin M, Gao V, Kahan J, et al. Covid-19 presenting with ophthalmoparesis from cranial nerve palsy. *Neurology*. 2020. https://doi.org/10.1212/WNL.0000000000009700 [Published online May 1].

18. Goh Y, Darius LL, DLL B, Makmur A, Somani J, Chan ACY. Pearls & oysters: facial nerve palsy as a neurological manifestation of Covid-19 infection. *Neurology*. 2020. https://doi.org/10.1212/WNL.0000000000009863.

19. Escalada Pellitero S, Garriga F-BL. Report of a patient with neurological symptoms as the sole manifestation of SARS-CoV-2 infection. *Neurologia*. 2020;35:271.

20. Glasmacher SA, Larraz J, Mehta AR, et al. The immediate impact of the COVID-19 pandemic on motor neuron disease services and mortality in Scotland. *J Neurol*. 2020. https://doi.org/10.1007/s00415-020-10207-9.

21. Lee S, Arcila-London X, Steijlen K, Newman D, Grover K. Case report of ALS patient with COVID-19 infection (5032). *Neurology*. 2021;96(15 Supplement):5032.

22. Miller C, O'Sullivan J, Jeffrey J, Power D. Brachial plexus neuropathies during the COVID-19 pandemic: a retrospective case series of 15 patients in critical care. *Phys Ther*. 2021;101(1). pzaa191.

23. Brugliera L, Filippi M, Del Carro U, Butera C, Bianchi F, et al. Nerve compression injuries after prolonged prone position ventilation in patients with SARS-CoV-2: a case series. *Arch Phys Med Rehabil*. 2020;102(3):359–362. https://doi.org/10.1016/j.apmr.2020.10.131. Epub ahead of print 33245939. PMC7685952.

24. Han CY, Tarr AM, Gewirtz AN, et al. Brachial plexopathy as a complication of COVID-19. *BMJ Case Rep*. 2021;14:e237459.

25. Ellul MA, Benjamin L, Singh B, et al. Neurological associations of COVID-19. *Lancet Neurol*. 2020. https://doi.org/10.1016/S1474-4422(20)30221-0.

26. Zhao H, Shen D, Zhou H, Liu J, Chen S. Guillain-Barré syndrome associated with SARS-CoV-2 infection: causality or coincidence? *Lancet Neurol*. 2020;19(5):383–384. https://doi.org/10.1016/S1474-4422(20)30109-5.

27. Gutiérrez-Ortiz C, et al. Miller Fisher syndrome and polyneuritis cranialis in COVID-19. *Neurology*. 2020. https://doi.org/10.1212/WNL.0000000000009619 87 [Published online April 17].

28. Toscano G, et al. Guillain–Barré syndrome associated with SARSCoV-2. *NEJM*. 2020. https://doi.org/10.1056/NEJMc2009191 [Published online April 17].

29. Arnaud S, et al. Post SARS-CoV-2 Guillain-Barré syndrome. *Clin Neurophysiol*. 2020;131(7):1652–1654. https://doi.org/10.1016/j.clinph.2020.05.003.

30. Ramaswamy SB, Govindarajan R. COVID-19 in refractory myasthenia Gravis—a case report of successful outcome. *J Neuromuscul Dis*. 2020;7(3):361–364. https://doi.org/10.3233/JND-200520.

31. Delly F, Syed MJ, Lisak RP, Deepti ZD. Myasthenic crisis in COVID-19. *J Neurol Sci*. 2020;414:116888.

32. Anand P, Slama MCC, Kaku M, et al. COVID-19 in patients with myasthenia gravis. *Muscle Nerve*. 2020;1–5. https://doi.org/10.1002/mus.26918.

33. International MG/COVID-19 Working Group, Jacob S, Muppidi S, Guidon A, et al. Guidance for the management of myasthenia gravis (MG) and Lambert-Eaton myasthenic syndrome (LEMS) during the COVID-19 pandemic. *J Neurol Sci*. 2020;412:116803. https://doi.org/10.1016/j.jns.2020.116803.

34. Wang D, Hu B, Hu C, et al. Clinical characteristics of 138 hospitalized patients with 2019 novel coronavirus-infected pneumonia in Wuhan, China. *JAMA*. 2020. https://doi.org/10.1001/jama.2020.1585.

35. Huang C, Wang Y, Li X, et al. Clinical features of patients infected with 2019 novel coronavirus in Wuhan, China. *Lancet*. 2020;395:497–506.

36. Chen N, Zhou M, Dong X, et al. Epidemiological and clinical characteristics of 99 cases of 2019 novel coronavirus pneumonia in Wuhan, China: a descriptive study. *Lancet*. 2020;395:507–513.

37. Ding Y, He L, Zhang Q, et al. Organ distribution of severe acute respiratory syndrome (SARS) associated coronavirus (SARS-CoV) in SARS patients: implications for pathogenesis and virus transmission pathways. *J Pathol*. 2004;203(2):622–630.

38. Guan W, Ni Z, Hu Y, et al. Clinical characteristics of coronavirus disease 2019 in China. *N Engl J Med*. 2020;382:1708–1720.

39. Suwanwongse K, Shabarek N. Rhabdomyolysis as a presentation of 2019 novel coronavirus disease. *Cureus*. 2020;12(4):e7561. https://doi.org/10.7759/cureus.7561.

40. Zhang Q, Shan KS, Minalyam A, O'Sullivan C, Nace T. A rare presentation of coronavirus disease 2019 (COVID-19) induced viral myositis with subsequent rhabdomyolysis. *Cureus*. 2020;12(5):e8074. https://doi.org/10.7759/cureus.8074.

41. Jin M, Tong Q. Rhabdomyolysis as potential late complication associated with COVID-19. *Emerg Infect Dis*. 2020. https://doi.org/10.3201/eid2607.200445. July.

42. Beydon M, Chevalier K, Al Tabaa O, et al. *Ann Rheum Dis*. 2020;1–2. https://doi.org/10.1136/annrheumdis-2020-217573.

CHAPTER 8

Pediatric Neurology and the COVID-19 Pandemic

GHADA A. MOHAMED[a] • JULES E.C. CONSTANTINOU[a,b]
[a]Department of Neurology, Henry Ford Health System, Detroit, MI, United States, [b]Wayne State University School of Medicine, Detroit, MI, United States

INTRODUCTION: THE REDUCED BURDEN OF COVID-19 ON CHILDHOOD

Because children with COVID-19 are often asymptomatic or exhibit respiratory illness of only mild-to-moderate degree, the extent of disease in childhood is difficult to define with accuracy.[1]

In reports skewed toward hospitalized and severely ill individuals from China, Italy, Spain, and the United States, children are found to comprise only 1%–2% of COVID-19 cases.[2–5] On the other hand, children constitute up to 5%–13.7% of cases in Korea, Iceland, and Canada where broad population-based screening has been carried out.[6–8]

Although it is uncertain why COVID-19 runs a mild course in most children, it is hypothesized that children may have higher antibody levels because of their frequent exposure to respiratory illnesses and that the pediatric immune system may respond differently to the virus.[9] In children, reduced expression and binding ability of the ACE2 receptor, which negotiates entry of SARS-CoV-2 into human cells, may play a role in the attenuated vulnerability of children to severe infection.

In a series of 2143 Chinese pediatric cases, symptoms were mild in 50.9%, moderate in 38.8%, and 4.2% were asymptomatic.[9] Severe disease was noted in only 2% of children and only 0.6% developed acute respiratory distress syndrome and multiorgan failure. This rate of critical illness was significantly lower than the 18.5% rate reported in adults.[10]

In a descriptive study of 130 children from 28 hospitals in Italy, 75.4% had asymptomatic or mild disease.[11] In all, 11.5% needed respiratory support and 6.9% were treated in an intensive care unit. There were no deaths. Of 57 children identified in a large community-based hospital system in the first 5 weeks of the Houston pandemic, the majority had the mild illness. Hospital admission was necessary for 14%.[12]

A 25 country European multicenter cohort study of 582 children with COVID-19 reiterated that COVID-19 is generally a mild disease in children and infants.[13] Only a small proportion of children required admission to ICU (8%) or mechanical ventilation (4%). Only 3% required inotropic support and only one child (<1%) necessitated extracorporeal membrane oxygenation (ECMO). Four children died (case fatality rate of 0.69%). The remaining 578 were alive and only 4% of them were still symptomatic or requiring some kind of respiratory support.

In a cross-sectional report of the clinical course of critically ill infants and children with COVID-19 at 46 pediatric hospitals in North America between March 14 and April 3, 2020, it was remarkable that only 35% of the hospitals participating in the study reported admissions of children with COVID-19 infection to the PICU.[14] Of the 48 children in this series, 38% required invasive ventilation, and all but two survived, reflecting the markedly decreased burden of disease from COVID-19 on children.

COVID-19 IN THE FETUS AND NEWBORN

COVID-19 may also affect the fetus and the newborn. A review of nine case series and two case reports from Wuhan described outcomes of maternal COVID-19 infection during pregnancy in 65 women and 67 neonates.[15] Two mothers (3%) were admitted to the ICU. Fetal distress was reported in 30% of pregnancies. Preterm birth occurred in 37% of the women. Neonatal complications included respiratory distress or pneumonia (18%), disseminated intravascular coagulation (3%), asphyxia (2%), and two perinatal deaths. Stringent measures to prevent transmission during delivery and separation of mother and child did not prevent infection in four neonates (three with pneumonia), suggesting the possibility of vertical transmission.

Neurological Care and the COVID-19 Pandemic. https://doi.org/10.1016/B978-0-323-82691-4.00001-7

RISK FACTORS FOR SEVERE DISEASE

Presenting symptoms of COVID-19 in childhood include cough (48%), fever (47%), and sore throat or pharyngitis (28.6%).[16] Other respiratory symptoms such as rhinorrhea, sneezing, and nasal congestion are less common. Vomiting or nausea occurs in 7.8% of cases and diarrhea in 10.1%.

Infants and preschool children are more likely to exhibit severe disease.[9] In a systematic review of the literature, 27% of children hospitalized because of COVID-19 were under 1 year of age.[16] As in adults, comorbidities such as chronic lung disease (asthma), cardiovascular disease, and immunosuppression may predispose to severe illness. In a CDC report, 28 of 37 (77%) hospitalized children had one or more underlying conditions.[5] In a multicenter cohort study from Europe, neurological comorbidities were noted in 26 among 582 children, nine of whom had epilepsy and eight had cerebral palsy. Ten other children had chromosomal abnormalities, eight of whom with trisomy 21.[13]

SEVERE MULTISYSTEM INFLAMMATORY SYNDROME

In reports from the UK, Italy, and the United States, COVID-19 has been linked to a severe multisystem inflammatory syndrome with mixed features of Kawasaki disease and toxic shock syndrome. A postinfectious mechanism is hypothesized given that cases cluster 3–4 weeks after the peak of community spread and that respiratory symptoms are not conspicuous.[17] Patients are often SARS-CoV-2 seropositive but PCR negative.

Symptoms include a persistent fever above 39 °C, nonpurulent conjunctivitis, dry cracked lips, rash, and edema of the hands and feet, and cervical lymphadenopathy.[18] Inflammatory markers including CRP, ferritin, and cytokines (IL-1, IL-6, and TNF alpha) are markedly elevated. In all, 50%–70% of the children require ICU admission mainly for cardiovascular insufficiency. Left ventricular ejection fraction is reduced and there are coronary artery abnormalities particularly ectatic dilated arteries.[19]

NEUROLOGIC COMPLICATIONS OF PEDIATRIC COVID-19

Neurological manifestations are an important component of the multiorgan involvement of COVID-19. In a seminal report from Wuhan, 36.4% of hospitalized patients with severe acute respiratory distress syndrome (ARDS) exhibited central nervous system involvement.[20] CNS disease may present with encephalopathy, encephalitis, meningitis, acute ischemic and hemorrhagic cerebrovascular disease, venous sinus thrombosis, and acute disseminated encephalomyelitis.[21, 22] Muscle disorders, Guillain-Barre, and Miller Fisher syndromes reflect peripheral nervous system involvement.

As discussed in Chapter 2, mechanisms of neural damage may include direct infection of the nervous system through hematogenous or retrograde neuronal routes, virus-mediated hyperinflammatory or hypercoagulable states, and postinfectious immune-mediated means.[21, 22] Impairment of taste and smell affects between 30% and 80% of adults with COVID-19,[21] likely through invasion of the neuro-olfactory epithelium.[23]

Despite the growing body of evidence in the predominantly adult literature, the prevalence of neurologic symptoms in children with COVID-19 is uncertain. Reports of anosmia or dysgeusia in children are scant, possibly because younger children may have difficulty elaborating on these symptoms.

An online survey of 212 child neurologists from 49 countries documented caring for 160 children without preexisting epilepsy who presented with COVID-19.[24] Seventeen of these children (10.6%) were reported to have acute symptomatic or febrile seizures. Encephalopathy was present in 7 (4.4%), while another 7 (4.4%) had other neurologic symptoms (headache, weakness, and muscle pain). Seven children (4.4%) had anosmia.

A few case reports detail the nervous system involvement which may be a feature of pediatric COVID-19. For instance, a 6-week-old term infant with symptoms of fever and cough presented with two seizure-like episodes consisting of altered responsiveness, sustained upgaze, and dystonic extension of the legs lasting 10–15 s.[25] EEG showed an excess of left temporal sharp waves but representative episodes were not captured so that the diagnosis of seizures could not be confirmed. A lumbar puncture showed an unremarkable CSF profile. Nasopharyngeal swab was positive for SARS-CoV-2 RNA and rhinovirus C and a note was made that coinfection is common in infants. SARS-CoV-2 RNA was not detected in blood or CSF and the baby made a quick recovery.

A case of encephalitis was reported in an 11-year-old boy with no respiratory symptoms. The symptomatology was dominated by fever, weakness, and status epilepticus requiring four anticonvulsant medications.[26] CSF evaluation showed mild pleocytosis with a normal protein and glucose. Nasopharyngeal swab was positive for COVID-19 as well as rhinovirus/enterovirus, but absent in cerebrospinal fluid. The child recovered without treatment in 6 days. Direct brain infection by the virus was proposed.

Ischemic stroke was described in a 12-year-old boy presenting with seizures, right-sided hemiparesis, and ataxia.[27] Fever and respiratory symptoms were not evident. SARS-CoV-2 RNA was detected in the nasopharynx and the CSF. MRI showed acute infarction affecting the left basal ganglia and the insula without microhemorrhages. Focal irregular narrowing and banding of the M1 segment of the left middle cerebral artery (MCA) were ascribed to a focal cerebral arteriopathy.

Neurological complications in severe forms of COVID-19 were outlined in a case series of 27 severely affected children from an ICU in Paris.[28] All the children exhibited acute organ dysfunction and/or respiratory distress. Preexisting neurological conditions like epileptic encephalopathy, genetic, or metabolic disorders were noted in seven patients. One 16-year-old boy without preexisting conditions or respiratory symptoms presented with aseptic meningitis associated with a Glasgow coma scale score of 11. Sphenoidal sinusitis and cavernous sinus thrombosis were noted on MRI. MCA stroke occurred on day 4, followed on day 7 by the development of severe coma as a result of progressive and fatal intracranial hypertension associated with progressive stenosis of the cerebral vasculature and ischemia. The time course of the illness suggested SARS-CoV2-mediated inflammatory injury to the cerebral vessels. Another 6-year-old girl required ECMO because of necrotizing pneumonia, refractory hypoxemia, and pericarditis. Acute neurological deterioration and brain death related to massive brain hemorrhage occurred on day 14.

NEUROLOGICAL COMPLICATIONS OF SEVERE MULTISYSTEM INFLAMMATORY SYNDROME

Neurological features, although not typical, have also been described in children with the severe multisystem inflammatory syndrome. In the Italian experience of 16 patients, signs included headaches (6/16), aseptic meningitis (3/16), and anosmia (1/16).[17]

A report from New York City draws attention to major neurologic disease in 2 of 145 suspected cases of pediatric multisystem inflammatory syndrome.[29] A 5-year-old boy presented with several days of fever, cough, and abdominal pain. He tested positive for COVID-19 antibodies and IL-6 levels were high. ECMO became necessary because of cardiopulmonary failure. After 5 days, the pupils became fixed and dilated

and brainstem reflexes were absent. CT scan showed brain edema, right MCA infarction, and contralateral subarachnoid hemorrhage. Brain death was confirmed 3 days later. The second patient was a 2-month-old boy who was placed on ECMO because of progressive respiratory failure after 8 days. Despite the clinical picture and high IL-6 antibodies, he tested negative for antibodies to COVID-19. Nonconvulsive status epilepticus, requiring 4 antiseizure medications, was noted on continuous EEG. An early CT scan showed bilateral MCA and posterior cerebral artery infarcts with hemorrhagic transformation. Poor seizure control continued for several weeks and interval MRI identified evolving hemorrhagic infarctions in the bilateral parieto-occipital lobes, left temporal and left frontal lobes, and stable bilateral subdural collections believed to be cardioembolic in origin. Sepsis-induced coagulopathy was thought to contribute to cerebrovascular disease.

IMPLICATIONS OF THE PANDEMIC FOR DELIVERY OF HEALTH CARE

The pandemic carries broad implications in terms of the delivery of health care to all children and especially those with acute or chronic neurological disorders. Access to in-person care, ancillary services, and therapies has been limited because of community mitigation strategies including quarantine and stay-at-home orders and because of restrictions to clinic visits and hospitalizations in order to minimize exposure. Treatment schedules for the administration of intravenous immunoglobulin, alglucosidase alpha (Pompe's disease), rituximab, and nusinersen (spinal muscular atrophy), and for neurostimulation procedures may be disturbed. Speech and physical therapies, and specialized behavioral interventions such as applied behavior analysis (ABA) for children with autism, have been directly impacted by the pandemic.

The worldwide survey of 212 child neurologists described above highlighted dramatic changes to pediatric epilepsy care with 91.5% reporting changes to outpatient care and 90.6% reduced access to EEG, 37.5% altered management of infantile spasms, 92.3% restrictions to initiation of the ketogenic diet, and 93.4% closed or reduced epilepsy monitoring units and availability of epilepsy surgery.[24] Care was provided exclusively by telemedicine by 24.7% of neurologists.

In a survey of 277 Spanish caregivers of children with epileptic encephalopathies including SCN1A, CDKL5, KCNQ2, and other disorders, increased seizure frequency was noted in 39 children (14%) and behavioral deterioration in 87 (30.3%).[30] There was one case of status epilepticus and nine patients who regressed developmentally. Factors that contributed to the declines were inability to reach the neurologist through telemedicine (62.8%), avoidance of emergency care owing to fear of COVID-19 (20.6%), anxiety or depression in the caregivers (68.7%), and loss of regular stimulation and physical therapies (51.8%).

Barriers to health-care delivery, whether inpatient or ambulatory, imposed by COVID-19 public health measures to contain the infection, have tangible untoward effects on the neurodevelopment of children affected by chronic neurological disorders, the full extent of which cannot be gauged at this time.

TELEMEDICINE/TELEHEALTH IN THE PANDEMIC

Increased utilization of telemedicine has become a necessary aspect of care during the pandemic. Effective programs have been described in the management of pediatric epilepsy and neurodevelopmental disabilities.[31] Toddlers and young children who, by nature, struggle with the demands of the formal neurological examination and in whom much of the clinical impression rests on visual observation are well adapted to video evaluation.[32] There is an opportunity to watch the child's verbal and nonverbal interactions, social play, and fine and gross motor movement patterns.

Subspecialties such as headache and movement disorders are also a good match for telemedicine. Telehealth can establish a multidisciplinary therapeutic alliance, assure continuity of care, and address aspects of the care of cerebral palsy such as managing medications and providing exercises in home environments, with increased participation of patients and families.[33] The ketogenic diet has been successfully initiated and maintained through telehealth.[34] Disadvantages of pediatric telemedicine, however, are not negligible and include the inability to measure head circumference, perform fundoscopy, and evaluate tone and reflexes.

The influence of telehealth on difficult discussions like new diagnoses and SUDEP is uncertain.[24] The demand for telehealth is likely to continue beyond the pandemic and there will be a need for vigilance to assure access to all and to minimize health-care disparities. It is important that neurology practitioners are educated in best practices for the delivery of resources.[35]

CRISIS STANDARDS FOR THE DELIVERY OF PEDIATRIC NEUROLOGICAL CARE

Crisis standards for the provision of care are beginning to emerge especially in the disciplines of pediatric

epilepsy and of pediatric neuromuscular disorders. Recommendations for the treatment of infantile spasms (IS) were released by the Child Neurology Society on April 6, 2020.[36,37] Enduring recommendations are considered to survive beyond the pandemic and include the performance of an initial visit for suspected IS by telemedicine.[36,37] Parents should provide videos of several consecutive habitual episodes. The skin must be examined for depigmented patches. EEG confirmation of the diagnosis with the capture of at least one sleep–wake cycle is strongly advised. MRI should be obtained if causation is uncertain to look at possibilities in relation to tuberous sclerosis (TS) or a structural brain anomaly. Limited recommendations which apply only through the duration of the pandemic favor outpatient EEG and treatment. Except in TS in which vigabatrin is the treatment of choice, treatment with high-dose prednisone (4–8 mg/kg/day), possibly more effective than lower dose prednisone, may avoid the complexities of treatment with ACTH. Weekly follow-up telehealth visits should be conducted.

A consensus statement addressing the care of spinal muscular atrophy (SMA) patients emphasizes that molecular treatments for SMA should not be considered elective.[38] Decisions about potential delays should balance the potential risks of COVID-19 exposure and the risks of treatment delays. Missed doses of nusinersen should be given as soon as possible to maximize therapeutic benefit. Requirements for laboratory monitoring for liver function abnormalities, elevated troponin, and thrombocytopenia after gene transfer therapy can be addressed with home blood draws. Insurance requirements for in-person physical therapy evaluations to monitor the effectiveness of treatment should be waived in favor of telehealth evaluation.

Steroids and other immunotherapies should be continued in children with neuromuscular disorders such as SMA, Duchenne muscular dystrophy, inflammatory myopathy, and myasthenia gravis.[39] Steroids should not be stopped if the child contracts COVID-19 and stress doses of steroids are advised.

Children receiving steroids, everolimus, and other immunotherapies are at high risk for the development of COVID-19 complications. Patients and their families should strictly adhere to recommendations in place for isolation, social distancing, the wearing of masks, and handwashing.[38,39] Special attention to these measures is also advised for those with neurologically based cardio-respiratory compromise and/or severe kyphoscoliosis.

Children with chronic neuromuscular disorders and COVID-19 should not be denied access to critical care.[40] The long-term outcome is more favorable than previously understood given improvements in multidisciplinary comprehensive care and new molecular therapies which change the outlook of the disease. Transparency and accessibility are keystone of triage pathways which foster the fair distribution of hospital and home-based services.

Targeted therapies used in critically ill children with COVID-19, most commonly include hydroxychloroquine, singly or in combination, azithromycin, remdesivir, tocilizumab, and occasionally steroids and intravenous immunoglobulin or convalescent plasma.[13, 14] Hydroxychloroquine and azithromycin which may affect transmission at the neuromuscular junction should be used cautiously in children with myasthenia.[39] Antiseizure medications such as phenobarbital, phenytoin, fosphenytoin, carbamazepine, eslicarbazepine, and rufinamide may reduce remdesivir levels through induction of CYP3A4. Prone positioning for severe respiratory distress may not be feasible in children with cerebral palsy or severe neuromuscular disorders.

ACADEMIC, SOCIAL, AND PSYCHOLOGICAL ASPECTS

The academic, social, and psychological burden of the pandemic on children and their families are considerable. Separation from friends and extended family, isolation at home, school closures, reduced access to teachers, school curricula and exercise, and illness of family and friends result in a psychological toll.[41] An increase in children and adolescents of clingy behavior, worry, irritability, with fear of asking questions, fatigue, sleep and appetite disturbances, distractibility, and inattention was documented by a symptom checklist in Shaanxi province at the height of the China pandemic.[42] Our clinic experience would suggest that children with background neurodevelopmental disorders such as autistic spectrum disorder and ADHD might be more vulnerable to heightened symptoms of anxiety and depression and increased behavioral dysregulation during the pandemic, but we are not able to find corroborative studies in the literature. Escalation of behaviors has been demonstrated in children with cerebral palsy, even though improved participation and equality can develop within the household in others.[33] Children may benefit from dialogue and discussion, collaborative games to address loneliness, exercise, and the modeling by parents of a positive mindset.[42]

SUMMARY

Neurologic expressions of severe pediatric COVID-19 include headache, weakness, muscle pain, acute symptomatic seizures, anosmia, aseptic meningitis, encephalitis, encephalopathy, ischemic, and hemorrhagic stroke. Telemedicine or telehealth is proving effective in addressing the care gap for children with acute or chronological disorders during the pandemic and beyond. Crisis standards for best practice care have been developed in infantile spasms and in pediatric neuromuscular disorders. The considerable scholastic and psychological burden of the pandemic on children and their families should be recognized by the pediatric neurologist.

REFERENCES

1. Rajapske K, Dixit D. Human and novel coronavirus infections in children: a review. *Paediatr Int Child Health.* 2020;382:2302–2315. NEJMoa2006100.2020 https://doi.org/10.1080/20469047.2020.1781356.
2. Zhu N, Zhang D, Wang W. A novel coronavirus from patients with pneumonia in China. *NEJM.* 2019;382:270–273.
3. Livingston E, Bucher K. Coronavirus disease in Italy. *JAMA.* 2020. Available from https://jamanetwork.com/journals/jama/fullarticle/2763401.
4. Tagarro A, Epalza C, Santos M. Screening and severity of coronavirus disease 2019 (COVID-19) in children in Madrid, Spain [manuscript published ahead of print 8 April 2020]. *JAMA Pediatr.* 2020. https://doi.org/10.1001/jamapediatrics.2020.13.
5. Centers for Disease Control and Prevention. Coronavirus disease 2019 in children-United States, February 12–April 2, 2020. *Morb Mortal Wkly Rep.* 2020;69:422–426. Available from: https://www.cdc.gov/mmwr/volumes/69/wr/mm6914e4.htm.
6. Shim E, Tariq A, Choi W, et al. Transmission potential and severity of COVID-19 in South Korea. *Int J Infect Dis.* 2020;93:339–344.
7. Gudbjartsson DF, Helgason A, Jonsson H, et al. Spread of SARS-CoV-2 in the icelandic population. *N Engl J Med.* 2020;382:2302–2315. NEJMoa2006100.
8. COVID-19 Alberta statistics. [cited 2020 May 25]. Available from: https://www.alberta.ca/stats/covid-19-alberta-statistics.htm.
9. Dong Y, Mo X, Hu Y. Epidemiological characteristics of 2143 pediatric patient with 2019 coronavirus disease in China. *Pediatrics.* 2020;1(45):1–10. https://aapublications.org/content/pediatrics/145/6/e20200702.full.pdf.
10. Wu Z, JM MG. Characteristics of and important lessons from the coronavirus 2019 (COVID-19) outbreak in China: summary of a report of 72,314 cases from the Chinese Center for Disease Control and Prevention. *JAMA.* 2020;323:1239. [cited 2020 Mar 21]. Available from: https://jamanetwork.com/journals/jama/fullarticle/2762130.
11. Parri N, Magista A, Marchetti F, et al. Characteristics of COVID-19 infection in pediatric patients: early findings from two Italian pediatric research networks. *Eur J Pediatr.* 2020 Jun;3:1–9. https://doi.org/10.1007/s00431-020-03683-8.

12. Ce F, Moulton EA, Munoz FM, et al. Coronavirus disease in children cared for at Texas Children's Hospital: initial clinical characteristics and outcome. *J Pediatr Infect Dis Soc.* 2020;1–5.

13. Gotzinger F, Santiago-Garcia B, Noguera-Julian A, et al. COVID-19 in children and adolescents in Europe: a multinational, multicenter cohort study. *Lancet Child Adolesc Health.* 2020. https://doi.org/10.1016/S2352-4642(20)30177-2. S2352-4642(20)30177-2.

14. Shekerdemian LS, Mahmood NR, Wolfe KW, et al. Characteristics and outcomes of children with coronavirus disease 2019 (COVID-19) infection admitted to US and Canadian pediatric intensive care units. *JAMA Pediatr.* 2020. https://doi.org/10.1001/jamapediatrics.2020.1948.

15. Zimmermann P, Curtis N. COVID-19 in children, pregnancy and neonates: a review of epidemiologic and clinical features. *Pediatr Infect Dis J.* 2020 June;39(6):469–477. https://doi.org/10.1097/INF.0000000000002700.

16. Patel NE. Pediatric COVID-19: Systematic review of the literature. *Am J Otolaryngol.* 2020. https://doi.org/10.1016/j.amjoto.2020.102573.

17. Verdoni L, Mazza A, Gervasoni A, et al. An outbreak of severe Kawasaki-like disease at the Italian epicenter of the SARS-CoV-2 epidemic-an observational cohort study. *Lancet.* 2020;395:1771–1778. https://doi.org/10.1016/S0140-6736(20)31103-X.o.

18. Pouletty M, Borocco C, Ouldali N, et al. Pediatric multisystem inflammatory syndrome temporally associated with SARS-CoV2 mimicking Kawasaki disease (Kawa-COVID-19): a multicenter cohort. *Ann Rheum Dis.* 2020;1–8. https://doi.org/10.1136/annrheumdis-2020-217960.

19. Ramcharan T, Nolan O, Lai CY, et al. Pediatric multisystem syndrome: temporally associated with SARS-CoV-2 (PIMS-TS) and short-term outcomes at a UK Tertiary Pediatric Hospital. *Pediatr Cardiol.* 2020. https://doi.org/10.1007/s00246-020-02391-2.

20. Mao L, Jin H, Wang M, et al. Neurologic manifestations of hospitalized patients with coronavirus disease 2019 in Wuhan, China. *JAMA Neurol.* 2020;77(6):1–9. https://doi.org/10.1001/jmaneurol.2020.1127.

21. Wang L, Shen Y, Li M, et al. Clinical manifestations and evidence of neurological involvement in 2019 novel coronavirus SAR-COV-2: a systematic review and meta-analysis. *J Neurol.* 2020;1–13. https://doi.org/10.1007/s00415-020-09974-2.

22. Kovalnik IJ, Tyler KL. COVID-19: a global threat to the nervous system. *Ann Neurol.* 2020;88:1–11. https://doi.org/10.1002/ana.25807.

23. Eliezer M, Hautefort C, Hamel AL, et al. Sudden and complete olfactory loss function as a possible symptom of COVID-19. *JAMA Otolaryngol Head Neck Surg.* 2020. https://doi.org/10.1001/jamaoto.2020.0832.

24. Wirrell EC, Grinspan ZM, Knupp K, et al. Care delivery for children with epilepsy during the COVID-19 pandemic: an international survey of clinicians. *J Child Neurol.* 2020 Jul 15. https://doi.org/10.1177/0883073820940189, 883073820940189.

25. Dugue R, Cay-Martinez K, Thakur KT, et al. Neurologic manifestations in an infant with COVID-19. *Neurology.* 2020;94:1–3. https://doi.org/10.1212/WNL.0000000000009653.

26. McAbee GN, Brosgol Y, Pavlakis M, et al. Encephalitis associated with COVID-19 infection in an 11-year-old child. *Pediatr Neurol.* 2020 Apr;24. https://doi.org/10.1016/j.pediatrneurol.2020.04.013. S0887-8994(20)30143-0.

27. Mirzaee SMM, Goncalves FG, Mohammadifard M, et al. Focal cerebral arteriopathy in a COVID-19 pediatric patient. *Radiology.* 2020 Jun;2:202197. https://doi.org/10.1148/radiol.2020202197.

28. Oualha M, Bedavid M, Berteloot L, et al. Severe and fatal forms of COVID-19 in children. *Arch Pediatr.* 2020 Jul;27(5):235–238. https://doi.org/10.1016/j.arcped.2020.05.010.

29. Schupper AJ, Yaeger KA, Morgenstern PF. Neurological manifestations of pediatric multi-system inflammatory syndrome potentially associated with COVID-19. *Childs Nerv Syst.* 2020;36(8):1579–1580. https://doi.org/10.1007/s00381-020-04755-8.

30. Aledo-Serrano A, Mingorance A, Jimenez-Huete A, et al. Genetic epilepsies and COVID-19 pandemic: lessons from the caregiver perspective. *Epilepsia.* 2020 Jun;61(6):1312–1314. https://doi.org/10.1111/epi.16537 [Epub 2020 May 18].

31. Lo MD, Gospe SM. Telemedicine and child neurology. *J Child Neurol.* 2019;34(1):22–26. https://doi.org/10.1177/0883073818807516.

32. Joshi C. Telemedicine in pediatric neurology. *Pediatr Neurol.* 2014;51:189–191.

33. Ben-Pazi H, Beni-Adani L, Lamdan R. Accelerating telemedicine for cerebral palsy during the COVID-19 pandemic and beyond. *Front Neurol.* 2020;11:746–749. https://doi.org/10.3389/fneurol.2020.00746.

34. Kossoff EH, Turner Z, Adams J, et al. Ketogenic diet therapy provision in the COVID-19 pandemic: dual center experience and recommendations. *Epilepsy Behav.* 2020;111:107181. https://doi.org/10.1016/j.yebeh.2020.107181.

35. Govindarajan R, Anderson ER, Hesselbrock RR, et al. Developing an outline for teleneurology curriculum: AAN telemedicine work group recommendations. *Neurology.* 2017;89(9):951–959.

36. Grinspan ZM, Mytinger JR, Baumer FM, et al, On behalf of the Child Neurology Society (Practice Committee and Executive Board) and the Pediatric Epilepsy Research Committee (Infantile Spasms Interest Group and Steering Committee). *J Child Neurol.* 2020. https://doi.org/10.1177/0883073820933739, 883073820933739.

37. Grinspan ZM, Mytinger JR, Baumer FM, et al, On behalf of the Child Neurology Society (Practice Committee and Executive Board) and the Pediatric Epilepsy Research Committee (Infantile Spasms Interest Group and Steering Committee). Crisis standard of care: management of infantile spasms during COVID-19. *Ann Neurol.* 2020. https://doi.org/10.1002/ana.25792.

38. Veerapandiyan A, Connolly A, Finkel RS, et al. Spinal muscular atrophy care in the COVID-19 pandemic era. *Muscle Nerve.* 2020 Jul;62(1):46–49. https://doi.org/10.1002/mus26903.Epub2020 May3.

39. Panda PK, Sharawat IK. COVID-19(SARS-CoV2 infection) and children: pediatric neurologist's perspective. *Indian J Pediatr.* July 2020;87(7):556–557.

40. Laventhal NT, Graham RJ, Rasmussen S, et al. Ethical decision-making for children with neuromuscular disorders in the COVID-19 crisis. *Neurology.* 2020. 10.121/WNL.0000000000009936.

41. Condie LO. Neurotropic mechanisms in COVID-19 and their potential influence on neuropsychological outcomes in children. *Child Neuropsychol.* 2020;26(5):577–596. https://doi.org/10.1080/09297049.2020.1763938.

42. Jiao WY, Wang LN, Liu J, et al. Behavioral and emotional disorders in children during the COVID-19 epidemic. *J Pediatr.* 2020;221:264–266.e1. https://doi.org/10.1016/j.jpeds.2020.03.013.

CHAPTER 9

Neuro-Oncologic Care During the COVID-19 Pandemic

JAMES M. SNYDER[a,b] • MOHAMMED F. REHMAN[a]
[a]Departments of Neurology and Neurosurgery, Henry Ford Hospital, Detroit, MI, United States,
[b]Hermelin Brain Tumor Center, Henry Ford Hospital, Detroit, MI, United States

INTRODUCTION

Neuro-oncology is a multidisciplinary specialty dedicated to caring for those faced with neoplasms in the nervous system. Neuro-oncologists are often fellowship-trained neurologists or medical oncologists. The bulk of care is directed at primary brain tumors of which the majority have no cure and limited effective treatments, metastatic cancer to the brain and spine, central nervous system (CNS) lymphoma, and complications of cancer or cancer treatment such as paraneoplastic syndromes and drug toxicities. Neuro-oncologists manage patients with primary CNS tumors from suspicion of diagnosis through end-of-life to survivorship. Neuro-oncologic care requires a coordinated effort by neurosurgeons, oncologists, radiation oncologists, neurologists, nurses, supportive services, and others. As COVID-19 takes the health-care system hostage, those faced with cancer are left with deviations in care and a greater need for supportive services while providers strive to maintain clinical operations in a time of previously unforeseen hazards and limited resources. Health-care providers, patients, and caregivers are scrambling to redesign health services during the pandemic resulting in new paradigms and opportunities to improve such as dependence on video visits from home upending traditional access to care barriers (yet introducing new barriers), decentralized access to specialized resources through isolated non-COVID-19 health centers, and reliance on subspecialty clinics to reduce emergency room and intensive care unit (ICU) utilization.

The risks of COVID-19 in vulnerable neuro-oncologic populations necessitate a balancing act of resource restrictions, mitigation of COVID-19 risks to patients and providers through the lens that every health-care contact is an infection risk, observation of altered therapy-related comorbidities, and potential undertreatment of incurable and devastating diseases.[1,2] If at all possible, standard of care (SOC) guidelines should be followed; however, this may not be feasible during a pandemic. Neuro-oncologists have an additional responsibility to advocate within the health system for prioritization of resources including ICU beds and operating room access for this population with the largely incurable disease but also tremendous variability in outcomes that may result in many years of high-quality life with appropriate interventions.[1]

Oncologic care reorganization is a dynamic and evolving process dictated by local circumstances. Treatment plans may be altered to reduce exposure to COVID-19 environments, de-escalate dependence on hospital resources, and prevent anticipated complications of anticancer therapy in the setting of potential COVID-19 infection.[3] In health systems that have multiple hospitals or regional federations of hospitals isolating non-COVID-19 cancer services to dedicated centers may reduce exposure. Our core neuro-oncologic services are anchored at the quaternary hospital with radiologic imaging, multidisciplinary subspecialty clinics, supportive services, and clinical trial staff in one location to facilitate an efficient patient experience. As hospital resources shifted toward COVID-19 management we decentralized operations. Clinical trial and routine oncologic care were provided at a smaller non-COVID-19 satellite center, video visits for nonessential care were used, we redesigned clinical trial protocols to maximize safety, and we obtained MRI imaging at a satellite center distant from COVID-19 caring facilities which reduced patient exposure. Neuro-oncology teams are typically small and may have only one or two providers within each subspecialty in a hospital or geographic region, thus efforts to limit exposure among the care team are also necessary to ensure the preservation of the program.[1]

Neurological Care and the COVID-19 Pandemic. https://doi.org/10.1016/B978-0-323-82691-4.00004-2

Brain tumors and CNS metastatic cancer have always been emotionally isolating conditions due to disease sequelae and social stigma but in the COVID-19 world where patients are undergoing brain surgery, chemotherapy, and treatment in isolation from family and friends—feelings of isolation and despair have increased.[4, 5] Behavioral health and supportive oncological resources for patients and caregivers need to be escalated and distance-based solutions such as virtual platforms of communication must be utilized. Caregivers for those faced with a neuro-oncologic condition are caring for someone with possible cancer, neurologic deficits that limit mobility or communication, executive function impairments, socioeconomic stressors, and mental health concerns.[6, 7] Increasing burden is placed on caregivers during COVID-19 due to social distancing practices, escalated emotional stressors, and fear of virus exposure that limits engagement with home care providers, therapists, and social support services. Clinicians should screen for caregiver health and provide resources to address emotional support and other caregiver needs.[8]

Anticipated risks between COVID-19 and disease-modifying agents such as immunotherapies and chemotherapies need to be factored into treatment recommendations. There is a void of high-level evidence for direction; however, international consensus recommendations are available in neuro-oncology to provide guidance. Adjustment toward less toxic therapies and reduced hospital exposures are common recommendations.[1-3] Alkylating chemotherapy with temozolomide (TMZ) or lomustine is SOC treatments for many primary brain tumors that often cause lymphopenia. In the general population, lymphopenia has been used to predict the severity of COVID-19 outcomes.[9] The relationship between chemotherapy-induced lymphopenia, brain tumors, and COVID-19 infection outcomes has yet to be elucidated. Immunotherapy agents that manipulate the immune system as a disease treatment are commonly used in solid tumors that are metastatic to the brain (melanoma, non-small cell lung cancer, renal carcinoma, others) and represent an active area for primary brain tumor clinical trials. Severe cases of COVID-19 are marked by a hyperinflammatory immune response and complications of immune-related adverse events, therefore agents such as checkpoint inhibitors that carry a rare risk of immune-related adverse events such as pneumonitis, or agents disrupting cytotoxic lymphocytes and natural killer cells which facilitate the body's control of a viral infection may pose uncertain additional risks during the COVID-19 pandemic.[10, 11]

ADVOCATING FOR PATIENTS IN RESOURCE-LIMITED SETTINGS

Prospective multidisciplinary cancer conferences (MCC) or tumor boards are a standard in neuro-oncology and should continue during the COVID-19 pandemic. Virtual technologies such as video conferencing provide an opportunity to reduce patient and provider exposure to COVID-19 which can also result in reduced barriers to MCC participation and perhaps a wider breadth of expertise at the meeting. MCCs should also be used to stratify therapy and exposure risk for patients with COVID-19. If there is a need to ration scarce resources in your institution (mechanical ventilation, operating room access) then this forum may be an effective way to document neuro-oncologic specific factors informative to your institution's ethical framework for rationing.[12]

Comprehensive neuro-oncology MCCs often include social work support and supportive oncology representation that provide important insight into barriers to care and health outcome disparities that need to be considered, particularly during COVID-19, a disease that disproportionately impacts specific communities.[13, 14] For example, does your recommendation for 6 weeks of radiation therapy change if the patient is taking a city bus to their appointments, or lives in assisted living that requires 14-day quarantine after each health system encounter? What is the health-related quality of life impact of these decisions? Guidance by a patient and patient-advocate advisory board when rendering treatment recommendations in this new health landscape is needed.

PRIMARY BRAIN TUMORS

The most common malignant primary brain tumor is glioblastoma (GBM) which is an incurable tumor with an average survival of less than 2 years despite the best available treatment.[15, 16] Glioblastoma is a World Health Organization (WHO) Grade IV glioma. It is conceivable that social distancing restrictions may be in place for the remainder of a person's life who is diagnosed with a GBM. The majority of gliomas have no cure and are treated with maximal safe resection followed by external beam radiation therapy (EBRT) typically delivered in 30 fractions over 6 weeks with additional chemotherapy. GBM SOC treatment includes oral TMZ alkylating chemotherapy concurrently with EBRT followed by adjuvant TMZ and a wearable tumor treatment field device that utilizes alternating low-frequency electric fields to disrupt mitosis.[16] Low-grade gliomas (LGGs), such as WHO grade II oligodendroglioma and astrocytoma, may also receive a fractionated course of EBRT followed by combination chemotherapy with Procarbazine, Lomustine, and Vincristine that has demonstrated median overall survival exceeding a decade in clinical trials.[17] Given the favorable long-term survival in the LGG population consensus recommendations during COVID-19 encourage MCC review to consider delayed therapy and/or surgery in some patients.[1, 2]

The average age of GBM diagnosis is 64 years and many GBM patients have additional comorbidities—thus this group faces significant morbidity from their primary disease as well as from COVID-19. Early reports revealed that people with advanced age and a cancer diagnosis have poorer outcomes when infected with COVID-19.[18, 19] Optimal GBM treatment for elderly or frail patients is an ongoing debate. There is a rationale to support hypofractionated radiation therapy, such as a 15 fraction 40 Gy course of EBRT with or without TMZ that may result in reduced virus exposure for this vulnerable population.[1, 2, 20] For advanced age patients, the benefits of TMZ chemotherapy are dependent on O6 methylguanine-DNA methyltransferase (*MGMT*) DNA repair methylation status, which influences whether or not to include TMZ in the treatment.[21] Epigenetic silencing of this DNA repair pathway results in improved response to alkylating chemotherapies such as TMZ. However, there is minimal to no benefit of TMZ in MGMT unmethylated elderly patients, which is even less appealing when considered in the context of additional COVID-19 risks.[2, 21, 22] In elderly patients with poor performance status who do not have MGMT methylation, omitting TMZ should be considered. For elderly patients with poor performance status harboring favorable MGMT promoter methylation, one may consider using TMZ alone without EBRT, depending on additional factors such as COVID-19 risk and comorbidities. This therapeutic complexity is compounded by COVID-19, however simulation models are being presented to provide some insight into the relationship between COVID-19 exposure risks, comorbidities, EBRT fractionation regimens, and the historical landscape of elderly GBM trial data to guide decision making and quantify relative risk.[22]

METASTATIC CNS CANCER

The incidence of metastatic cancer to the CNS is much greater than primary CNS tumors. When CNS metastatic cancer is identified, any acute neurologic emergencies should be addressed which may necessitate surgery and/or radiation in addition, (re)staging of the primary disease is warranted. Brain and spine metastatic lesions with a known solid tumor source are typically treated with surgical resection for large lesions or those with impending neurologic consequences, followed by radiation with either stereotactic radiosurgery (SRS) or fractionated whole-brain radiation therapy (WBRT). Stereotactic radiosurgery can be an outpatient procedure that does not require inpatient or ICU management and requires less in-person health system exposures than other radiation modalities or surgery, thus if possible SRS is preferred.[23] In some situations, such as leptomeningeal metastatic disease, large lesions, multiple lesions, or situations where microseeding is suspected, WBRT is clearly indicated and should be pursued. Neurologic complications of metastatic disease should be closely monitored and addressed early to prevent hospital admission. These interventions may include corticosteroids for CNS edema, seizure management, and education of the neurocognitive consequences of disease, treatment, and therapy.

COMPLICATIONS OF CANCER

Complications of cancer may range from chemotherapy-induced neuropathy to elusive paraneoplastic syndromes that require tremendous ICU resources such as anti-*N*-methyl D-aspartate (NMDA) receptor encephalitis. Neuro-oncologists may provide a unique insight in managing these patients, which may reduce patient exposure and resource utilization. Some patients must be examined in person with a comprehensive neurologic exam as the level of detail required is not possible through a video visit with current technology.

NEUROSURGICAL MANAGEMENT

Neurosurgery is of paramount value in neuro-oncology as a diagnostic and therapeutic intervention. Surgery provides histologic and therapy-defining molecular diagnosis, cytoreduction, and can be lifesaving. Centers for Medicaid and Medicare Services (CMS) provided guidelines for elective surgery during the COVID-19 pandemic with most oncologic neurosurgical procedures receiving a grade of 3A declaring that surgery should not be postponed.[24] For high-grade glioma, maximal safe resection is a SOC that results in prolonged survival and should be pursued if at all possible.[1, 25] Institutional and regional factors in the setting of a pandemic may limit procedures that require ICU resources and thus alternative methods of surgery that utilize reduced resources may also be considered. Laser interstitial thermal ablation therapy with biopsy rarely requires ICU care and is one such approach despite limited evidence that this intervention is as effective as conventional surgery.[26] Staged surgery with the delay of larger resections requiring prolonged ICU care may also be considered, however, limited data supports this approach. It should be stressed that if a patient is undergoing a biopsy for diagnosis, enough tissue should be harvested to facilitate molecular tumor profiling which is critical to guiding care and integral to diagnosis.

PERIOPERATIVE AND INPATIENT NEURO-ONCOLOGICAL CARE

It is imperative that providers with expertise in neuro-oncology (neurosurgeons, neuro-oncologists, medical oncologists, neuro-intensivists, nurse coordinators) work collaboratively to ensure timely and adjudicated care.[27] Cohesive clinical care teams along with hospital administrative teams should provide transparent reporting on available resources locally and regionally based on available real-time information. Daily resource huddles addressing bed availability, personal protection equipment (PPE) availability, and status of patient screening processes are critical to execute timely care for neuro-oncologic patients. For procedures, the bare minimum of staff and Graduate Medical Education (GME) trainees (if any) should be permitted into the operating room and ICUs to minimize staff and patient exposure and to conserve PPE. Patients should receive COVID testing prior to their procedures to inform discussions about relative risks to patients and providers. Procedures in COVID-19 positive patients should be done only for true emergencies stratified by relative risk and resource availability. Patients with considerable risk factors or lab abnormalities that might decrease their immune response (including severe pancytopenia) should be individually evaluated in detail to determine whether surgical intervention is advisable.

In preparation for any surgery, preoperative testing should include COVID-19 testing within 1 day of hospital admission or surgical intervention to minimize patient and provider exposure. Operating room sterilization processes should be closely monitored with the utilization of a negative pressure environment, if available. Due to the high likelihood of aerosolization during intubation and extubation, strict restrictions on the number of medical personnel in the operating room or any space where such procedures are undertaken should be observed. It is recommended that all surgical and non-surgical care team members in the room remain in PPE during the duration of care. Surgical/ Frozen specimens should be utilized only when the

information will change intraoperative management to help minimize the risk of staff exposure and contamination of the operating rooms. Tissue banking procedures should be modified such that minimal necessary staff is required to complete the tissue procurement activities. Intraoperative neuromonitoring should be utilized only if absolutely necessary.

Postoperative care should be provided in areas designated as COVID-19 positive or COVID-19 free environments depending on the patient's COVID-19 test status. Whenever possible, ICU bed utilization should be avoided for simple craniotomies or spine surgeries to help conserve the much-needed resources of ICUs for those in most need which includes access to ventilators that have been in short supply during the pandemic.[28] All efforts should be undertaken to facilitate patient discharge to their home rather than subacute nursing facilities or rehabilitation centers given the observed increased COVID-19 exposure in these health-care settings.[29] Considerable attention should be paid to reducing the length of stay for hospitalized neuro-oncology patients to help reduce in-hospital patient exposure and reduce strain on health-care institutions.

RADIATION THERAPY

Patients at risk of progressive neurologic compromise from spinal cord lesions or multiple brain metastatic lesions should be prioritized for radiation treatment.[23] For metastatic spine lesions, a combined approach with neurosurgical intervention and/or radiation therapy should be considered that prioritizes single fraction radiation over conventional regimens if possible.[23, 30] For patients with high-grade glioma and excellent performance status, SOC EBRT should be attempted.[2] For patients with significantly compromised functional status and/or age greater than 70 short-course EBRT should be considered.[2, 20] Meningiomas are extremely heterogeneous, particularly atypical and anaplastic meningiomas that can follow a malignant course. Meningiomas have no SOC systemic therapy and are managed with surgery or radiation. Atypical meningiomas and other rare CNS tumors should be risk stratified and managed under the guidance of an MCC. For low-risk LGG and benign tumors that are not at risk for neurologic compromise, delayed radiation therapy should be considered.[1, 23]

Patients with metastatic brain disease and favorable prognosis may consider SRS with attention to lesions of highest morbidity.[23] In cases with multiple metastatic lesions or leptomeningeal disease, whole-brain radiation is typically indicated; however, it may be reasonable to consider a five fraction regimen, possibly with memantine to mitigate neurocognitive sequelae, as opposed to the standard 10 fraction course in hopes of limiting patient and staff exposure.[23]

CLINICAL TRIALS

Most neuro-oncologic conditions are incurable and many have no approved therapies therefore clinical trials which provide high-quality evidence that leads to new SOC treatments are prioritized in this population. GBM is notoriously treatment-resistant with dismal outcomes thus national guidelines recommend participation in a clinical trial over SOC.[31] The pandemic fractured clinical trial systems and halted neuro-oncology research. During the pandemic, therapeutic clinical trials that offer the most patient benefit are prioritized as every in-person encounter carries some level of comorbid risk. For example, therapeutic trials targeting diseases where there are no effective therapies such as in recurrent GBM or anaplastic meningioma, and later-phase trials investigating efficacy which have the most promise of directly benefiting patients are prioritized. Clinical trials are designed in phases to answer specific questions, with some trials using hybrid designs that overlap traditional phases. Phase 0 studies investigate how the drug works in the body and if the agent gets to the target which may require surgery to evaluate the tumor tissue for the desired response. Phase 1 studies investigate dose safety, phase 2 studies evaluate the efficacy, and Phase 3 trials are designed to answer how the agent compares to standard therapies.[32] Therapeutic clinical trials are rigorously monitored under the direction of an Institutional Review Board (IRB) that requires approval before any protocol changes are implemented.

Changes in therapeutic clinical trials are dictated by pandemic conditions. At many centers, patients already enrolled in clinical trials are prioritized to continue with modifications to maximize safety and patient benefit.[33] During surging pandemic conditions many centers halted new clinical trial enrollment with the implementation of a staged IRB-guided reopening plan. Any opportunity to preserve patient and healthcare personal safety should be exercised. Obtaining key study endpoints for outcome analysis should be prioritized with the evaluation of the risks/value of obtaining exploratory endpoints. Alternate methods of measuring outcomes should be employed to mitigate risks, such as virtual tools to reduce exposure.[33] Clinical trials are integral to neuro-oncology patient care and every effort should be made to retain access to therapies that offer patient benefit, however, modifications are needed to ensure safety, and these should be undertaken under the approval of an IRB. Despite the world's attention on the pandemic, devastating neuro-oncologic diseases like GBM continue to march forward and clinical trials are the path toward innovative new therapies that will result in improved health outcomes.

TRAGEDY AS A STIMULUS FOR PROGRESS

The approach to care for patients with cancer during COVID-19 has been largely based on expert opinion and extrapolations from clinical trials designed to answer other questions. This is a stern deviation from the evidence-based-medicine philosophy that is ingrained in oncology. Clinical trial protocols are becoming less restrictive, yet the historical trials we use to guide care during COVID-19 were often restricted to younger patients with limited comorbidities in an effort to maximize internal validity.[34] It is becoming clear through the COVID-19 crisis that older adults with comorbidities have the greatest risk from COVID-19, unfortunately these are also the patients that harbor the most uncertainty as to how existing clinical trial data applies. Neuro-oncology care teams and patients are faced with risk versus benefit analysis of toxic interventions that are rarely curative and now have new layers of uncertainty as to their impact on COVID-19 outcomes. For decades, the Institute of Medicine has gravitated toward a *"learning health system"* where key attributes are routinely recorded that inform care decisions at the point-of-care by capitalizing on the power of computational advances.[35] To do so requires a seismic shift in how health data is recorded.[36] For rare diseases that cannot power a statistically significant clinical trial, such systems are gaining steam. Had such a system been adopted prior to the current pandemic, we may have had greater insight into the impact of care decisions, particularly for our most vulnerable patients that may not have access to a clinical trial, perhaps due to the same comorbidities or socioeconomic factors that carry the greatest risk with COVID-19.[14, 18, 34]

Through the tragedy of this pandemic, there is hope that a new health landscape will emerge. COVID-19 has forced rapid adoption of virtual resources which may reduce geographic and functional access to care barriers in neuro-oncology, increasing patient exposure to specialized multidisciplinary services and clinical trials. Clinical trials have been deconstructed and rebuilt in ways that will provide insight to develop the next generation of trials that is more inclusive and takes advantage of newly adopted tools that reduce patient burden.

The paucity of high-level data to guide the management of patients with significant comorbidities will lead the health-care system toward the utilization of computational advances. These advances have reformatted other industries and hold the promise of doing the same to clinical care through the pursuit of *learning health systems* enabled at the point-of-care that approach every patient as an N-of-1. The greatest impact may be that the health-care system better incorporates the patient experience and social determinants of health into the care we provide.

REFERENCES

1. Bernhardt D, Wick W, Weiss SE, et al. Neuro-oncology management during the COVID-19 pandemic with a focus on WHO grades III and IV gliomas. *Neuro Oncol.* 2020;22(7):928–935.   https://doi.org/10.1093/neuonc/noaa113.

2. Mohile NA, Blakeley JO, Gatson NTN, et al. Urgent considerations for the neuro-oncologic treatment of patients with gliomas during the COVID-19 pandemic. *Neuro Oncol.* 2020;22(7):912–917.   https://doi.org/10.1093/neuonc/noaa090.

3. van de Haar J, Hoes LR, Coles CE, et al. Caring for patients with cancer in the COVID-19 era. *Nat Med.* 2020;26(5):665–671. https://doi.org/10.1038/s41591-020-0874-8.

4. Lucas MR. Psychosocial implications for the patient with a high-grade glioma. *J Neurosci Nurs.* 2010;42(2):104–108. https://doi.org/10.1097/JNN.0b013e3181ce5a34.

5. Pfefferbaum B, North CS. Mental health and the Covid-19 pandemic. *N Engl J Med.* 2020. https://doi.org/10.1056/NEJMp2008017.

6. Walbert T, Chasteen K. Palliative and supportive care for glioma patients. In: Raizer J, Parsa A, eds. *Current Understanding and Treatment of Gliomas. Cancer Treatment and Research.* Springer International Publishing; 2015:171–184. https://doi.org/10.1007/978-3-319-12048-5_11.

7. Bevans M, Sternberg EM. Caregiving burden, stress, and health effects among family caregivers of adult cancer patients. *JAMA.* 2012;307(4):398–403. https://doi.org/10.1001/jama.2012.29.

8. Longacre ML, Applebaum AJ, Buzaglo JS, et al. Reducing informal caregiver burden in cancer: evidence-based programs in practice. *Transl Behav Med.* 2018;8(2):145–155. https://doi.org/10.1093/tbm/ibx028.

9. Zhao Q, Meng M, Kumar R, et al. Lymphopenia is associated with severe coronavirus disease 2019 (COVID-19) infections: a systemic review and meta-analysis. *Int J Infect Dis.* 2020;96:131–135. https://doi.org/10.1016/j.ijid.2020.04.086.

10. Delaunay M, Prévot G, Collot S, Guilleminault L, Didier A, Mazières J. Management of pulmonary toxicity associated with immune checkpoint inhibitors. *Eur Respir Rev.* 2019;28(154). https://doi.org/10.1183/16000617.0012-2019.

11. Zheng M, Gao Y, Wang G, et al. Functional exhaustion of antiviral lymphocytes in COVID-19 patients. *Cell Mol Immunol.* 2020;17(5):533–535. https://doi.org/10.1038/s41423-020-0402-2.

12. Emanuel EJ, Persad G, Upshur R, et al. Fair allocation of scarce medical resources in the time of Covid-19. *N Engl J Med.* 2020;382(21):2049–2055. https://doi.org/10.1056/NEJMsb2005114.

13. Curry WT, Barker FG. Racial, ethnic and socioeconomic disparities in the treatment of brain tumors. *J Neurooncol.* 2009;93(1):25.   https://doi.org/10.1007/s11060-009-9840-5.

14. Hooper MW, Nápoles AM, Pérez-Stable EJ. COVID-19 and racial/ethnic disparities. *JAMA.* 2020;323(24):2466–2467. https://doi.org/10.1001/jama.2020.8598.

15. Ostrom QT, Gittleman H, Xu J, et al. CBTRUS statistical report: primary brain and other central nervous system tumors diagnosed in the United States in 2009–2013. *Neuro Oncol.* 2016;18(Suppl 5):v1–v75. https://doi.org/10.1093/neuonc/now207.

16. Stupp R, Taillibert S, Kanner AA, et al. Maintenance therapy with tumor-treating fields plus Temozolomide vs Temozolomide alone for glioblastoma: a randomized clinical trial. *JAMA.* 2015;314(23):2535–2543. https://doi.org/10.1001/jama.2015.16669.

17. Buckner JC, Shaw EG, Pugh SL, et al. Radiation plus Procarbazine, CCNU, and vincristine in low-grade glioma. *N Engl J Med.* 2016;374(14):1344–1355. https://doi.org/10.1056/NEJMoa1500925.

18. Wu Z, McGoogan JM. Characteristics of and important lessons from the coronavirus disease 2019 (COVID-19) outbreak in China: summary of a report of 72314 cases from the Chinese Center for Disease Control and Prevention. *JAMA.* 2020. https://doi.org/10.1001/jama.2020.2648.

19. Zhang L, Zhu F, Xie L, et al. Clinical characteristics of COVID-19-infected cancer patients: a retrospective case study in three hospitals within Wuhan, China. *Ann Oncol.* 2020;31(7):894–901.   https://doi.org/10.1016/j.annonc.2020.03.296.

20. Perry JR, Laperriere N, O'Callaghan CJ, et al. Short-course radiation plus Temozolomide in elderly patients with glioblastoma. *N Engl J Med.* 2017;376(11):1027–1037. https://doi.org/10.1056/NEJMoa1611977.

21. Hegi ME, Diserens A-C, Gorlia T, et al. MGMT gene silencing and benefit from Temozolomide in glioblastoma. *N Engl J Med.* 2005;352(10):997–1003. https://doi.org/10.1056/NEJMoa043331.

22. Tabrizi S, Trippa L, Cagney D, et al. A quantitative framework for modeling COVID-19 risk during adjuvant therapy using published randomized trials of glioblastoma in the elderly. *Neuro Oncol.* 2020;22(7):918–927. https://doi.org/10.1093/neuonc/noaa111.

23. Yerramilli D, Xu AJ, Gillespie EF, et al. Palliative radiation therapy for oncologic emergencies in the setting of COVID-19: approaches to balancing risks and benefits. *Adv Radiat Oncol.* 2020. https://doi.org/10.1016/j.adro.2020.04.001.

24. CMS releases recommendations on adult elective surgeries, non-essential medical, surgical, and dental procedures during COVID-19 response. https://www.cms.gov/files/document/cms-non-emergent-elective-medical-recommendations.pdf.

25. Brown PD, Maurer MJ, Rummans TA, et al. A prospective study of quality of life in adults with newly diagnosed high-grade gliomas: the impact of the extent of resection on quality of life and survival. *Neurosurgery.* 2005;57(3):495–504. https://doi.org/10.1227/01.NEU.0000170562.25335.C7.

26. Mohammadi AM, Hawasli AH, Rodriguez A, et al. The role of laser interstitial thermal therapy in enhancing progression-free survival of difficult-to-access high-grade gliomas: a multicenter study. *Cancer Med.* 2014;3(4):971–979. https://doi.org/10.1002/cam4.266.

27. Ramakrishna R, Zadeh G, Sheehan JP, Aghi MK. Inpatient and outpatient case prioritization for patients with neuro-oncologic disease amid the COVID-19 pandemic: general guidance for neuro-oncology practitioners from the AANS/CNS Tumor Section and Society for Neuro-Oncology. *J Neurooncol.* 2020;147(3):525–529. https://doi.org/10.1007/s11060-020-03488-7.

28. Florman JE, Cushing D, Keller LA, Rughani AI. A protocol for postoperative admission of elective craniotomy patients to a non-ICU or step-down setting. *J Neurosurg.* 2017;127(6):1392–1397. https://doi.org/10.3171/2016.10.JNS16954.

29. Barnett ML, Grabowski DC. Nursing homes are ground zero for COVID-19 pandemic. *JAMA Health Forum.* 2020;1(3):e200369. https://doi.org/10.1001/jamahealthforum.2020.0369.

30. Laufer I, Rubin DG, Lis E, et al. The NOMS framework: approach to the treatment of spinal metastatic tumors. *Oncologist.* 2013;18(6):744–751. https://doi.org/10.1634/theoncologist.2012-0293.

31. National Comprehensive Cancer Network. NCCN Clinical Practice Guidelines in Oncology. Central Nervous System Cancers. Version 1.2016. nccn.org. Accessed 10/17/2016.

32. What are the phases of clinical trials? Accessed August 2, 2020. https://www.cancer.org/treatment/treatments-and-side-effects/clinical-trials/what-you-need-to-know/phases-of-clinical-trials.html.

33. McDermott MM, Newman AB. Preserving clinical trial integrity during the coronavirus pandemic. *JAMA.* 2020;323(21):2135–2136. https://doi.org/10.1001/jama.2020.4689.

34. Unger JM, Cook E, Tai E, Bleyer A. Role of clinical trial participation in cancer research: barriers, evidence, and strategies. *Am Soc Clin Oncol Educ Book Am Soc Clin Oncol Meet.* 2016;35:185–198. https://doi.org/10.14694/EDBK_156686.

35. Smith MD, Institute of Medicine (U.S.), eds. *Best Care at Lower Cost: The Path to Continuously Learning Health Care in America.* National Academies Press; 2013.

36. Snyder JM, Pawloski JA, Poisson LM. Developing real-world evidence-ready datasets: time for clinician engagement. *Curr Oncol Rep.* 2020;22(5). https://doi.org/10.1007/s11912-020-00904-z.

CHAPTER 10

COVID-19 Infection: Impaired Olfaction, Movement Disorders, Encephalopathy, and Neuropsychiatric Manifestations

TESSA M. LEWITT[a,b] • HANNAH KOPINSKY[a,b] • PETER A. LEWITT[a,c]

[a]Department of Neurology, Henry Ford Hospital, Detroit, MI, United States, [b]Wayne State University School of Medicine, Detroit, MI, United States, [c]Department of Neurology, Wayne State University, Detroit, MI, United States

INTRODUCTION

Beyond the possibility of life-threatening consequences of pulmonary invasion and respiratory failure, COVID-19 infection imparts a wide range of neurological and neuropsychiatric consequences for many infected persons. This chapter reviews several of the problems that arise from central nervous system (CNS) involvement in patients with COVID-19. The emerging clinical experience and its medical literature have revealed several common and a few rare neurological outcomes caused by the virus, whose mode of entry into the CNS is still a matter of contention. Several possible pathways—hematogenous spread with direct invasion through blood-brain barrier, retrograde dissemination via trigeminal nerve, and passage through the cribriform plate into the olfactory bulb or cerebrospinal fluid—have been proposed. Possibly, each of them can be an explanation.

One of the most prominent neurological consequences of COVID-19, a decline in sense of smell, can be the sole manifestation of infection or can be the prelude to more serious systemic or CNS involvement. Other neurological features, like the few reported instances of movement disorders, seem to be relatively rare occurrences. An intensive neuropathological analysis of the effects of COVID-19 on the brain is still a work in progress throughout the medical community. In one of the few available autopsy reports from a well-characterized COVID-19 case, widespread CNS damage was found, with extensive white matter infarcts and hemorrhagic changes. No neuronal necrosis was found in cortical or subcortical gray matter (including the olfactory bulb).[1] We are also limited in our understanding of what's ahead in upcoming months and years for those who sustained COVID-19 infection (including those with relatively mild pulmonary symptoms). Fortunately, several programs including ours will be following long-term neurological and neuropsychiatric outcomes for persons who have encountered and survived COVID-19. There is considerable evidence that neurological symptomatology may be among the persisting health problems long after the course of the initial presentation of the viral illness. New neurological manifestations are also being recognized as COVID-19 cases undergo increased scrutiny, For example, one report among Northern Italian patients found 16% experienced vertigo (and at approximately 60 days afterwards, these symptoms persisted for 6.7% of the 143 patients evaluated).[2]

Although up to date at the time of publication, this chapter should be viewed as a work in progress whose further perspectives will be enhanced by neuropathological study of human cases, discovery of relevant biomarkers, and possibly, the development of animal models. Topics to be considered including smell and taste impairments, movement disorders, encephalopathy, and neuropsychiatric manifestations.

DISORDERS OF OLFACTION AND TASTE FROM COVID-19 INFECTION

Anosmia, hyposmia, ageusia, and hypogeusia have been well documented in the recent medical literature describing the COVID-19.[3–5] Though mentioned only rarely in the Chinese literature during the first weeks of the pandemic, subsequent studies published throughout Europe and the United States have emphasized its role as an early symptom of illness.[5, 6] In addition, these unique sensory deficits constitute a window into the pathophysiology of COVID-19 infection as it affects the CNS.

Between January and February 2020, Mao et al. retrospectively studied 214 hospitalized COVID-19-positive patients in Wuhan, China.[5] Of these patients, 36.4% had neurologic manifestations of this disease; 5.1% reported olfactory dysfunction (OD) and 5.6% reported gustatory dysfunction (GD).[5] Within a few weeks, further reporting from emerging cohorts of affected patients made it clear that this initial report likely underestimated the prevalence of OD and GD as neurological symptoms of COVID-19.[3, 4, 6, 7]

In a large multicenter cohort of 2013 COVID-19-positive patients in Europe, 87% reported impaired sense of smell and 56% reported impaired sense of taste.[8] Similarly, a group in Italy noted that 74.2% of COVID-19-positive patients reported impaired sense of smell, taste, or both.[9] This symptomatology in studies reporting relatively large populations of COVID-19-infected patients are outlined in Table 10.1.

Interestingly, Lechien et al. noted that among those with subjective reports of either anosmia or hyposmia, many did not meet objective criteria for OD.[15] In fact, 38% of those who reported complete anosmia were normosmic upon testing with a validated and highly reproducible bedside test, the Sniffin' Sticks.[15, 16] Further, Lechien et al. found no significant correlation between either subjective nasal obstruction or rhinorrhea with either objective hyposmia or anosmia.[15] On the other hand, Vaira et al. found that 30% of patients whose history included no subjective report of OD nonetheless proved, upon Connecticut Chemosensory Clinical Research Center testing, to be hyposmic.[17-19] These conflicting conclusions highlight the disparities that can occur with subjective olfaction reporting and emphasize the need for objective testing for OD.

Gustatory function can be evaluated objectively by patient- or operator-prepared solutions (salty, sweet, sour, and bitter).[17, 20, 21] Patients are asked to rate quality of taste perception from 0 (complete ageusia) to 10 (normal taste perception) for each solution.[17, 20, 21] Similar to olfactory testing, this validated tool can help clinicians distinguish between subjective and objective GD, and can differentiate OD-induced taste dysfunction from true GD.

Many of the common pathogens causing upper respiratory infections are known to impair the sense of smell in infected patients.[15] OD in these cases is often secondary to an inflammatory process within the nasal mucosa that ultimately manifests as rhinitis and sometimes, nasal obstruction.[15] Several groups have reported a lack of relationship between symptoms of nasal inflammation and objective OD, indicating that COVID-19-induced OD might require an alternate explanation.[12, 15, 22-24]

CNS viral invasion has been described in the literature covering other viruses including parainfluenza virus, influenza A virus, and adenovirus, as well as other coronavirus strains, including Middle Eastern respiratory syndrome (MERS) and severe acute respiratory syndrome (SARS).[12, 22-24] In fact, a mouse model of SARS demonstrated the virus' transneuronal pathway through the olfactory bulb.[24] The mechanism of OD in COVID-19 may be similar. There is evidence that the virus may travel trans-synaptically in a retrograde direction across the cribriform plate of the ethmoid bone into the neuroepithelium and olfactory bulb.[25, 26]

Viral invasion into the olfactory bulb may induce reactive astrogliosis, activation of microglia, and ultimately, direct damage to the primary organs of olfaction, olfactory receptors.[12, 22, 25, 26] In accordance with this theory, a similar path may be taken by the virus to injure gustatory receptors in GD.[25, 27] Neurological damage caused by the virus may explain one study's findings that 20% of COVID-19 patients with anosmia did not recover within 2-months following the onset of OD.[28]

The "neurotropic" hypothesis does not involve the angiotensin-converting enzyme-2 (ACE-2) receptor, the site known to interact with the virus and facilitate its fusion with the host cell.[25, 26] Therefore, an alternate hypothesis has been posed to explain the relationship between GD and COVID-19. ACE-2 receptors are prevalent in the oral cavity, with highest density on the tongue. Viral entry into cells via the ACE-2 receptor and subsequent inflammation may disrupt perception of taste signals as well as the renewal of taste buds.[14, 29]

A second hypothesis proposes that the virus enters the CNS via a hematogenous route. According to this mechanism, CNS manifestations arise from direct viral entry into the CNS because of an abnormally permeable blood-brain barrier. This hypothesis, however, does not readily explain anosmia or ageusia.[30]

Anosmia and ageusia are intimately linked with respect to the processing of their respective sensory modalities in the CNS. A report by Speth et al. determined that the severity of OD was closely correlated with the presence of GD.[29, 31] The sense of smell and taste share regions in the brain that are dedicated to identifying, interpreting, and integrating these senses. Viral-induced inflammatory damage to the frontobasal region of the brain may partially explain OD and GD,

TABLE 10.1

Prevalence of Anosmia, Hyposmia, Ageusia, and Hypogeusia in COVID-19.

Source	Country	Date	Patient Population	COVID-19 Testing	OD N (%)	GD N (%)	Mode of Testing Symptoms	Comments
Magnavita et al.[10]	Italy	March-April 2020	N=82 COVID-19 + health-care workers	RT-PCR	35 (42.7)	31 (37.8)	Self-reported	Of the 10 patients with anosmia and myalgias, nine tested positive for COVID-19
Tostmann et al.[11]	The Netherlands	March 2020	N=79 symptomatic COVID-19 + health-care workers	RT-PCR	37 (46.8)	Not reported	Self-reported	
Lechien et al.[8]	Belgium, France, Spain, Italy, Canada, Switzerland	Not reported	N=417 COVID-19 + patients with mild-to-moderate symptoms	RT-PCR	357 (85.6)	342 (82.0)	Taste and smell component of sQOD-NS, NHANES	There was a significant association between OD and GD. OD appeared before other symptoms in 11.8% of cases
Lee et al.[12]	South Korea	March 2020	N=3191 COVID-19+ patients	RT-PCR	389 (12.2)	353 (11.1)	Self-reported	
Mao et al.[5]	China	January-February 2020	N=214 hospitalized COVID-19+ patients	RT-PCR	11 (5.1)	12 (5.6)	Retrospective chart review	
Vaira et al.[9]	Italy	Not reported	N=345 nonhospitalized and hospitalized COVID-19+ patients	RT-PCR	241 (69.9)	155 (44.9)	Self-reported, CCCRC, validated gustatory function test	30.1% of patients who reported normosmia proved objectively hyposmic upon CCCRC testing
Güner et al.[13]	Turkey	March-April 2020	N=222 hospitalized COVID-19+ patients	RT-PCR	19 (8.6)	17 (7.7)	Retrospective chart review	
Lechien et al.[14]	France	March-April 2020	N=2013 nonhospitalized and hospitalized COVID-19+ patients	RT-PCR	1754 (87.1)	1136 (56.4)	NHANES, Sniffin' Sticks	
Kaye et al.[6]	United States	March-April 2020	N=237 COVID-19+ patients	Presumed in some cases	172 (72.6)		American Academy Otolaryngology Head and Neck Surgery's COVID-19 Anosmia Reporting Tool for Clinicians	Anosmia was reported by 73% of patients prior to COVID-19 diagnosis. Anosmia was the earliest symptom in 26.6% of patients

RT-PCR, real-time polymerase chain reaction; *sQOD-NS*, short version of the Questionnaire of Olfactory Disorders-Negative Statements; *NHANES*, National Health and Nutrition Examination Survey; *CCCRC*, Connecticut Chemosensory Clinical Research Center.

as this region lies close to the olfactory bulb and expresses ACE-2 receptors.[29, 31]

Most patients with COVID-19-induced OD and GD recover within 3 weeks, with a median recovery time of 1 week. However, Li et al. found that in some cases, dysosmia may linger for 95 days or longer.[9, 12, 29, 32] In a single-center review of 143 COVID-19-infected patients in Northern Italy, 43% experienced anosmia and 13% persisted in this symptomatology at a mean of 60 days after the acute infection.[2] Recovery from anosmia may reflect viral damage to basal cells, as invasion of these precursor cells can halt their progression to olfactory epithelium. Under normal circumstances, the recovery cycle for olfactory basal cells takes between 28 and 30 days.[9, 12] Therefore, reports of shorter "recovery" times may reflect partial return of the sense of smell rather than a complete objective recovery from anosmia. Regarding dysgeusia, a single-center study of 143 Northern Italian patients found that 48% were affected during the acute infection; the persistence of impaired taste at approximately 60 days later was 7%.[2]

Conflicting data have been reported about GD. The rate of turnover for taste receptors cells is only 7–10 days. However, subjective GD may be unreliable as taste perception is intimately tied to accompanying aromas (requiring the input of olfactory function, whose recovery might be on a different time course).[33]

Though cranial nerve 1 (olfactory) evaluation is often foregone in neurologic examinations performed by health-care providers, there are important lessons to be learned from acute anosmia and ageusia that often arise in the setting of COVID-19. First, these symptoms can represent the earliest or sole manifestations of disease in some cases.[6, 32] It is, therefore, critical to realize that COVID-19 can present with OD or GD in paucisymptomatic, afebrile patients (especially women and younger adults).[3, 12] In a study by Speth et al., OD presented, on average, around day 3 after infection, but onset in the study population ranged from day 1 to 12 of symptomatic illness.[31] Ageusia is not routinely tested in the neurological examinations of some practitioners, but the medical literature on this topic would suggest that positive screening with this examination might be indicative of COVID-19 infection.[3, 8, 14]

Because they can be sensitive and early indicators of COVID-19 infection, impairment of both sense of smell and taste can serve as important clues for patients to perform self-isolation or seek COVID-19 testing. This is especially important since an estimated 40%–50% of COVID-19-positive patients are expected to be asymptomatic at initial positive polymerase chain reaction testing.[34–36]

Early reports of prevalence may have underrepresented the true occurrence of OD and GD, as these manifestations may have been deemed too mild to be reported or documented in the electronic medical record of hospitalized patients. Further, patients may not have been inclined to report their OD or GD unless directly asked, and bedside examination of ill patients may skip detailed neurological testing that would otherwise detect such problems. Nonetheless, as subjective OD may not always indicate objective OD and vice versa, objective testing with odorants and taste solutions may be important to adopt.[15–21] A proposed approach for the assessment and management of COVID-19-related OD, published in The Journal of the American Medical Association, recommends a full otolaryngologic examination which includes a three-pass nasendoscopy when appropriate PPE is available. It also recommends CT to assess the paranasal sinuses, and MRI brain to examine brain and olfactory tracts.[37] A psychophysical assessment using validated tests of odorants/tastants should complement the subjective assessment. Treatment may be needed in persistent OD, i.e., lasting for 2 weeks or more. This includes olfactory training by sniffing specific odorants such as rose, lemon, cloves, and eucalyptus, at least twice daily for at least 3 months. Other promising therapies which work in postinfectious OD include intranasal vitamin A and systemic omega-3 but have not been tested in COVID-19 specifically. Corticosteroids, on the other hand, whether oral or intranasal, are not recommended due to lacking evidence of benefit and potential harm.

It is becoming increasingly evident that OD and GD can be helpful at recognizing possible COVID-19 infection and encouraging steps like self-isolation.[35, 36] Both anosmia and ageusia often present early in the course of the disease, especially in women and in younger adults. They can also be the only manifestation of COVID-19 infection.[6] Asking patients if they have experienced these symptoms may be useful in triage settings, as affirmative answers should heighten suspicion for COVID-19 infection. The Centers for Disease Control and Prevention included "new loss of taste or smell" to its overview of common symptomatology.[38]

MOVEMENT DISORDERS AND COVID-19 INFECTION

Review of the emerging medical literature and the author's (PAL) personal experience do not point to disorders of movement as common features of COVID-19 infection. Among persons who have tested positive for nasopharyngeal presence of the virus, who have been ill but not hospitalized, and who have had serious pulmonary or other systemic manifestations, the majority have been spared any signs or symptoms of motor impairment or involuntary movements. Development or exacerbation of restless limb syndrome (the most common movement disorder in the general population) hasn't been reported. The same can be said about the second most common movement disorder, the syndrome of essential tremor. Parkinson disease, which affects 1% or more of the general population over the age of 60 years, doesn't impart increased vulnerability for symptomatic worsening in those with COVID-19 infection.[32] A case-controlled survey during the pandemic period was conducted by telephone interview of 1486 advanced PD patients in Lombardy (region of the highest incidence of infection in Italy) and 1207 of their family members.[39] The results indicated no increased risk of acquiring or developing different COVID-19 signs or symptoms than the general population, which at the time had more than a 7% prevalence of COVID-19 positivity. PD patients and their family control did not differ in mortality from the viral infection. The COVID-19 PD group had, in general, fewer instances of dyspnea and lower rates of subsequent hospitalization. Despite the lack of increased risk from medical consequences of COVID-19, persons with PD may be particularly vulnerable to the stress of isolation and other social consequences of quarantine.[40] Some of the health costs for the PD patient include reduced opportunity for physical exercise and management of other daily activities that can be important for counteracting the physical disabilities of PD. For the patient with PD disabilities, various countermeasures that have been recommended include educational measures to enhance self-management strategies for stress reduction (such as mindfulness training), increase coping skills (such as participation in cognitive behavioral therapy), and developing alternatives for physical exercise in isolation at home (such as internet exercise guidance).

The major category of CNS consequences from COVID-19 infection, as demonstrated by neuropathological and radiological findings, are small hemorrhages and infarctions.[1] Consequently, brain injury in key locations can lead to distinctive movement disorders. For example, damage to white matter pathways in or out of the subthalamic nucleus (or the nucleus itself) can bring out contralateral ballistic movements, sometimes with choreic or dystonic features. Infarcts or hemorrhages in the outflow pathway from the dentate nucleus of the cerebellum through the red nucleus of the midbrain and on to the thalamus can generate action tremor. Another vulnerable pathway extending

from the substantia nigra pars compacta to the putamen and caudate nuclei can be the source of contralateral Parkinsonism if a destructive lesion occurs from circulatory damage. A much wider region of motor pathways in the corticospinal system (from cerebral motor and supplementary motor cortex), descending through the internal capsule and through the brainstem, provides territory in which paresis and paralysis can develop with vascular occlusion or bleeding.

The medical literature does provide a few examples of movement disorders in documented COVID-19 infections. One case report describes a 73-year-old man presenting with ataxic gait and mild encephalopathy beginning 4 days before the diagnosis of COVID-19 infection.[41] In another report, a 70-year-old man with a typical COVID-19 respiratory infection developed 4-limb postural and action (not resting) tremors, tremulous voice, and shaking that developed in his legs while standing (orthostatic tremor).[42] The patient's gait was unstable and ataxic; Romberg's sign was absent. Slight symptomatic improvement came from the use of clonazepam and by 1 month later, there was gradual recovery reported. Another report of a hyperkinetic movement disorder described three instances of generalized myoclonus developing early during otherwise typical acute pulmonary infections with COVID-19. Apart from the pulmonary and systemic consequences of COVID-19, there were no other identified causes of acquired myoclonus including liver failure, metabolic disturbance, or hypoxic episodes.[43] In each of the cases, there were bilateral manifestations of positive and negative myoclonus affecting upper extremity, shoulder, and facial regions. The myoclonic movements occurred spontaneously. They also were elicited during voluntary movements and after stimulation (startle, tactile, and auditory). The three patients went on to partial recovery from this movement disorder. Generalized myoclonus has also been reported in two patients suspected of developing *serotonin syndrome*. In these cases, the hyperkinetic movements were regarded as the consequence of interaction between an administered antiviral drug combination, lopinavir/ritonavir, and coadministration of psychiatric medications affecting CNS serotonin neurotransmission (the selective serotonin reuptake inhibitor duloxetine in one patient and the antipsychotic risperidone in the other).[44]

The spectrum of motor impairment reported in COVID-19 infection can include problems that aren't genuine movement disorders and instead are determined to be a category termed *functional* (sometimes alternatively classified as "feigned" or "psychogenic"). Functional movement disorders require considerable effort to achieve diagnostic certainty, as they are generally diagnoses of exclusion. One instance of COVID-19-related functional movement disorder was published in which the patient was affected with a relatively mild COVID-19 nasopharyngeal infection and anosmia. This patient had no prior episodes of functional movement disorder or psychiatric illness. She eventually exhibited several patterns of motor impairment bilaterally, including action tremors, other jerking movements, and ataxic gait. Features against the diagnosis of a genuine movement disorder included their atypical presentation, distractibility, and the absence of signs indicating neurological dysfunction. As a result, the treating physicians concluded that the motor abnormalities were functional in origin.[45] Clinicians should be aware that functional movement disorders are not rare and sometimes arise in the context of obvious psychological stress or some manner of secondary gain (including seeking medical care). Functional movement disorders also appear without any obvious explanation of what might be triggering them, and in the absence of insight by the affected person. Given the enormous stresses and altered normalcy of life imposed by the COVID-19 pandemic, it should not be surprising if the prevalence of functional movement disorders might increase in persons sick with, harboring, or just fearing this potentially deadly viral infection.

Finally, there has been some discussion in the medical literature about movement disorders that arose widely throughout the world in the aftermath of the last major pandemic caused by influenza in 1918. In the years following the spread of influenza, a novel disorder evolved that was variably characterized by Parkinsonism, tics, dystonia, and other persisting neurological deficits. This disorder, encephalitis lethargica, affected hundreds of thousands of young and old alike over more than one decade following the pandemic (though its etiological relationship to influenza remains unclear).[46] An analogy to the 1918 influenza pandemic and increasing evidence for COVID-19 dissemination to the brain[47] have raised concerns that similar postinfection neurological syndromes might arise in the future. Fortunately, no evidence for this possibility has been detected so far with COVID-19 or with other coronavirus infections.

ENCEPHALOPATHY AND NEUROPSYCHIATRIC MANIFESTATIONS OF COVID-19

Neuropsychiatric manifestations have been increasingly recognized in the medical literature appearing as COVID-19 unfolds in the worldwide population affected.[48, 49] Its prevalence was emphasized in one study that found that nearly 60% of all patients hospitalized with COVID-19 developed one or more neuropsychiatric symptoms. These included anxiety, depression, and insomnia as well as more serious neurological impairments such as delirium.[50] These findings are not surprising given the severity and stress imposed by the acute pulmonary disease and its other complications such as hypoxia and multiorgan failure. These acute manifestations lay themselves on top of a preexistent heightened stress level that is fueled by the distressing psychological and economic impacts the pandemic has had on societies and mental health. Other coronavirus infections imposing respiratory and other systemic manifestations, such as SARS-CoV and MERS-CoV, have also manifested a variety of neuropsychiatric manifestation seen during past coronavirus outbreaks.[51] Short- and long-term sequelae of COVID-19 are increasingly undergoing categorization reporting in the emerging medical literature about the worldwide population affected by this viral pandemic.

Acute Neuropsychiatric Symptomatology During COVID-19 Infection

The most commonly reported neuropsychiatric symptoms during acute COVID-19 infection are confusion, altered consciousness, insomnia, and impaired attention, features that have been collectively classified in the spectrum of delirium.[51] In some reviews, the severity of delirium has been associated with the extent of pulmonary disease.[52] The severity of delirium in serious neurocritical illnesses has also been associated with the likelihood of persisting neurocognitive deficits.[53]

In addition to delirium, a more profound encephalopathic state can develop acutely with COVID-19.[54–56] In a retrospective study from Wuhan, China, approximately one-fifth of hospitalized COVID-19-infected individuals were classified as encephalopathic.[57] One analysis of 125 patients with COVID-19 and acute neurologic or psychiatric symptoms revealed that 31% of patients suffered from altered mental status, and of which 13% were encephalopathic.[58] This has been attributed to wide range of physiological insults acutely resulting from COVID-19 infection, including hypoxia, fluid-electrolyte imbalance, and cardiovascular complications. Another explanation might be CNS invasion by the virus. In another study, approximately two-thirds of patients experiencing the COVID-19 acute respiratory distress syndrome were categorized as encephalopathic.[59]

Beyond the spectrum of neurological impairments constituting a continuum from confusional state to coma, behavioral and psychiatric dimensions of COVID-19 infection have been increasingly recognized. Several studies have reported high prevalence of mood disorders diagnosed in patients with COVID-19, both during the acute infection and arising in the postinfection period. In the abovementioned analysis of 125 patients with COVID-19 acute neurologic or psychiatric symptoms, 8% of patients presented with psychosis and 3% with an affective disorder.[58] Hu et al.[60] surveyed COVID-19-hospitalized patients and found high proportions of patients experiencing depression (45.9%), anxiety (38.8%), and insomnia (54.1%). In addition, those patients manifesting these neuropsychiatric problems typically underwent more extended disease duration, a longer hospital stay, and a greater self-perceived severity of illness. Another investigation of hospitalized COVID-19 patients found that 96.2% of patients reported the presence of symptoms meeting criteria for a posttraumatic stress disorder.[61] Not surprisingly, patients going through infection with COVID-19 who had a preexisting psychiatric illness were at increased risk for worsening of their psychiatric symptoms.[48, 62]

Long-Term Neuropsychiatric Symptoms of COVID-19 Infection

To date, there is limited published data on long-term neuropsychiatric sequelae of COVID-19. However, several possible outcomes can be predicted from reports of postillness neuropsychiatric complications that evolved from prior coronavirus outbreaks. A systematic review and metaanalysis by Rogers and colleagues[51] determined that, in the postillness period of both SARS and MERS epidemics, the most common neuropsychiatric sequelae were depression, anxiety, fatigue, and posttraumatic stress disorder. The time period for the development of these conditions ranged from 1 month[63, 64] to 30 or more months postinfection.[65, 66]

Pathogenesis

Several hypotheses have arisen for explaining why neuropsychiatric manifestations develop with COVID-19 infections. One of the leading considerations is that the neuropsychiatric spectrum of problems arise from the heightened inflammatory response generated by COVID-19.[50, 51, 59] Prominent immunological abnormalities evolve in many critically ill patients with COVID-19, including elevated serum C-reactive protein, reduced total blood lymphocyte counts, and the elevation of pro-inflammatory cytokines (described as a "cytokine storm").[67] The surge of pro-inflammatory cytokines may precipitate neuropsychiatric symptoms

through a compromised blood-brain barrier resulting from localized neuroinflammatory changes, permitting immune cell migration into the CNS. The consequences of such a mechanism could range from disruption of neurotransmission to cellular damage. The nature and extent of such CNS involvement could govern the reversibility of the observed clinical problems.[67, 68]

Other possible mechanisms for explaining neuropsychiatric complications associated with COVID-19 include direct viral infiltration of the CNS, cerebral hypoxic injury, dysfunction in mechanisms associated with angiotensin-converting enzyme 2 (whose receptors may serve in the process of intracellular uptake of the virus), postinfectious autoimmune reactions, and immunomodulatory treatments used (such as corticosteroids).[30, 68] Ultimately, the pathogenesis of neuropsychiatric diseases both during and after infection from COVID-19 is likely due to a combination of biological and psychosocial factors. Autopsy evidence to date is limited in providing explanations. One case of CNS consequences from COVID-19 infection showed extensive small hemorrhages and white matter infarctions.[1] A more detailed account of the various pathogenic mechanisms underlying the neurological manifestations of COVID-19 can be found in Chapter 2.

CONCLUSIONS

The ongoing COVID-19 pandemic is placing an enormous psychological burden on both patients infected with the virus and the general public, especially those with friends and relatives affected. Given the high incidence of neuropsychiatric problems arising acutely and chronically, there is a need for increasing awareness of the problems in both the hospitalized patient and in their aftercare. As for other patients surviving neurocritical management in life-threatening circumstances, the clinical team managing COVID-19 infections needs to plan for the emergence of neurological and psychiatric consequences both in the acute and chronic care settings. This is especially important for patients with preexisting psychiatric conditions.[48, 49]

REFERENCES

1. Reichard RR, Kashani KB, Boire NA, et al. Neuropathology of COVID-19: a spectrum of vascular and acute disseminated encephalomyelitis (ADEM)-like pathology. *Acta Neuropathol.* 2020;140:1–6. https://doi.org/10.1007/s00401-020-02166-2.
2. Carfì A, Brnabei R, Landi F, et al. Persistent symptoms in patients after acute COVID-19. *JAMA.* 2020;324(6):603–605. https://doi.org/10.1001/jama.2020.12603.

3. Vaira LA, Salzano G, Deiana G, De Riu G. Anosmia and ageusia: common findings in COVID-19 patients. *Laryngoscope*. 2020;130(7):1787. https://doi.org/10.1002/lary.28692.

4. Eliezer M, Hautefort C, Hamel A-L, Verillaud B, Herman P, Houdart E. Sudden and complete olfactory loss function as a possible symptom of COVID-19. *JAMA Otolaryngol Head Neck Surg*. 2020;146(7):674–675. https://doi.org/10.1001/jamaoto.2020.0832.

5. Mao L, Wang M, Chen S, He Q, Chang J, Hong C. Neurological manifestations of hospitalized patients with COVID-19 in Wuhan, China: a retrospective case series study. *medRxiv*. 2020;77(6):683–690. https://doi.org/10.1001/jamaneurol.2020.1127.

6. Kaye R, Chang CWD, Kazahaya K, Brereton J, Denneny JC. COVID-19 anosmia reporting tool: Initial findings. *Otolaryngol Head Neck Surg*. 2020;163(1):132–134. https://doi.org/10.1177/0194599820922992.

7. Joffily L, Ungierowicz A, David AG, et al. The close relationship between sudden loss of smell and COVID-19. *Braz J Otorhinolaryngol*. 2020;86(5):632–638. https://doi.org/10.1016/j.bjorl.2020.05.002.

8. Lechien JR, Chiesa-Estomba CM, De Siati DR, et al. Olfactory and gustatory dysfunctions as a clinical presentation of mild-to-moderate forms of the coronavirus disease (COVID-19): a multicenter European study. *Eur Arch Otorhinolaryngol*. 2020;277(8):2251–2261. https://doi.org/10.1007/s00405-020-05965-1.

9. Vaira LA, Hopkins C, Salzano G, et al. Olfactory and gustatory function impairment in COVID-19 patients: Italian objective multicenter-study. *Head Neck*. 2020;42(7):1560–1569. https://doi.org/10.1002/hed.26269.

10. Magnavita N, Tripepi G, Di Prinzio RR. Symptoms in health care workers during the COVID-19 epidemic. A cross-sectional survey. *Int J Environ Res Public Health*. 2020;17(14):5218. https://doi.org/10.3390/ijerph17145218.

11. Tostmann A, Bradley J, Bousema T, et al. Strong associations and moderate predictive value of early symptoms for SARS-CoV-2 test positivity among healthcare workers, the Netherlands, March 2020. *Eurosurveillance*. 2020;25(16):2000508. https://doi.org/10.2807/1560-7917.ES.2020.25.16.2000508.

12. Lee Y, Min P, Lee S, Kim SW. Prevalence and duration of acute loss of smell or taste in COVID-19 patients. *J Korean Med Sci*. 2020;35(18):e174. https://doi.org/10.3346/jkms.2020.35.e174.

13. Güner R, Hasanoğlu İ, Kayaaslan B, et al. COVID-19 experience of the major pandemic response center in the capital: Results of the pandemic's first month in Turkey. *Turk J Med Sci*. 2020;50(8):1801–1809. https://doi.org/10.3906/sag-2006-164.

14. Lechien JR, Chiesa-Estomba CM, Hans S, Barillari MR, Jouffe L, Saussez S. Loss of smell and taste in 2013 European patients with mild to moderate COVID-19. *Ann Intern Med*. 2020;173(8):672–675. https://doi.org/10.7326/M20-2428.

15. Lechien JR, Cabaraux P, Chiesa-Estomba CM, et al. Objective olfactory evaluation of self-reported loss of smell in a case series of 86 COVID-19 patients. *Head Neck*. 2020;42(7):1583–1590. https://doi.org/10.1002/hed.26279.

16. Kobal G, Hummel T, Sekinger B, Barz S, Roscher S, Wolf S. "Sniffin' sticks": screening of olfactory performance. *Rhinology*. 1996;34(4):222–226.

17. Vaira LA, Salzano G, Petrocelli M, Deiana G, Salzano FA, De Riu G. Validation of a self-administered olfactory and gustatory test for the remotely evaluation of COVID-19 patients in home quarantine. *Head Neck*. 2020;42(7):1570–1576. https://doi.org/10.1002/hed.26228.

18. Cain WS, Gent J, Catalanotto FA, Goodspeed RB. Clinical evaluation of olfaction. *Am J Otolaryngol*. 1983;4(4):252–256. https://doi.org/10.1016/s0196-0709(83)80068-4.

19. Cain WS, Gent JF, Goodspeed RB, Leonard G. Evaluation of olfactory dysfunction in the Connecticut chemosensory clinical research center. *Laryngoscope*. 1998;98(1):83–88. https://doi.org/10.1288/00005537-198801000-00017.

20. Massarelli O, Vaira LA, Biglio A, Gobbi R, Dell'aversana Orabona G, De Riu G. Sensory recovery of myomucosal flap oral cavity reconstructions. *Head Neck*. 2018;40(3):467–474. https://doi.org/10.1002/hed.25000.

21. Pingel J, Ostwald J, Pau HW, Hummel T, Just T. Normative data for a solution-based taste test. *Eur Arch Otorhinolaryngol*. 2010;267(12):1911–1917. https://doi.org/10.1007/s00405-010-1276-1.

22. van Riel D, Verdijk R, Kuiken T. The olfactory nerve: a shortcut for influenza and other viral diseases into the central nervous system. *J Pathol*. 2015;235(2):277–287. https://doi.org/10.1002/path.4461.

23. Hummel T, Landis BN, Hüttenbrink K-B. Smell and taste disorders. *GMS Curr Top Otorhinolaryngol Head Neck Surg*. 2012;10:Doc04. https://doi.org/10.3205/cto000077.

24. Netland J, Meyerholz DK, Moore S, Cassell M, Perlman S. Severe acute respiratory syndrome coronavirus infection causes neuronal death in the absence of encephalitis in mice transgenic for human ACE2. *J Virol*. 2008;82(15):7264–7275. https://doi.org/10.1128/JVI.00737-08.

25. Steardo L, Steardo L, Zorec R, Verkhratsky A. Neuroinfection may contribute to pathophysiology and clinical manifestations of COVID-19. *Acta Physiol*. 2020;229:e13473. https://doi.org/10.1111/apha.13473.

26. Sheraton M, Deo N, Kashyap R, Surani S. A review of neurological complications of COVID-19. *Cureus*. 2020;12(5):e8192. https://doi.org/10.7759/cureus.8192.

27. Xu H, Zhong L, Deng J, et al. High expression of ACE2 receptor of 2019-nCoV on the epithelial cells of oral mucosa. *Int J Oral Sci*. 2020;12(1):8. https://doi.org/10.1038/s41368-020-0074-x.

28. Lechien JR, Journe F, Beckers E, et al. Severity of anosmia as early symptom of COVID-19 infection may predict lasting loss of smell. *Front Med (Lausanne)*. 2020;7:582802. https://doi.org/10.3389/fmed.2020.582802.

29. Bigiani A. Gustatory dysfunctions in COVID-19 patients: possible involvement of taste renin-angiotensin system

(RAS). *Eur Arch Otorhinolaryngol.* 2020;277(8):2395. https://doi.org/10.1007/s00405-020-06054-z.

30. Wu Y, Xu X, Chen Z, et al. Nervous system involvement after infection with COVID-19 and other coronaviruses. *Brain Behav Immun.* 2020;87:18–22. https://doi.org/10.1016/j.bbi.2020.03.031.

31. Speth MM, Singer-Cornelius T, Oberle M, Gengler I, Brockmeier SJ, Sedaghat AR. Olfactory dysfunction and sinonasal symptomatology in COVID-19: prevalence, severity, timing, and associated characteristics. *Otolaryngol Head Neck Surg.* 2020;163(1):114–120. https://doi.org/10.1177/0194599820929185.

32. Papa SM, Brundin P, Fung VSC, et al. Impact of the COVID-19 pandemic on Parkinson's disease and movement disorders. *Mov Disord.* 2020;35:711–715.

33. Oakley B, Riddle DR. Receptor cell regeneration and connectivity in olfaction and taste. *Exp Neurol.* 1992;115(1):50–54. https://doi.org/10.1016/0014-4886(92)90220-k.

34. Vaira LA, Deiana G, Foid AG, et al. Objective evaluation of anosmia and ageusia in COVID-19 patients: single-center experience on 72 cases. *Head Neck.* 2020;42(6):1252–1258. https://doi.org/10.1002/hed.26204.

35. Yousaf AR, Duca LM, Chu V, et al. A prospective cohort study in non-hospitalized household contacts with SARS-CoV-2 infection: symptom profiles and symptom change over time. *Clin Infect Dis.* 2020;ciaa1072. https://doi.org/10.1093/cid/ciaa1072. Online ahead of print.

36. Oran DP, Topol EJ. Prevalence of asymptomatic SARS-CoV-2 infection: a narrative review. *Ann Intern Med.* 2020;173(5):362–367. https://doi.org/10.7326/M20-3012.

37. Whitcroft KL, Hummel T. Olfactory dysfunction in COVID-19: diagnosis and management. *JAMA.* 2020;323(24):2512–2514. https://doi.org/10.1001/jama.2020.8391 [published online 2020 May 20].

38. Coelho DH, Kons ZA, Costanzo RM, Reiter ER. Subjective changes in smell and taste during the COVID-19 pandemic: a national survey-preliminary results. *Otolaryngol Head Neck Surg.* 2020;163(2):302–306. https://doi.org/10.1177/0194599820929957 [published online ahead of print, 2020 May 19].

39. Fasano A, Cereda E, Barichella M, et al. COVID-19 in Parkinson's disease patients living in Lombardy, Italy. *Mov Disord.* 2020;35(7):1089–1093. https://doi.org/10.1002/mds.28176.

40. Helmich RC, Bloem BR. The impact of the COVID-19 pandemic on Parkinson's disease: hidden sorrows and emerging opportunities. *J Parkinsons Dis.* 2020;10(2):351–354. https://doi.org/10.3233/JPD-202038.

41. Balestrino R, Rizzone M, Zibetti M, et al. Onset of Covid-19 with impaired consciousness and ataxia: a case report. *J Neurol.* 2020;267(10):2797–2798. https://doi.org/10.1007/s00415-020-09879-0.

42. Diezma-Martín AM, Morales-Married MI, García-Alvarado N, et al. Temblor y ataxia en COVID-19. *Neurologia.* 2020;35(6):409–410. https://doi.org/10.1016/j.nrl.2020.06.005.

43. Rábano-Suárez P, Bermejo-Guerrero L, Méndez-Guerrero A, et al. Generalized myoclonus in COVID-19. *Neurology.* 2020;95(6):e767–e772. https://doi.org/10.1212/WNL.0000000000009829. May 21.

44. Serranoa MM, Pérez-Sánchez JR, Portela Sánchez S, et al. Serotonin syndrome in two COVID-19 patients treated with lopinavir/ritonavir. *J Neurol Sci.* 2020;415:116944. https://doi.org/10.1016/j.jns.2020.116944.

45. Piscitelli D, Perin C, Tremolizzo L. Functional movement disorders in a patient with COVID-19. *Neurol Sci.* 2020;41(9):2343–2344. https://doi.org/10.1007/s10072-020-04593-1.

46. Hoffman LA, Vilensky JA. Encephalitis lethargica: 100 years after the epidemic. *Brain.* 2017;140(8):2246–2251. https://doi.org/10.1093/brain/awx177.

47. Giordano A, Schwarz G, Cacciaguerra L, et al. COVID-19: can we learn from encephalitis lethargica? *Lancet Neurol.* 2020;19(7):570. https://doi.org/10.1016/S1474-4422(20)30189-7.

48. Kang L, Li Y, Hu S, et al. The mental health of medical workers in Wuhan, China dealing with the 2019 novel coronavirus. *Lancet Psychiatry.* 2020;7(3):e14. https://doi.org/10.1016/S2215-0366(20)30047-X.

49. Holmes EA, O'Connor RC, Perry VH, et al. Multidisciplinary research priorities for the COVID-19 pandemic: a call for action for mental health science. *Lancet Psychiatry.* 2020;7(6):547–560. https://doi.org/10.1016/S2215-0366(20)30168-1.

50. Romero-Sanchez CM, Diaz-Maroto I, Fernandez-Diaz E, et al. Neurologic manifestations in hospitalized patients with COVID-19: the ALBACOVID registry. *Neurology.* 2020;95(8):e1060–e1070. https://doi.org/10.1212/WNL.0000000000009937.

51. Rogers JP, Chesney E, Oliver D, et al. Psychiatric and neuropsychiatric presentations associated with severe coronavirus infections: a systematic review and meta-analysis with comparison to the COVID-19 pandemic. *Lancet Psychiatry.* 2020;7(7):611–627. https://doi.org/10.1016/S2215-0366(20)30203-0.

52. Kotfis K, Williams Roberson S, Wilson JE, et al. COVID-19: ICU delirium management during SARS-CoV-2 pandemic. *Crit Care.* 2020;24(1):176. https://doi.org/10.1186/s13054-020-02882-x.

53. Salluh JI, Wang H, Schneider EB, et al. Outcome of delirium in critically ill patients: systematic review and meta-analysis. *BMJ.* 2015;350:h2538. https://doi.org/10.1136/bmj.h2538.

54. Karimi N, Razavi AS, Rouhani N. Frequent convulsive seizures in an adult patient with COVID-19 : a case report. *Iran Red Crescent Med J.* 2020;22(3):e102828.

55. Filatov A, Sharma P, Hindi F, et al. Neurological complications of coronavirus disease (COVID-19): encephalopathy. *Cureus.* 2020;12(3):e7352. https://doi.org/10.7759/cureus.7352.

56. Pilotto A, Odolini S, Masciocchi S, et al. Steroid-responsive encephalitis in coronavirus disease. *Ann Neurol.* 2019;88(2):423–427. https://doi.org/10.1002/ana.25783.

57. Chen T, Wu D, Chen H, et al. Clinical characteristics of 113 deceased patients with coronavirus disease 2019: retrospective study. *BMJ.* 2020;368:m1091. https://doi.org/10.1136/bmj.m1091.

58. Varatharaj A, Thomas N, Ellul MA, et al. Neurological and neuropsychiatric complications of COVID-19 in 153 patients: a UK-wide surveillance study. *Lancet Psychiatry.* 2020;7(10):875–882. https://doi.org/10.1016/s2215-0366(20)30287-x.

59. Helms J, Kremer S, Merdji H, et al. Neurologic features in severe SARS-CoV-2 infection. *N Engl J Med.* 2020;382(23):2268–2270. https://doi.org/10.1056/NEJMc2008597.

60. Hu Y, Chen Y, Zheng Y, et al. Factors related to mental health of inpatients with COVID-19 in Wuhan, China. *Brain Behav Immun.* 2020;89:587–593. https://doi.org/10.1016/j.bbi.2020.07.016.

61. Bo HX, Li W, Yang Y, et al. Posttraumatic stress symptoms and attitude toward crisis mental health services among clinically stable patients with COVID-19 in China. *Psychol Med.* 2020;51(6):1052–1053. https://doi.org/10.1017/S0033291720000999.

62. Zhou J, Liu L, Xue P, et al. Mental health response to the COVID-19 outbreak in China. *Am J Psychiatry.* 2020;177(7):574–575. https://doi.org/10.1176/appi.ajp.2020.20030304.

63. Cheng SK, Wong CW, Tsang J, et al. Psychological distress and negative appraisals in survivors of severe acute respiratory syndrome (SARS). *Psychol Med.* 2004;34(7):1187–1195. https://doi.org/10.1017/s0033291704002272.

64. Wu KK, Chan SK, Ma TM. Posttraumatic stress, anxiety, and depression in survivors of severe acute respiratory syndrome (SARS). *J Trauma Stress.* 2005;18(1):39–42. https://doi.org/10.1002/jts.20004.

65. Mak IW, Chu CM, Pan PC, et al. Long-term psychiatric morbidities among SARS survivors. *Gen Hosp Psychiatry.* 2009;31(4):318–326. https://doi.org/10.1016/j.genhosppsych.2009.03.001.

66. Lam MH, Wing YK, Yu MW, et al. Mental morbidities and chronic fatigue in severe acute respiratory syndrome survivors: long-term follow-up. *Arch Intern Med.* 2009;169(22):2142–2147. https://doi.org/10.1001/archinternmed.2009.384.

67. Troyer EA, Kohn JN, Hong S. Are we facing a crashing wave of neuropsychiatric sequelae of COVID-19? Neuropsychiatric symptoms and potential immunologic mechanisms. *Brain Behav Immun.* 2020;87:34–39. https://doi.org/10.1016/j.bbi.2020.04.027.

68. Dantzer R. Neuroimmune interactions: from the brain to the immune system and vice versa. *Physiol Rev.* 2018;98(1):477–504. https://doi.org/10.1152/physrev.00039.2016.

CHAPTER 11

COVID-19 and Headache Disorders

AARUSHI SUNEJA[a] • ASHHAR ALI[b,c] • AHMAD RIAD RAMADAN[d]
[a]Department of Neurology, Cleveland Clinic, Cleveland, OH, United States, [b]Department of Neurology, Henry Ford Hospital, Detroit, MI, United States, [c]Department of Neurology, Wayne State University School of Medicine, Detroit, MI, United States, [d]Neurologist, Stroke and Neurocritical Care, Henry Ford Neuroscience Institute, Henry Ford Hospital, Detroit, MI, United States

Headache is the most common neurological symptom presenting in patients infected with COVID-19. In large retrospective studies of international populations, the incidence of headache is greater than 70%.[1] Understanding, diagnosing, and treating these patients remain a challenge.

EPIDEMIOLOGY

Headache is the fifth most common COVID-19 symptom after fever, cough, myalgia/fatigue, and dyspnea, and the most frequent neurological manifestation.[2, 3] The prevalence of headache in COVID-19 patients is reported highest in the young (< age 50) and in female patients with mild-to-moderate disease—in both hospitalized and nonhospitalized patients.[2] Studies show that headache appears to be the presenting symptom for 6%–10% of patients globally with or without other signs of systemic involvement.[3] This prevalence is markedly lower than that in SARS in which headache was recorded as a symptom in 20%–56% of infected individuals,[4] but similar to MERS in which it appeared in 11% of patients.[5] Interestingly, health-care professionals also had a high incidence (> 80%) of self-reported headaches during the COVID-19 pandemic, which is thought to be related to high stress work environments and long hours of PPE use.[6] In one study, the presence of headache was associated with, and predictive of, a shorter clinical course of COVID-19 (23.9 days for those with headache vs 31.2 days for those without headache).[7] Risk factors associated with the incidence of headaches include a history of primary headache disorders, comorbidities, fever, and dehydration.[8]

CLINICAL SYNDROMES

Several phenotypes of headaches are found in patients with COVID-19 and the nature and type of headache may evolve during the course of the illness in affected individuals. In one study reporting on the characteristics of headaches in 172 patients with COVID-19, the majority of headaches were holocephalic (52.9%) and pressure-type (40.7%).[8] Fever but also anosmia and ageusia were frequently associated with more severe headaches.[8, 9] While the pressure type seems to be the predominant phenotype, migrainous features were more frequent in patients with a prior history of migraines. When headaches are prodromal, i.e., when they happen as the first COVID-19 manifestation, before the emergence of respiratory symptoms, they tend to be more severe than those who arise later in the course of the disease. This characteristic is important as these prodromal headaches heralded a protracted course of cephalalgia, lingering for up to 6 weeks in a third of the cases in one series.[7]

PATHOPHYSIOLOGY

While the pathophysiology of headache in these patients is yet to be understood, one study reports that patients who did have symptoms of headache and fever and were considered initially negative for COVID-19 based on normal blood work and a negative CT head without contrast, several days later, developed typical COVID-19 symptoms and eventually tested positive for the disease.[2] In another study, two patients with a history of migraine presented with headache as the presenting symptom of COVID-19.[10] These studies may imply that headache can occur prior to, during, or after the presence of other systemic signs of the infection including fever and respiratory illness. One theory is that, similarly to the development of anosmia and ageusia, there is a direct invasion of the trigeminal nerve endings in the nasal cavity by SARS-CoV-2 binding to and internalizing ACE2 receptors. This, in turn, downregulates their functions, which include degradation of angiotensin II and circulating levels of the neuropeptide *calcitonin gene-related peptide* (CGRP), a potent

Neurological Care and the COVID-19 Pandemic. https://doi.org/10.1016/B978-0-323-82691-4.00002-9

vasodilator and nociception mediator which plays a central role in the pathogenesis of migraine.[11] Another theory advances a vascular mechanism through the involvement of endothelial cells with high expression of ACE2 receptors leading to trigeminovascular activation and subsequently headache and migraine secondary to the release of proinflammatory mediators and cytokines.[12]

WORKUP

Evaluation of COVID-19 patients' headaches should include a thorough history and physical examination paying special attention to red flags and ruling out secondary causes while ordering the appropriate neuroimaging as indicated. Classifying the headache pattern, frequency, and characterization is crucial for appropriately diagnosing and treating patients. Patients without a history of a primary headache disorder who are infected with COVID-19 are presumed to have a secondary headache disorder related to the virus. The development of primary headache disorders following recovery from the virus is yet to be reported. Currently, the use of neuroimaging, lumbar puncture, and additional testing is provider-dependent and not standardized for patients who present with headache and COVID-19.

TREATMENT

Treatment options include standard preventive and abortive therapies used for chronic tension-type or chronic migraine headache types. Those patients who go on to develop primary headache syndromes after recovering from the COVID-19 pandemic are also candidates for outpatient preventive and abortive oral medications, CGRP antibodies and onabotulinumtoxinA therapy.

(a) NSAIDs: The use of nonsteroidal antiinflammatories (NSAIDs) in patients infected with COVID-19 remains an area of controversy and generated a lot of media attention earlier in the pandemic over the potential risks associated with taking NSAIDs. Anecdotal evidence cites worsening of COVID-19 symptoms as a result of taking NSAIDs. Both the CDC and FDA agree on the lack of association between intake of NSAIDs and exacerbation of the clinical course.[13] The WHO, which initially cautioned against the use of NSAIDs in patients with COVID-19, later retracted this statement due to the lack of supporting evidence.[14, 15] The British National Health Services (NHS) and the

European Medicines Agency have assumed a similar stance on the matter.[16, 17] The concern over the use of NSAIDs stems from theoretical concerns that NSAIDs can mask the initial COVID-19 symptoms, delaying its detection and contributing to the spread of the disease. There have also been concerns that renal hypoperfusion, a recognized side effect of NSAIDs, could lead to worsening pulmonary edema in COVID-19 cases.[18] Another potential complication of the use of NSAIDs is their effects on lowering body temperature and on impairing the recruitment of neutrophils via inhibition of cyclooxygenase-1 and 2 (COX-1 and COX-2), thereby delaying resolution of inflammation.[19] NSAIDs are also thought to upregulate the expression of the ACE2 receptor, the prime cellular entry point for SARS-CoV-2 virions, making the human host more vulnerable to the virus and its replicative potential. This effect is related to the inhibited synthesis of prostaglandins PGE2 and PGI2 which leads to an increase in systemic vascular resistance and decreased renal perfusion. As a compensatory mechanism, the nephron upregulates ACE2 so it can catalyze the conversion of angiotensin II (Ang II) to angiotensin 1–7 (Ang 1–7), thereby reducing renal vasoconstriction and restoring renal perfusion.[20, 21] The observational French study, RISC (NCT04383899) is currently enrolling patients and studying the effect of ibuprofen on the severity of COVID-19.[22] Another French study, this time a randomized controlled trial, ENACOVID (NCT04325633), is still in the preparatory stage and will be assessing the efficacy of naproxen in treating severe COVID-19.[23]

(b) Steroids: The use of corticosteroids for the specific treatment of headache in patients with COVID-19 has not been studied and therefore data is scant. Although not generally indicated for viral pneumonia due to the risk of prolonged viral shedding, the only recommendation for the use of steroids in COVID-19 thus far is in patients with severe disease, i.e., on mechanical ventilation, where it has shown to reduce mortality.[24]

(c) Other therapies: At this time, there is no contraindication for using triptans in this patient population if the patient's headache-type fits the International Classification of Headache Disorders, 3rd edition (ICHD-3) migraine criteria (add ICHD 3 reference). Inpatient management of headache includes options of intravenous antiemetics (i.e., prochlorperazine and ondansetron), antihistamines, magnesium, valproic acid, and dihydroergotamine, if necessary. The use of opioids in this patient population, like most other headache syndromes, is not recommended.

IMPACT OF THE PANDEMIC ON HEADACHE MANAGEMENT

Headache management for chronic headache patients in the COVID-19 era has been significantly altered due to the development of exclusive telehealth measures implementing outpatient management plans and alternative plans for procedural interventions such as onabotulinumtoxinA injections.[25] Specifically, the management of migraine has been dramatically impacted by the pandemic. In a web-based survey of 1018 patients with migraine during the pandemic in Kuwait, 59.6% reported an increase in the frequency of their headaches, while 10.3% experienced chronification of their migraines.[26] An impressive 61.5% did not maintain communication with their neurologist and 58.7% reported overusing analgesics during this period. Of those patients receiving onabotulinumtoxinA injections, 66.1% reported worsening of their migraines due to the cancelation of their injections. Bridging therapies and the use of CGRP antagonists administered at home may be options to consider during a local virus outbreak.[25, 27]

REFERENCES

1. Lechien JR, Chiesa-Estomba CM, Place S, et al. Clinical and epidemiological characteristics of 1420 European patients with mild-to-moderate coronavirus disease 2019. *J Intern Med.* 2020;288(3):335–344. https://doi.org/10.1111/joim.13089.
2. Mao L, Jin H, Wang M, et al. Neurologic manifestations of hospitalized patients with coronavirus disease 2019 in Wuhan, China. *JAMA Neurol.* 2020. https://doi.org/10.1001/jamaneurol.2020.1127. Published online April 10.
3. Borges do Nascimento IJ, Cacic N, Abdulazeem HM, et al. Novel coronavirus infection (COVID-19) in humans: a scoping review and meta-analysis. *J Clin Med.* 2020;9:E941.
4. Hui DS, Wong PC, Wang C. SARS: clinical features and diagnosis. *Respirology.* 2003;8:S20–S24.
5. Shehata MM, Gomaa MR, Ali MA, Kayali G. Middle East respiratory syndrome coronavirus: a comprehensive review. *Front Med.* 2016;10:120–136.
6. Ong JJY, Bharatendu C, Goh Y, et al. Headaches associated with personal protective equipment—a cross-sectional study among frontline healthcare workers during COVID-19. *Headache.* 2020;60(5):864–877. https://doi.org/10.1111/head.13811.
7. Caronna E, Ballvé A, Llauradó A, et al. Headache: a striking prodromal and persistent symptom, predictive of COVID-19 clinical evolution. *Cephalalgia.* 2020;40(13):1410–1421. https://doi.org/10.1177/0333102420965157.
8. Magdy R, Hussein M, Ragaie C, et al. Characteristics of headache attributed to COVID-19 infection and predictors of its frequency and intensity: a cross sectional study. *Cephalalgia.* 2020;40(13):1422–1431. https://doi.org/10.1177/0333102420965140.
9. Rocha-Filho PAS, Magalhães JE. Headache associated with COVID-19: frequency, characteristics and association with anosmia and ageusia. *Cephalalgia.* 2020;40(13):1443–1451. https://doi.org/10.1177/0333102420966770.
10. Bolay H, Gül A, Baykan B. COVID-19 is a real headache! *Headache.* 2020;60(7):1415–1421. https://doi.org/10.1111/head.13856.
11. Xu P, et al. ACE2/ANG-(1–7)/Mas pathway in the brain: the axis of good. *Am J Physiol Regul Integr Comp Physiol.* 2011;**300**:R804–R817.
12. Patil J, et al. Intraneuronal angiotensinergic system in rat and human dorsal root ganglia. *Regul Pept.* 2010;162:90–98.
13. Maddipatla M. FDA says no scientific evidence that ibuprofen worsens coronavirus. *Reuters.* 2020. Thomson Reuters, 19 March www.reuters.com/article/us-health-coronavirus-usa-fda/fda-says-no-scientific-evidence-that-ibuprofen-worsens-coronavirus-idUSKBN21645S.
14. World Health Organization. *Could Ibuprofen Worsen Disease for People With COVID-19?* Geneva: World Health Organization; 2020.
15. *The Use of Non-Steroidal Anti-Inflammatory Drugs (NSAIDs) in Patients With COVID-19.* World Health Organization; 19 April 2020. www.who.int/news-room/commentaries/detail/the-use-of-non-steroidal-anti-inflammatory-drugs-(nsaids)-in-patients-with-covid-19.
16. Francisco EM. *EMA Gives Advice on the Use of Non-Steroidal Anti-Inflammatories for COVID-19.* European Medicines Agency; 19 June 2020. www.ema.europa.eu/en/news/ema-gives-advice-use-non-steroidal-anti-inflammatories-covid-19.
17. *NHS Guidance on NSAIDs in COVID-19.* Guidelines; 5 November 2020. www.guidelines.co.uk/infection/nhs-guidance-on-nsaids-in-covid-19/455488.article.
18. Li XC, Zhang J, Zhuo JL. The vasoprotective axes of the renin-angiotensin system: physiological relevance and therapeutic implications in cardiovascular, hypertensive and kidney diseases. *Pharmacol Res.* 2017;125(Pt A):21–38. https://doi.org/10.1016/j.phrs.2017.06.005.
19. Fukunaga K, Kohli P, Bonnans C, Fredenburgh LE, Levy BD. Cyclooxygenase 2 plays a pivotal role in the resolution of acute lung injury. *J Immunol.* 2005;174:5033–5039.
20. Tikellis C, Thomas MC. Angiotensin-converting enzyme 2 (ACE2) is a key modulator of the renin angiotensin system in health and disease. *Int J Pept.* 2012;2012:256294. https://doi.org/10.1155/2012/256294.
21. Cabbab ILN, Manalo RVM. Anti-inflammatory drugs and the renin-angiotensin-aldosterone system: current knowledge and potential effects on early SARS-CoV-2 infection. *Virus Res.* 2021;291:198190. https://doi.org/10.1016/j.virusres.2020.198190012.

22. *Role of Ibuprofen and Other Medicines on Severity of Coronavirus Disease 2019—Full Text View.* ClinicalTrials.gov; 11 June 2020. clinicaltrials.gov/ct2/show/NCT04383899.

23. *Efficacy of Addition of Naproxen in the Treatment of Critically Ill Patients Hospitalized for COVID-19 Infection—Full Text View.* ClinicalTrials.gov; 14 April 2020. clinicaltrials.gov/ct2/show/NCT04325633.

24. RECOVERY Collaborative Group, Horby P, Lim WS, et al. Dexamethasone in hospitalized patients with covid-19—preliminary report. *N Engl J Med.* 2020. https://doi.org/10.1056/NEJMoa2021436. NEJMoa2021436. [published online ahead of print, 2020 Jul 17].

25. Ali A. Delay in onabotulinumtoxin A treatment during the COVID-19 pandemic-perspectives from a virus hotspot. *Headache.* 2020. https://doi.org/10.1111/head.13830.

26. Al-Hashel JY, Ismail II. Impact of coronavirus disease 2019 (COVID-19) pandemic on patients with migraine: a web-based survey study. *J Headache Pain.* 2020;21:115. https://doi.org/10.1186/s10194-020-01183-6.

27. Silvestro M, Tessitore A, Tedeschi G, Russo A. Migraine in the time of COVID-19. *Headache.* 2020;60:988–989. https://doi.org/10.1111/head.13803.

CHAPTER 12

Treatment Approach, Pharmacological Agents and Vaccines

QUINTON J. TAFOYA[a] • VICTORIA WATSON[b] • JACOB PAWLOSKI[c] • GHADA A. MOHAMED[d] • AHMAD RIAD RAMADAN[e]
[a]Department of Pharmacy, Veterans Affairs, San Antonio, TX, United States, [b]Department of Neurosurgery, Southern Illinois University, Springfield, IL, United States, [c]Department of Neurosurgery, Henry Ford Hospital, Detroit, MI, United States, [d]Department of Neurology, Henry Ford Health System, Detroit, MI, United States, [e]Neurologist, Stroke and Neurocritical Care, Henry Ford Neuroscience Institute, Henry Ford Hospital, Detroit, MI, United States

TREATMENT APPROACH FOR THE HOSPITALIZED PATIENT WITH COVID-19

Introduction

The goal of this chapter is to inform the neurologist of the disease-specific treatments that exist and are recommended for the patient with COVID-19. The proposed approach to management is tiered according to the severity of illness and encompasses medications that are recommended by several notable organizations, such as the National Institute of Health (NIH) and the Society of Critical Care Medicine (SCCM), according to their most recent guidelines. Treatment of severe COVID-19 is complex and requires expertise in critical care medicine including hemodynamic and ventilatory support, topics that are beyond the scope of this book. An appendix grouping several medications related to the care of patients with COVID-19 is provided at the end of this book (Appendix: Medication). We also present a summary table of the various treatments with a particular mention of the neurological complications and considerations for each one of them (Table 12.1).

Treatment Approach for Patients With COVID-19

The approach more commonly adopted to caring for the hospitalized patient with COVID-19 depends on the degree of severity of the illness. Therefore defining severity in COVID-19 is important and one of the first steps in managing such patients. Dyspnea is the key in categorizing patients with suspected or confirmed COVID-19. Patients with no dyspnea but with other symptoms such as fever, chills, cough, malaise, anosmia, headaches, and upper respiratory symptoms are considered nonsevere and rarely require hospitalization. Once dyspnea is observed and the patient requires supplemental oxygen, the patient's condition is deemed severe.[5] The *Surviving Sepsis Campaign Guidelines on the Management of Adults with Coronavirus Disease 2019 (COVID-19) in the ICU*, for instance, further differentiates severe from critical disease. Severe disease concerns patients with clinical signs of pneumonia (e.g., tachypnea, dyspnea, fever, and cough) and one of the following: respiratory rate greater than 30 breaths per minute, severe respiratory distress, or oxygen saturation of less than 90% on room air. Critical disease identifies patients with acute respiratory distress syndrome (ARDS) or respiratory distress requiring mechanical ventilation, sepsis, or septic shock.[5] The *NIH Panel on COVID-19 Treatment Guidelines* published a pharmacological management based on disease severity, which can be found in Fig. 12.1.[6]

In general terms:

1. Only supportive treatment and monitoring is recommended for patients with nonsevere disease.
2. Anti-SARS-CoV-2 monoclonal antibody combinations, such as bamlanivimab plus etesevimab, or casirivimab plus imdevimab, should be considered for nonhospitalized patients or patients with mild COVID-19 hospitalized for reasons other than COVID-19 who are at high risk of disease progression.
3. Dexamethasone is strongly recommended in patients who require any amount of supplemental oxygen and/or mechanical ventilation or extracorporeal membrane oxygenation (ECMO).
4. Remdesivir is the only FDA-approved medication for the treatment of COVID-19. It is recommended in patients on supplemental oxygen but not in patients who present to the hospital needing mechanical ventilation or ECMO, since their condition is considered too advanced to derive any significant

Neurological Care and the COVID-19 Pandemic. https://doi.org/10.1016/B978-0-323-82691-4.00015-7

TABLE 12.1
Selected COVID-19-Specific Treatments in Use in the United States and Other Countries.

Name	Mechanism of Action	Efficacy	Safety	Neurologic Considerations
Bamlanivimab + etesevimab	Bamlanivimab (also known as LY-CoV555 and LY3819253) is a neutralizing monoclonal antibody that targets the RBD of the S protein of SARS-CoV-2. Etesevimab (also known as LY-CoV016 and LY3832479) is another neutralizing monoclonal antibody that binds to a different but overlapping epitope in the RBD of the SARS-CoV-2 S protein.	Authorized for use in outpatient cases at high risk of progression to severe COVID-19. 70% relative risk reduction of hospitalization or death compared to placebo. Not authorized for hospitalized patients or those requiring oxygen supplementation except in special circumstances.	Associated with few and mainly low-grade toxic effects. BLAZE-1 trial data demonstrated nausea, diarrhea, dizziness, and headaches as most common side effects. 1% of patients experienced hypersensitivity reactions.[1]	No significant reported neurologic complications or considerations to date.
Baricitinib	Selective inhibitor of JAK-1 and −2 and causes inhibition of the intracellular signaling pathway of cytokines known to be elevated in severe Covid-19 including IL-2 and IL-6.	ACT-2 Trial compared Baricitinib + remdesivir to remdesivir alone with 30% improvement in time to recovery and clinical status in the combination group. Results were more positive in patients receiving high-flow oxygen and noninvasive BIPAP.[2]	Adverse events were less common in combination therapy arm than in the remdesivir alone arm. Most common side effects include upper respiratory infections, headaches, and nasopharyngitis. Dose-related neutropenia and lymphopenia have been observed.	No major neurologic complications reported. 20% CNS penetration (higher than most other reported COVID-19 treatments)
Casirivimab + imdevimab	Casirivimab (previously REGN10933) and imdevimab (previously REGN10987) are recombinant human monoclonal antibodies that bind to nonoverlapping epitopes of the S protein RBD of SARS-CoV-2.	Available through FDA emergency use authorization for mild-moderate COVID-19 cases at high risk of progression to severe disease. 71% relative risk reduction of hospitalization or death compared to placebo. Not authorized for hospital patients or those requiring oxygen supplementation except in special circumstances.	Associated with few and mainly low-grade toxic effects. Percentages of patients with hypersensitivity reactions, infusion-related reactions, and other adverse events were similar in the combined REGN-COV2 dose groups and the placebo group.[3]	No significant reported neurologic complications or considerations to date.
Convalescent Plasma	Pooled human IgG antibodies from COVID-19 survivors contain IgG with a high titer (1:1000) of anti-SARS-CoV-2 S protein	15% reduction in progression to severe COVID-19 when given in the first 72-h of symptom onset.	No major adverse events in largest COVID-19 trial, although transfusions may be associated with fluid overload, transfusion associated lung injury (TRALI), and allergic reaction	No significant reported neurologic complications or considerations to date.

Drug	Mechanism	Efficacy/Use	Side effects	Neurologic effects/CNS penetration
Corticosteroids	Physiologic activity to reduce systemic inflammatory responses via effects on cytokine production, potentially reducing inflammation-related lung damage	Reduction in death rates when administered to hospital patients receiving supplemental O_2 or mechanical ventilation (RECOVERY trial).[4]	High doses associated with metabolic derangement, increased infection risk, increased viral replication, delayed viral clearance.	Protracted use can contribute to myopathy, neuromuscular weakness, delirium, and psychiatric symptoms.
Hydroxychloroquine/chloroquine	Impacts viral entry into cells and effects viral protein synthesis through multiple pathways.	Conflicting results; most randomized studies conclude no clinical benefit when HCQ is added to standard of care. Not recommended for treatment of inpatient or outpatient COVID-19.	Narrow therapeutic index; can cause QT prolongation, torsade de pointes, bone marrow suppression, seizure, retinopathy, and myopathy.	Mood disorders, psychosis. At high doses can cause ototoxicity leading to hearing loss, tinnitus, and imbalance. 21% CNS penetration.
Immunoglobulin (IVIG)	Pooled human IgG antibodies consisting of Fab fragment and Fc fragment which aid in antigen recognition and immune system response. Used in a variety of autoimmune and inflammatory disorders as well as tested in bacterial, viral and fungal infections.	Significant reduction of in-hospital mortality in small randomized, controlled trials of IVIG versus placebo. Has been studied specifically in lymphopenic patients	Risks similar to the expected risks of plasma transfusion and transfusion reactions. Infusions must be done slowly over several days.	Headache and dizziness. Thromboembolic events (TIA, stroke, CVST). Rare reports of aseptic meningitis and acute encephalopathy following IVIG infusion have been suggested from immunoallergic reaction from entry of IgG into CSF spaces
Ivermectin	Inhibits viral replication; also used in *strongyloides* and *onchocerca* infections	Decreases SARS-CoV-2 replication in vitro, but failed to improve time to resolution of symptoms in humans	Common side effects include rash, muscle aches, headache, fever	Dizziness, vertigo, tremor, lethargy. Encephalopathy, stupor or coma in individuals with mdr-1 gene mutations or when combined with CYP-3A4 inhibitors.
Lopinavir +/− ritonavir	HIV-1 protease inhibitor + ritonavir booster (inhibits lopinavir metabolism). Also effective in treating SARS-CoV.	Some reports of efficacy in individual cases, but more studies are needed.	Most common side effects include renal tubular acidosis, AKI, dermatitis.	Used in a case of COVID-19-associated cerebritis with significant improvement. 0.02% CNS penetration.
Remdesivir	Adenosine analog, incorporates into viral RNA, disrupts transcription	Shortens time to recovery when administered within 1 day of symptom onset	Associated with AKI or transaminitis	No neurologic adverse events reported. <5% CNS penetration.
Tocilizumab	Recombinant anti-IL-6 receptor monoclonal antibody which can limit cytokine-related pulmonary injury from cytokine storm. Used in treatment of rheumatoid arthritis.	Has demonstrated efficacy in improving fevers, oxygen requirements, and CT findings in patients with severe COVID-19 pneumonia. 12% reduction in mortality in meta-analysis of use in COVID-19 patients.	Associated with infections (skin, cellulitis), gastrointestinal disorders and transfusion reactions.	Few case reports of cerebral microangiopathy and leukoencephalopathy when used in patients with pre-existing rheumatologic conditions. 0.1% CNS penetration

DISEASE SEVERITY

PANEL'S RECOMMENDATIONS

Disease Severity	Panel's Recommendations
Not Hospitalized, Mild to Moderate COVID-19	For patients who are not at high risk for disease progression, provide supportive care and symptomatic management **(AIII)**. For patients who are at high risk of disease progression (as defined by the FDA EUA criteria for treatment with anti-SARS-CoV-2 monoclonal antibodies), use one of the following combinations: • **Bamlanivimab plus etesevimab (AIIa)** • **Casirivimab plus imdevimab (AIIa)**
Hospitalized but Does Not Require Supplemental Oxygen	Thera are insufficient data to recommend either for or against the routine use of remdesivir. For patients at high risk of disease progression, the use of remdesivir may be appropriate.
Hospitalized and Requires Supplemental Oxygen	Use one of the following options: • **Remdesivir**[a,b] (e.g., for patients who require minimal supplemental oxygen) **(BIIa)** • **Dexamethasone**[c] **plus remdesivir**[a,b] (e.g., for patients who require increasing amounts of supplemental oxygen) **(BIII)**[d,e] • **Dexamethasone**[c] (e.g., when combination therapy with remdesivir cannot be used or is not available) **(BI)**
Hospitalized and Requires Oxygen Delivery Through a High-Flow Device or Noninvasive Ventilation	Use one of the following options: • **Dexamethasone**[c] **(AI)**[e] • **Dexamethasone**[c] **plus remdesivir**[a,b] **(BIII)**[d,e] For patients who were recently hospitalized[f] with rapidly increasing oxygen needs and systemic inflammation: • Add **tocilizumab**[g] to one of the two options above **(BIIa)**
Hospitalized and Requires Invasive Mechanical Ventilation or ECMO	• **Dexamethasone**[c] **(AI)**[h] For patients who are within 24 hours of admission to the ICU: • **Dexamethasone**[c] **plus tocilizumab**[g] **(BIIa)**

Rating of Recommendations: A = Strong; B = Moderate; C = Optional
Rating of Evidence: I = One or more randomized trials without major limitations; IIa = Other randomized trials or subgroup analyses of randomized trials; IIb = Nonrandomized trials or observational cohort studies; III = Expert opinion

FIG. 12.1 Pharmacological management guide of patients with COVID-19 based on disease severity. (From COVID-19 Treatment Guidelines Panel. Coronavirus Disease 2019 (COVID-19) Treatment Guidelines. National Institutes of Health. Available at https://www.covid19treatmentguidelines.nih.gov/. Accessed May 8, 2021.)

benefit from the antiviral. The combination dexamethasone/remdesivir has not been studied in patients requiring mechanical ventilation.

5. Interleukin-6 antagonists, such as tocilizumab, can be added to dexamethasone in patients who display evidence of systemic inflammation or whose respiratory condition rapidly decompensates, requiring escalating levels of oxygen, increasing settings on noninvasive ventilation, or mechanical ventilation.

Importantly, several societies and organizations now recommend against the use of hydroxychloroquine or chloroquine (with or without azithromycin), for either hospitalized or nonhospitalized patients with COVID-19.[6, 7] Also, due to poor-quality data, insufficient data, or lack of benefit, the use of convalescent plasma or intravenous immunoglobulin (IVIG) is not authorized for use in nonhospitalized patients.[6] The NIH Panel on COVID-19 Treatment Guidelines recommends against its use in patients with severe disease who are mechanically ventilated, or those who are hospitalized but not on mechanical ventilation, except in the context of a clinical trial. It is however authorized under the EAU for use in hospitalized patients with immune deficiencies.[6] Additionally, due to lack of evidence, the guidelines recommend neither for nor against the routine use of therapeutic anticoagulation for hospitalized patients with COVID-19 who do not have confirmed venous thromboembolic disease.[5, 6]

Special Considerations for COVID-19-Specific Treatments in Patients With Neurological Conditions

In this section, we provide information about the neurological considerations of drugs used for the specific treatment of COVID-19. These drugs and a summary of their neurotoxicities can be found in Table 12.1. We hope that neurologists consulting on hospitalized patients with COVID-19 will find this data relevant and useful.

Corticosteroids. Corticosteroids can have a plethora of complications depending on their route of administration, dose, and duration of use. In addition to hyperglycemia which can worsen encephalopathy, delay wound healing and independently worsen outcomes in patients with stroke or cerebral edema, these drugs have other more direct effects on central and peripheral nervous systems. Mood disturbances are the most pervasive and can occur with a few days of treatment, usually causing early euphoria and anxiety. Depression can set in with more prolonged therapy.[7] Memory impairment also occurs with more protracted treatment and usually happens with increased frequency and more rapidly in elderly patients (3 months as opposed to 1 year).[8] Psychosis also tends to happen with prolonged therapy and is therefore not expected in steroid therapy used for COVID-19 infection.[9] Delirium, sleep disturbances, and akathisia (psychomotor restlessness) are typical central nervous side effects of corticosteroids. In addition to their central complications, steroids can lead to ICU-acquired weakness, ICUAW (also known as critical care myopathy and neuropathy), especially when co-administered with neuromuscular blocking agents, a combination that is commonly used for the treatment of severe ARDS in patients with COVID-19. The association between steroids and ICUAW is almost twofold.[10] Other important risk factors for ICUAW are mechanical ventilation, prolonged ICU stay, and sepsis and septic shock.[11] Finally, although a ubiquitous treatment for it, steroids can initially worsen a myasthenic crisis and need to be started or increased with caution in patients with a confirmed or suspected diagnosis of MG. IVIG or plasmapheresis may be needed as a bridge to steroids when the symptoms get worse with treatment.[12]

Hydroxychloroquine/chloroquine. The antimalarial drugs are associated with a high risk of retinopathy which is dose and duration dependent (7.5%).[13] Ototoxicity in the form of sensorineural hearing loss, tinnitus, and imbalance can happen with both chloroquine and hydroxychloroquine and tends to happen more abruptly with the former and more insidiously with the latter. The ototoxicity risk at the doses used in COVID-19 infection is however not known.[14] Furthermore, these drugs can also prolong the QT interval, making the choice of antipsychotics in delirious patients with COVID-19 more challenging.[15] They have been linked to several psychiatric manifestations such as mania, depression, and psychosis as well as central nervous side effects like insomnia, dizziness, and headache in 4%–6% of patients.[15] Although seizure is listed in the package insert for both drugs, it is a very rare occurrence and data is limited to case reports and case series, without any causal relationship firmly established.[16]

Immunoglobulins. Thromboembolic events after IVIG can occur within hours to days of treatment for arterial clots and days to weeks for venous ones.[17] They can lead to acute coronary syndromes, transient ischemic attacks (TIA) and stroke, cerebral venous sinus thrombosis, pulmonary embolism, and deep venous thrombosis (DVT). Adequate hydration, slowing down the rate or breaking down the infusion into several smaller doses can help prevent this complication. Discontinuing the treatment is likely the safest approach in cases of thromboembolic events. Aseptic meningitis is another neurological complication of IVIG. It occurs in about 1% of patients and its pathophysiology is poorly understood. It is a self-limiting condition and resolves by slowing down the rate of infusion along with symptomatic care including use of proper hydration, analgesics, antipyretics, and antihistamines.[18]

Ivermectin. The anthelmintic is not used or recommended for use in COVID-19 outside of clinical trials in the United States. It is used in countries like India, South Africa, Zimbabwe, or Mexico. This drug is known to cause dizziness (2.8%), vertigo, tremor, and lethargy (<1%). Although coma and encephalopathy were reported in patients treated with ivermectin for *Onchocerciasis volvulus* in Africa, many of these cases were thought to be due to concomitant infection with *Loa loa* (loiasis). Cotreatment with drugs that inhibit the CYP3A4 enzyme can also predispose to higher neurotoxicity from ivermectin.[19]

Tocilizumab. Headaches (7%) and dizziness (3%) are the most commonly reported nervous side effects of tocilizumab. A case of multifocal cerebral microangiopathy arising shortly after a single infusion of the medication in a patient with rheumatoid arthritis was reported and was believed to be an immune-mediated vasculitic process.[20] Additionally, two cases of leukoencephalopathy in patients with rheumatoid arthritis treated with tocilizumab were reported.[21, 22] One of them was associated with limbic encephalitis and both cases showed symptoms several months following treatment with the IL-6 antagonist. These are believed to be exceedingly rare occurrences.

COVID-19 VACCINES

Introduction

Due to the rapid spread and devastating effects caused by SARS-CoV-2 on the human loss of life and livelihood, the need for vaccine development has been an unrivaled priority.[23] Publication of the viral genome in January 2020 enabled many pharmaceutical companies around the world to start developing a variety of vaccines against the pathogen.[24]

Vaccines have to go through a rigorous series of steps before being approved for marketing.[25] After research, discovery, and development, the vaccine is tested in animals (preclinical stage). In all, 77 COVID-19 vaccines are currently undergoing animal trials.[26] If the vaccine passes this first checkpoint, it proceeds to phase 1 clinical trials. In this phase, the safety of the vaccine using various doses is determined by testing it in a small group of healthy volunteers (20–100 subjects).[25] There are currently 49 COVID-19 vaccines in phase 1 trials.[26] Phase 2 trials are randomized, controlled, and recruit hundreds of patients at risk for developing the condition. The goal is to measure the vaccine's immunogenicity (i.e., the ability of the vaccine to elicit an immune response) and determine its tolerability and safety.[25] A total of 37 COVID-19 vaccines are currently in phase 2 trials.[26] Phase 3 aims at gathering more information on the effectiveness of the vaccine and detecting less common side effects by recruiting a much larger cohort of subjects (usually, thousands) and randomizing them to vaccine or placebo arm.[25] For vaccine approval, the United States FDA generally recommends that there be at least a 50% reduction in the primary endpoint of the phase 3 trial, which is usually effective in vaccine development.[25] In all, 27 COVID-19 vaccines are presently in this third stage of the study.[26] In the United States, three vaccines (BNT162b2, mRNA-1273, and Ad26. COV2·S) have received authorization for emergency use by the FDA but are not yet fully approved.[26] Four vaccine trials were ultimately abandoned due to lack of effectiveness.[26]

Further complicating the matter are the naturally occurring sporadic mutations of the virus leading to regional variants that are more transmissible, evade the traditional detection assays, and make vaccine development more challenging. Among the many SARS-CoV-2 virus mutants present across the world, five are of specific concern in the United States because they lead to more severe disease, greater transmissibility, and decreased neutralization by antibodies acquired via infection or vaccination: the United Kingdom, the South African, the Brazilian, and the two California variants.[27, 28]

Of note, none of these vaccines has been studied in human pregnancy or children, although some trials are currently underway in these populations. Long-term effects are still not known due to a lack of data but are presumed to be few. All currently used vaccines are in the form of intramuscular injection although there are several nasal mist vaccines in development.[29]

At the time of writing, at the end of the first week of May 2021, approximately 257 million vaccines have been administered in the United States, with 34% of the population being fully vaccinated and 46% having received at least one dose. Pfizer-BioNTech's vaccine leads in the number of doses administered followed closely by Moderna's mRNA-1273. Johnson & Johnson/Janssen's Ad26.COV2·S vaccine trails behind others due to the later issuance of emergency use authorization by the FDA.[30]

Types of SARS-CoV-2 Vaccines

Most human antibodies produced in response to SARS-CoV-2 are in the form of neutralizing antibodies directed against the receptor-binding domain of the spike protein, which is located on the surface of the viral envelope and acts as the portal of viral entry into the host cells (Chapter 2).[31] Variants of SARS-CoV-2 generally carry a mutation in the receptor-binding domain of the spike protein.[28] Although most mutations make the virus less infectious, some of them, like D614G present in all the variants of interest mentioned above, have been shown to increase the virus' affinity to the ACE2 receptor, evade the host's neutralizing antibodies, and jeopardize vaccine effectiveness since the vast majority of vaccines target the spike protein.[32, 33]

Vaccines currently developed for COVID-19 come in different flavors, such as mRNA, adenoviral vector, protein subunit, DNA, or inactivated viruses. Each vaccine type is associated with a different mechanism of action, delivery method, advantages, and disadvantages. Here, we give a brief overview of the various types along with a description of a few pharmaceutical products in use around the world for each category. Table 12.2 gives a summary of the efficacy, regimen, and neurological complications of some of the marketed vaccines in use around the world.

TABLE 12.2
Selected COVID-19 Vaccines With Emergency Use Authorization Around the World.

Name	Company	Vaccine Type	Reported Efficacy (%)	Regimen	Notable Neurological Side Effects[a]
BNT162b2	Pfizer/BioNTech	mRNA	95	2 doses; 3 weeks apart	
mRNA-1273	Moderna	mRNA	94.5	2 doses; 4 weeks apart	
Ad26.COV2-S	Johnson & Johnson/ Janssen	Adenovirus vector	61–72	1 dose	CVST (VITT/TTS)
Sputnik V	Gamaleya Research Institute of Epidemiology and Microbiology	Adenovirus vector	91.6	2 doses; 3 weeks apart	
AZD1222	Oxford/ Astrazeneca	Adenovirus vector	79	2 doses; 8–12 weeks apart	- CVST (VITT/TTS) - Transverse myelitis (1 case)
ZF2001	Anhui Zhifei/ Longcom Institute of Medical Biology at the Chinese Academy of Medical Sciences	Protein subunit	Unknown	3 doses; 4 weeks apart	
BBIBP-CorV	Sinopharm	Attenuated	79.34	2 doses; 3 weeks apart	
CoronaVac	Sinovac	Attenuated	50.38–83.5	2 doses; 2 weeks apart	
BBV152	Bharat Biotech	Attenuated	80.6	2 doses; 4 weeks apart	

[a] Only those neurological side effects that were probably related to vaccination are noted here. No causal relationship was found between the reported cases of Bell's palsy in mRNA vaccine recipients, or GBS in J&J/Janssen vaccine recipients. Dizziness and headaches are mild neurological side effects reported with many of the vaccines included in this table.

mRNA Vaccines

The COVID-19 pandemic has been the stage for the rise of a novel type of vaccine, the mRNA vaccine. These vaccines were first investigated in the 1990s after Wolff reported an effective direct gene transfer via mRNA inoculation.[34, 35]

The DNA template of the gene of choice, i.e., the receptor-binding domain of the spike protein in SARS-CoV-2, is cloned into the DNA template plasmid.[36] The desired sequence is flanked by a terminal 5' cap structure and a 40–120 adenosine residue 3' poly-A tail.[36–38] After the mRNA is safely and effectively delivered to the cytosol of the cell, the resulting proteins are translated.[35] There is no need for the mRNA to access the cell's nucleus which simplifies drug delivery to some degree.[39] Since they are RNA-based molecules, there is no risk of incorporation into and modification of the host genome since humans do not possess reverse transcriptase.[35] There is also no risk of infection from the parent virus, as the delivered mRNA does not code for the proteins that are essential for viral replication. It was traditionally thought that mRNA vaccines did not confer significant stimulation of the immune system, but this has since been disproven.[40]

The problem with mRNA vaccines is their expeditious degradation once they are in the human body by mRNases.[41] Additionally, the mRNA itself is immunogenic and functions as a pathogen-associated molecular pattern (PAMP) which is recognized by the innate immune system.[42] For this reason, mRNA technology had not been widely used until the current pandemic. In order to circumvent the abovementioned issues, the mRNA vaccines have been embedded in lipid nanoparticles, protecting them from quick degradation and inadvertent activation of the innate immune system.[23] The lipid layer of the lipid nanoparticle facilitates binding and endocytosis into the cell.[39] The nanoparticles also contain polyethylene glycol (PEG), which increases the half-life of the molecule.[43] PEG has never before been used in an approved vaccine, although it is present in other types of medications. Allergists and immunologists have, at times, raised concerns that the substance can cause anaphylaxis, due to the high numbers of circulating antibodies to PEG in some individuals.[43]

There are several distinct advantages to mRNA vaccines. First, it is considered to be safer than DNA-derived vaccines, as there is no interaction with the genetic makeup of the cell. It is also much easier to deliver, as the mRNA does not need to penetrate the nuclear envelope as does a DNA-based vaccine.[39] The proteins are transcribed in the cytosol of the cell and are expressed only transiently. Disadvantages of the mRNA vaccines include the novelty and lack of long-term data regarding their use, the need for deep refrigeration for storage stability (in the case of the BNT162b2 vaccine), and their higher cost of production. We discuss here the two mRNA viruses marketed in the United States and other countries.

BNT162b2/tozinameran

The first vaccine approved for human use was the Pfizer-BioNTech vaccine by the name of BNT162b2.[26] The immune response consists of antibodies to the receptor-binding domain.[24] Its efficacy was announced at 95% on November 9, 2020, and it was authorized for emergency use by the FDA a month later, on December 11, making it the first vaccine to be authorized in the United States.[44, 45] It is a two-dose regimen, with the doses administered 3 weeks apart.

The initial downside of this vaccine is the fact that it must be stored in special freezers at −70° Celsius.[44] Many locations did not have the required equipment, but on February 19, 2021, the company announced that it is safe to store at a higher temperature.[45] Other countries have authorized its use such as Bahrain, Brazil, New Zealand, Saudi Arabia, and Switzerland.[26] It has also received emergency use validation from the WHO.[46]

In January, the discovery of more transmissible disease variants was a concern for vaccine development. BNT162b2 was tested against the Brazilian variant P.1 and demonstrated an effective response. However, the antibodies were found to be less effective against the South African variant B.1.351.[47] In February, Pfizer-BioNTech announced a trial that will investigate a booster vaccine against the South African variant.[48]

While there are no published studies involving pregnant women, Pfizer and BioNTech announced the registration of a trial looking into vaccine safety and effectiveness in this population. A report published in the *New England Journal of Medicine* did not reveal a preliminary safety concern for pregnant women who received an mRNA vaccine.[49] In March 2021, Pzifer and BioNTech announced that the vaccine is very effective in the 12–15 years of age group.[48] Two months later, in May 2021, the FDA authorized the BNT162b2 vaccine for emergency use in adolescents.[50]

mRNA-1273

Moderna's mRNA-1273 was approved for emergency use in adults by the FDA on December 18, 2020, after its efficacy was announced at 94.1%.[51] It was the second vaccine to gain authorization from the US FDA. Encoded in the mRNA are antibodies to the S-2 P antigen.[24] The two 100 μg doses are given 4 weeks apart.

It differs from the Pfizer vaccine in that it does not need to be stored in a special freezer.[52] It is authorized for use in Canada, Israel, the European Union, Switzerland, and the United Kingdom.[53] In December of 2020, the company announced a trial to test the vaccine in patients aged 12–18 years. Further testing in babies and younger children was announced in March of 2021.[54]

Another similar vaccine, also produced by Moderna, is named mRNA-1273.351. This vaccine is currently in phase 1 clinical trials and targets the South African variant B.1.351 SARS CoV. The study is led by the National Institute for Allergy and Infectious Disease and is looking to enroll 210 adult participants in the cities of Seattle, Nashville, Atlanta, and Cincinnati.[55]

Adenovirus Vector Vaccines

Human double-stranded DNA adenoviruses are a common entity, with several versions of the common cold or gastroenteritis developing from this strain of pathogens. Adenoviruses differ from other viruses in that the genome is well known and relatively easy to manipulate due to its small size.[56] By deleting the initial E1A unit of the genome, the virus is prevented from replicating and infecting human cells.[56] It is generally believed that vaccines developed via this method are superior to other forms of vaccines in terms of responsiveness.[57–59]

One disadvantage to this method of vaccine development is the presence of preexisting immunity to adenoviruses. Because adenoviral diseases are common, the average adult has immunity to the more common strains such as AdHu5. This complicates the use of this vector for vaccination, as it would require antibody testing prior to vaccination to ensure that one lacks preexisting immunity.[56]

Ad26.COV2.S

The vaccine produced by Johnson & Johnson/Janssen is the first single-dose vaccine to be authorized by the US FDA on February 27, 2021, making it the third vaccine authorized for use in the United States. The background for the vaccine came from work done at Beth Israel Deaconess Medical Center (BIDMC), as researchers were developing a vaccine for SARS-CoV-2 using Adenovirus 26. Johnson & Johnson had utilized this technology to engineer vaccines for Ebola and announced their collaboration with BIDMC in January 2020. Its efficacy was found to be 72% in the United States, with lower rates in South Africa and Latin American countries as a result of the variants in those locations.[60] It has received emergency use validation from the WHO and has emergency use authorization in many other countries. It can be stored in the refrigerator but will last longer if kept frozen.[61] The most common adverse events in trials were mild, such as fatigue, headache, myalgia, and injection site pain.

A November 2020 announcement was made for a second phase 3 trial, this time with two doses of the vaccine rather than one. Additionally, the company announced plans to begin trials in pregnant women and children.[62]

Sputnik V/Gam-Covid-Vac

Sputnik V, also known as Gam-Covid-Vac, is a recombinant adenovirus vaccine that was approved for use in Russia in August of 2020 but was not officially released to the Russian public until November of that year.[63] It is produced by the Russian Ministry of Health's Gamaleya Research Institute and is a combination of two different adenovirus strains. Its efficacy of 91.6% was published in February 2021 in The Lancet.[63] The phase 3 trial for Sputnik V occurred across 25 clinical sites in Russia and was randomized, placebo-controlled, and double-blinded. A total of 19,866 participants were included, and 7966 total adverse events were recorded. Of these adverse events, most were mild. None of the serious adverse events was linked to vaccination. There were a total of four deaths during the study period, but none was attributed to vaccination.[63]

It must currently be stored in the freezer; however, there is an ongoing development of a version that may be refrigerated. Two doses are given, and they are timed 3 weeks apart.[63]

In December 2020, the Gamaleya Institute announced a collaboration with AstraZeneca. The two companies planned to combine their own adenovirus vaccines in order to increase the efficacy of the AstraZeneca agent. This trial began in February 2021.

AZD1222

The University of Oxford and AstraZeneca partnered to develop AZD1222, formerly known as ChAdOx1 nCoV-19. This vaccine has not been approved for use in the United States but is actively being used in many countries including the United Kingdom and the European Union. It is stable in refrigerator storage for up to 6 months.[64] Two doses are administered at an interval of 8–12 weeks with a reported efficacy of 79% in the US studies.[64] It is approved for use in Brazil and has emergency use status in many other countries. Additionally, it has received emergency use validation from the WHO as of February 2020 in those patients above 18 years of age. It is endorsed by the Africa Regulatory Taskforce and recommended for emergency use by the Caribbean Regulatory System.[64]

Variants of the novel coronavirus greatly impacted the rollout of this vaccine in South Africa, as a study did not demonstrate efficacy toward the South African variant.[64] The doses that had been planned for the South African people were halted in February of 2021. There is a current study underway looking into a vaccine for this variant, as well as another investigating the feasibility of delivery of this vaccine via nasal mist. As discussed below, reports of venous thromboembolism and specifically cerebral venous sinus thrombosis in association with the vaccine further contributed to the slow and interrupted rollout of the vaccine across Europe.

Protein Subunit Vaccines

These vaccines do not contain any genetic material of the novel coronavirus, only the proteins that are expressed by the virions. By injecting spike proteins that have been assembled into nanoparticles, the immune system is able to recognize host cells expressing these cell surface receptors. This process begins with antigen-presenting cells phagocytosing the vaccine and presenting the proteins to other immune cells. When this spike protein is recognized by T helper cells, they become activated and start recruiting other immune cells, such as B cells which, in turn, become activated, and manufacture and release antibodies against the spike protein.

One of the benefits of protein-based vaccines is the fact that they do not require access to the nucleus of the human cell to alter genetic activity and activate their immune response. This simplifies vaccine creation and delivery, as the virus does not require incorporation of both outer cell membrane and inner nuclear membrane targeting proteins. As with mRNA vaccines, there is no risk of genetic mutation or alteration of the host's genetic material. Here, we only discuss one of the protein subunit vaccines, the Chinese ZF2001.

ZF2001

Anhui Zhifei Longcom and the Institute of Medical Biology at the Chinese Academy of Medical Sciences joined forces to create ZF2001.[65] This vaccine is derived from proteins, with the antigen being the receptor-binding domain of the spike protein.[66] Phase 1 and 2 trials were both placebo-controlled, randomized, and double-blinded, and found that three doses of the vaccine generated neutralizing antibody titers in 93%–100% of participants. No serious adverse events were considered to be related to the vaccine.[66] China and Uzbekistan authorized emergency use of this vaccine on March 15, 2021. This vaccine is a three-dose regimen, with each dose being administered at 4 week intervals.

Its efficacy is currently unknown, but phase 3 trials began in December 2020. Data has not yet been released.

DNA-Based Vaccines

DNA-based vaccines use DNA plasmids as vectors to deliver the genes encoding antigenic proteins to the host cell. These vaccines require access to the nucleus of the cell in order to exert their effect. After cell entry, the particles are released into the cytoplasm. The nuclear membrane receptors then recognize the viral particle and allow it into the nucleus. There, it is able to transcribe the DNA information it carries into messenger RNA, which leaves the nucleus and is translated into proteins in the cytoplasm. These proteins usually encode the spike protein of the novel coronavirus, and these proteins are expressed on the outer cell membrane for immune system recognition by T helper cells. The T helper cells then allow the remainder of the immune system to initiate the response against the intruder. When B cells interact with the novel coronavirus and T cell complex, they recognize the complex and begin producing antibodies, or particles that will essentially neutralize the virus. These particles recognize the cell surface proteins of the virus and label them for degradation by the immune system.

Advantages of this type of vaccine include stimulation of both humoral and cellular immunity for a broader immunogenicity, capability to deliver several genes using a single plasmid leading to the production of multiple viral antigens thereby enhancing the elicited immune response to the vaccine, low cost, and high-temperature stability. The latter is important as these vaccines are more heat-stable than mRNA vaccines and do not require deep refrigeration, facilitating their transport and storage. Currently, several DNA vaccines are in Phase 1 or 2 clinical trials (ClinicalTrials.gov NCT04788459, NCT04715997, NCT04445389, NCT04591184, NCT04673149) and many others are in the preplanning stages.

Inactivated Vaccines

These vaccines are made of whole virus particles that have been inactivated but retain their immunogenic potential. They may induce in general a weaker immune response and therefore usually require additional booster doses. This technique of vaccine development has been extensively used in the past and is the basis for polio, hepatitis A, rabies, and most influenza vaccines. They are considered safe to use in immunocompromised hosts. The main advantages of this type of vaccine are the extensive familiarity with the methodology and the low cost enabling large-scale production.

BBIBP-CorV

The Beijing Institute of Biological Products, in combination with Sinopharm, developed the BBIBP-CorV vaccine that has been approved for use in China, Bahrain, and the United Arab Emirates. It has an efficacy of 79.34% and is given in two doses, 3 weeks apart.[67] The data from phase 3 trials that began in July has yet to be published. This vaccine was also tested against the South African B.1.351 variant and was found to be only slightly weaker in terms of immune response compared to the wild-type virus. Data from this study is not yet available.

CoronaVac

Sinovac's CoronaVac, formerly known as PiCoVacc, has been approved for use in China but has received emergency approval in numerous other countries. It is a two-dose regimen, with the doses given 2 weeks apart from one another. A Brazilian trial demonstrated an efficacy of 50.38%, while a trial in Turkey revealed an efficacy of 83.5%.[68]

BBV152

Bharat Biotech partnered with the Indian Council of Medical Research and the National Institute of Virology to create BBV152. It is a two-dose regimen, with the two doses being administered 4 weeks apart.[69] Its efficacy is reported to be 80.6%, and it can be stored at room temperature. There were no serious adverse events in clinical trials. In December 2020, Bharat Biotech announced that it was partnering with US-based Ocugen to develop the vaccine for the United States. It has been granted emergency use authorization in India, Iran, Mauritius, Nepal, and Zimbabwe.

Vaccine Hesitancy

It is difficult to discuss immunization for the pandemic at large without mentioning the vaccine hesitancy that seems to have arisen in the United States. A growing number of people are hesitant to receive vaccinations, especially a vaccine against the novel coronavirus. This is evidenced by outbreaks of diseases in the developed world that are prevented by vaccination, such as measles or pertussis.[70] A Canadian study discovered that parents feel as though children receive too many vaccinations and that the newer vaccines are less safe than those that are older.[62] Current estimates are that up to 5%–10% of the population feels strongly against vaccination.[71] Presumably, a larger proportion of the population is hesitant to receive vaccines.

This hesitancy can originate from many different factors, and can even vary by type of vaccine. In the 1990s, a reported association between multiple sclerosis and the hepatitis B vaccine halted the vaccination distribution, even after this association was disproven.[72] The measles-mumps-rubella vaccine, on the other hand, was reported to be associated with autism, causing many parents to decline this vaccine for their children. Fear of developing autism is still a commonly cited fear from parents regarding the vaccination of their children.[73, 74]

Neurological Complications of COVID-19 Vaccines

Common side effects experienced as a result of vaccination for COVID-19 include fever, chills, myalgias, lymphadenopathy, injection site pain and swelling, fatigue, headache, and nausea. By May 6, 2021, more than 1.23 billion vaccine doses have been administered worldwide and none of the marketed vaccines has been associated with a high incidence of serious neurological complications.[75] Nonetheless, it is important for neurologists and other health-care providers to remain up-to-date with the evolving body of evidence surrounding the safety of COVID-19 vaccines, as communicated in a statement released by the American Academy of Neurology.[76]

Demyelinating complications. In the Oxford AstraZeneca vaccine trial, out of 12,174 recipients of the ChAdOx1 nCoV-19 vaccine, only one case of transverse myelitis was considered to be probably related to the vaccine and occurred 14 days after the second injection, while another case arose 10 days after initial injection and was attributed to preexisting multiple sclerosis and not the vaccine.[77] Another case of transverse myelitis, this one after Sinopharm's BBIBP-CorV vaccine, resulted in a 2-day interruption of the trial with subsequent resumption when the complication was deemed to be unrelated to vaccination.

Cranial neuropathies. Facial palsies are known to occur after viral vaccine administration, including the influenza vaccine. In the phase 3 trials leading to the commercialization of the two mRNA vaccines, Pfizer's BNT162b2 and Moderna's mRNA-1273, seven cases of Bell's palsy were observed in the vaccine groups (four in Pfizer's vaccine and three in Moderna's) compared to one in the placebo groups. Renoud et al. published a disproportionality analysis in JAMA Internal Medicine to study whether the postmarketing cases of facial palsy after mRNA vaccine administration occurred with higher frequency than with other viral vaccines or the influenza vaccines.[78] In doing this, they used the World Health Organization pharmacovigilance database, VigiBase, to gather their data. By the publication date in early May 2021, more than 320 million COVID-19 vaccine doses had already been administered around the world. The authors found no higher incidence of facial palsy after mRNA vaccine administration (0.6% of all reported adverse reactions) compared to other viral vaccines (0.5%) or influenza vaccines (0.7%). The CDC released a statement saying that, although cases of Bell's palsy have been reported in trials of COVID-19 vaccination, there was no causal relationship found between vaccination and cranial neuropathies since the incidence was no higher than the rate expected in the general population.[75]

Guillain-Barré syndrome (GBS). GBS deserves special mention as it has been associated with vaccination against the influenza virus. Although GBS has been reported in cases of SARS-CoV-2 infection, it has not been found to develop at a higher rate postvaccination for COVID-19 compared to the general population. A case report published in Neurology describes the case of two subjects, one in each arm of Johnson & Johnson's Ad26.COV2·S trial, who developed GBS after receiving vaccine and placebo.[79] Notably, there are no reports, thus far, of cases of GBS associated with the mRNA vaccines. In its "Vaccine Considerations for People with Underlying Medical Conditions" report, the CDC states that patients with a prior history of GBS may still receive a COVID-19 vaccine, due to the low risk of recurrence postvaccination.[75]

Thrombophilias. Recent and rare reports of thrombotic events and more specifically cerebral venous sinus thrombosis (CVST) *with thrombocytopenia* have raised concerns among the general public and the scientific community and led to the temporary suspension of Janssen's Ad26.COV2·S and AstraZeneca's ChAdOx1 nCoV-19 vaccines in the United States and Europe, respectively. As of April 23, no cases of thrombosis with thrombocytopenia have been reported with the mRNA vaccines.[80] By the end of April, six cases of CVST among 7 million recipients of the Janssen vaccine in the United States, and 169 possible cases of CVST among 34 million recipients of the AstraZeneca vaccine across Europe had been reported.[81] It is important to recognize, however, that it is six times more likely to develop CVST as a result of COVID-19 infection than after vaccination against the virus, and that the latter occurs with a relatively low frequency (one case per 100,000 vaccine exposures).[82]

Pathogenetically, DNA fragments released from adenovirus-infected cells trigger the production of autoantibodies that bind platelet factor 4 (PF4).[83] The latter is the same antigen that leads to the development of heparin-induced thrombocytopenia (HIT), a condition that results from exposure to heparin and causes

potentially life-threatening arteriovenous thrombosis and thrombocytopenia. In the case of adenovirus-based vaccines, the related condition is referred to as vaccine-induced immune thrombotic thrombocytopenia (VITT), or thrombosis with thrombocytopenia syndrome (TTS), and occurs irrespective of an exposure to heparin.

The initial cases have occurred mostly in women younger than 50 years of age (mean age in the 30s) who were relatively healthy, some of whom were on hormonal replacement therapy or oral contraceptives. In addition to CVST, patients often had thromboses in other sites including deep veins, pulmonary arteries, and splanchnic vessels. The most common symptom related to CVST has been headaches. Other symptoms have been visual changes, nausea, vomiting, bruising, abdominal pain, back pain, leg swelling, and shortness of breath. Mortality is high (40%), usually owing to ischemic strokes and/or hemorrhagic transformations.[81] The symptoms have arisen 6–13 days after administration of the Janssen vaccine and 5–24 days after the first AstraZeneca vaccine shot.[84]

The diagnosis is made when all four criteria are met: COVID-19 vaccination (Janssen or AstraZeneca) 4–30 days prior to symptom onset, development of venous or arterial thrombosis, thrombocytopenia (median platelet count: 20,000–30,000, range: 10,000–100,000) and a positive PF4 ELISA (to be tested before the start of treatment). Non-ELISA immunoassays for HIT should not be used as they are neither specific nor sensitive for VITT/TTS.

Rapid institution of therapy is key to curb the high mortality associated with the condition. The two main treatments are intravenous immunoglobulin (IVIG) 1 g/kg daily for 2 days and treatment-intensity nonheparin anticoagulation such as argatroban, fondaparinux, bivalirudin, direct oral anticoagulants, or danaparoid, until VITT/TTS is ruled out. Steroids and plasmapheresis are not routinely recommended but could have value in refractory cases. Similarly, platelet transfusions should be avoided, unless severe bleeding occurs along with profound thrombocytopenia. The American Heart Association and the American Society of Hematology also recommend consultation with experts in vascular neurology, hematology, and vascular medicine.[84, 85]

Functional neurological disorder. Since the beginning of vaccine campaign rollouts, several videos have been circulated on social media showing people displaying abnormal movements of trunk, limbs, and gait after receiving COVID-19 vaccine injections.[86] Review of many of these videos by The Functional Neurological Disorder Society led to the issuance of a statement by the society that these movements were indeed consistent with a functional neurological disorder (FND), a newer and broader term encompassing conversion disorder.[87] These videos have contributed to fueling the already rampant vaccine hesitancy around the world. The appropriate treatment approach for this disorder is centered around physical rehabilitation, cognitive behavioral therapy, and educating patients about the signs and symptoms of FND.[88]

Special Considerations for COVID-19 Vaccines in Patients With Neurological Conditions

There has been overwhelming support in favor of vaccination initiatives from various neurological societies worldwide and the United States. They have, one after the other, released statements urging patients with chronic neurological conditions to get vaccinated expeditiously. Patients with neurological conditions are at risk for severe COVID-19 either by virtue of their underlying disease or the therapies they receive for it. For instance, patients with demyelinating or neuromuscular diseases may be on immunosuppressant therapies, making them particularly vulnerable to COVID-19 infection. Therefore, vaccinating these at-risk patient populations is of paramount importance. The current evidence shows that vaccinating patients with epilepsy, dementia, cerebrovascular diseases, multiple sclerosis or neuromuscular diseases is safe and that the risk of developing transient side effects from the vaccine (such as a fever) far outweighs the risk of contracting the disease. Nonetheless, vaccinating patients on immunosuppressive or immunomodulatory therapies should always be carefully considered especially when it comes to the choice of vaccine type (avoid live attenuated viruses at all cost) and timing of vaccine administration in relationship to immunotherapy because the latter can reduce the former's effectiveness if administered too close in time.

The National Multiple Sclerosis Society encourages all patients with MS to get vaccinated, stating that the vaccine is safe for them and can be given with their disease-modifying therapies (DMT) unless advised otherwise by their neurologists.[89] The limited data we have suggests that the rate of MS relapses after vaccination is similar to that in nonvaccinated patients during the same study period.[90] Also, it is important for patients to consult with their treating physician when it comes to interaction between vaccination and DMT. Although we do not have specific data for the COVID-19 vaccines, by extrapolating from our prior experience with other vaccines (e.g., the influenza vaccines), we know that

some DMT can blunt vaccine effectiveness. This is particularly true of anti-CD20 monoclonal antibody therapies such as rituximab and ocrelizumab. Some milder degrees of vaccine effectiveness reduction was seen with teriflunomide, glatiramer acetate, natalizumab, fingolimod, and other sphingosine-1-phosphate receptor modulators. No significant effect was seen with beta-interferons and dimethyl fumarate.[91] Responses will likely vary with the different types and dosing regimens of COVID-19 vaccines. Until we have more data regarding these interactions, neurologists will need to apply clinical judgment in choosing a particular MS therapy as well as the timing of vaccination relative to DMT administration. Timing of vaccine administration is also important in patients with myasthenia gravis (MG) on monoclonal antibody therapy like rituximab. For instance, the Conquer Myasthenia Gravis Foundation recommends waiting for 6 weeks after the first vaccine dose before getting a rituximab treatment and 4 weeks after the second dose before the next treatment. Furthermore, little is known about the effect of plasmapheresis or IVIG, commonly used as part of the treatment of patients with MG, MS, and GBS, on the effectiveness of COVID-19 vaccines. The concern is that plasma exchange and IVIG can reduce the anti-SARS-CoV-2 antibody titers and make patients less protected against the virus after vaccination. This is, however, not substantiated, and prior data of plasmapheresis after vaccination for other diseases show that protective antibody titers are not significantly affected post plasma exchange.[92] Therefore, the recommendation is to not hold plasmapheresis in the patient vaccinated for COVID-19 and, conversely, to not hold COVID-19 vaccination in the patient who receives plasmapheresis.

The American Heart Association/American Stroke Association holds a similar stance on vaccination, and although there have been rare reports of CVST (see above) after administration of adenovirus-vectored vaccines, the organization's position remains the same, urging all stroke survivors to get vaccinated.[93]

Similarly, the International League Against Epilepsy has released a statement, encouraging all patients with epilepsy to get vaccinated since vaccines appear to be safe and the risk of developing a transient fever that could transiently lower seizure threshold outweighs the risk of getting infected.[94] Although not specifically known for COVID-19 vaccines, there may be potential interactions between these vaccines and antiseizure medications, specifically those that are metabolized by a cohort of cytochrome P450 (CYP) enzymes: CYP 1A2, CYP 2C8, CYP 3A4, CYP 2B6, and CYP 2E1.[95] The reason for this is that COVID-19 vaccines elicit a strong production of interferons-gamma which are known to dampen the expression of CYP enzymes.[96, 97] Antiseizure medications at higher risk for theoretical toxicity as a result of such interaction would be carbamazepine, clonazepam, ethosuximide, felbamate, phenytoin, tiagabine, and zonisamide.[98] Again, this is pure extrapolation and data is needed to ascertain the safety and interaction of antiseizure medications with COVID-19 vaccines.

It is important to note that COVID-19 vaccines are not approved yet for children under the age of 16 years of age. It is also worthwhile noting that vaccination is not compulsory and consent, either by the patient him/herself or if not consentable, by the legally authorized representative must be sought prior to vaccination.

ACKNOWLEDGMENT

We acknowledge the contribution by Dr. Mayur Ramesh of the Infection Diseases Service at Henry Ford Hospital, Detroit, Michigan, USA.

REFERENCES

1. Chen P, Nirula A, Heller B, et al. SARS-CoV-2 neutralizing antibody LY-CoV555 in outpatients with Covid-19. *N Engl J Med.* 2021;384(3):229–237. https://doi.org/10.1056/NEJMoa2029849.

2. Kalil AC, Patterson TF, Mehta AK, et al. Baricitinib plus Remdesivir for hospitalized adults with Covid-19. *N Engl J Med.* 2021;384(9):795–807. https://doi.org/10.1056/NEJMoa2031994.

3. Weinreich DM, Sivapalasingam S, Norton T, et al. REGN-COV2, a neutralizing antibody cocktail, in outpatients with Covid-19. *N Engl J Med.* 2021;384(3):238–251. https://doi.org/10.1056/NEJMoa2035002.

4. RECOVERY Collaborative Group, Horby P, Lim WS, et al. Dexamethasone in hospitalized patients with Covid-19. *N Engl J Med.* 2021;384(8):693–704. https://doi.org/10.1056/NEJMoa2021436.

5. Alhazzani W, Evans L, Alshamsi F, et al. Surviving sepsis campaign guidelines on the management of adults with coronavirus disease 2019 (COVID-19) in the ICU: first update. *Crit Care Med.* 2021;49(3):e219–e234. https://doi.org/10.1097/CCM.0000000000004899.

6. Coronavirus Disease 2019 (COVID-19) Treatment Guidelines. *National Institute of Health;* 2021. https://files.covid19treatmentguidelines.nih.gov/guidelines/covid19treatmentguidelines.pdf. Published 2021. Accessed May 11.

7. Brown ES, Chandler PA. Mood and cognitive changes during systemic corticosteroid therapy. *Prim Care Companion J Clin Psychiatry.* 2001;3(1):17–21. https://doi.org/10.4088/pcc.v03n0104.

8. Keenan PA, Jacobson MW, Soleymani RM, Mayes MD, Stress ME, Yaldoo DT. The effect on memory of chronic

9. Dubovsky AN, Arvikar S, Stern TA, Axelrod L. The neuropsychiatric complications of glucocorticoid use: steroid psychosis revisited. *Psychosomatics.* 2012;53(2):103–115. https://doi.org/10.1016/j.psym.2011.12.007.

10. Yang T, Li Z, Jiang L, Xi X. Corticosteroid use and intensive care unit-acquired weakness: a systematic review and meta-analysis. *Crit Care.* 2018;22(1):187. Published 2018 Aug 3 https://doi.org/10.1186/s13054-018-2111-0.

11. de Jonghe B, Lacherade JC, Sharshar T, Outin H. Intensive care unit-acquired weakness: risk factors and prevention. *Crit Care Med.* 2009;37(10 Suppl):S309–S315. https://doi.org/10.1097/CCM.0b013e3181b6e64c.

12. Kim JY, Park KD, Richman DP. Treatment of myasthenia gravis based on its immunopathogenesis. *J Clin Neurol.* 2011;7(4):173–183. https://doi.org/10.3988/jcn.2011.7.4.173.

13. Melles RB, Marmor MF. The risk of toxic retinopathy in patients on long-term hydroxychloroquine therapy [published correction appears in JAMA Ophthalmol. 2014 Dec;132(12):1493]. *JAMA Ophthalmol.* 2014;132(12):1453–1460. https://doi.org/10.1001/jamaophthalmol.2014.3459.

14. Prayuenyong P, Kasbekar AV, Baguley DM. Clinical implications of chloroquine and hydroxychloroquine ototoxicity for COVID-19 treatment: a mini-review. *Front Public Health.* 2020;8:252. Published 2020 May 29 https://doi.org/10.3389/fpubh.2020.00252.

15. Hamm BS, Rosenthal LJ. Psychiatric aspects of chloroquine and hydroxychloroquine treatment in the wake of coronavirus disease-2019: psychopharmacological interactions and neuropsychiatric sequelae. *Psychosomatics.* 2020;61(6):597–606. https://doi.org/10.1016/j.psym.2020.06.022.

16. Pati S, Houston T. Assessing the risk of seizures with chloroquine or hydroxychloroquine therapy for COVID-19 in persons with epilepsy. *Epilepsy Res.* 2020;165:106399. https://doi.org/10.1016/j.eplepsyres.2020.106399.

17. Stiehm ER. Adverse effects of human immunoglobulin therapy. *Transfus Med Rev.* 2013;27(3):171–178. https://doi.org/10.1016/j.tmrv.2013.05.004.

18. Jain RS, Kumar S, Aggarwal R, Kookna JC. Acute aseptic meningitis due to intravenous immunoglobulin therapy in Guillain-Barré syndrome. *Oxf Med Case Reports.* 2014;2014(7):132–134. Published 2014 Oct 29 https://doi.org/10.1093/omcr/omu051.

19. Chandler RE. Serious neurological adverse events after Ivermectin-do they occur beyond the indication of onchocerciasis? *Am J Trop Med Hyg.* 2018;98(2):382–388. https://doi.org/10.4269/ajtmh.17-0042.

20. Jewell P, Ansorge O, Kuker W, Irani SR, Zamboni G. Tocilizumab-associated multifocal cerebral thrombotic microangiopathy. *Neurol Clin Pract.* 2016;6(3):e24–e26. https://doi.org/10.1212/CPJ.0000000000000220.

21. Yamaguchi Y, Furukawa K, Yamamoto T, Takahashi Y, Tanaka K, Takahashi M. Multifocal encephalopathy and

autoimmune-mediated limbic encephalitis following tocilizumab therapy. *Intern Med.* 2014;53(8):879–882. https://doi.org/10.2169/internalmedicine.53.0615.

22. Kobayashi K, Okamoto Y, Inoue H, et al. Leukoencephalopathy with cognitive impairment following tocilizumab for the treatment of rheumatoid arthritis (RA). *Intern Med.* 2009;48(15):1307–1309. https://doi.org/10.2169/internalmedicine.48.1926.

23. Izda V, Jeffries MA, Sawalha AH. COVID-19: a review of therapeutic strategies and vaccine candidates. *Clin Immunol.* 2021;222:108634. https://doi.org/10.1016/j.clim.2020.108634.

24. Grigoryan L, Pulendran B. The immunology of SARS-CoV-2 infections and vaccines. *Semin Immunol.* 2020;50:101422. https://doi.org/10.1016/j.smim.2020.101422.

25. Vaccine Development – 101. U.S. Food and Drug Administration. https://www.fda.gov/vaccines-blood-biologics/development-approval-process-cber/vaccine-development-101. Published 2021. Accessed May 11, 2021.

26. Coronavirus Vaccine Tracker. *The New York Times*; 2021. https://www.nytimes.com/interactive/2020/science/coronavirus-vaccine-tracker.html. Published 2021. Accessed May 11.

27. SARS-CoV-2 Variant Classifications and Definitions. *Centers for Disease Control and Prevention*; 2021. https://www.cdc.gov/coronavirus/2019-ncov/cases-updates/variant-surveillance/variant-info.html. Published 2021. Accessed May 11.

28. Kared H, Redd AD, Bloch EM, et al. SARS-CoV-2-specific CD8+ T cell responses in convalescent COVID-19 individuals. *J Clin Invest.* 2021;131(5). https://doi.org/10.1172/JCI145476, e145476.

29. Palca J, What A. *Nasal Spray Vaccine Against COVID-19 Might Do Even Better Than a Shot.* NPR; 2021. https://www.npr.org/sections/health-shots/2020/08/28/906797539/what-a-nasal-spray-vaccine-against-covid-19-might-do-even-better-than-a-shot. Published 2021. Accessed May 11.

30. COVID Data Tracker. *Centers for Disease Control and Prevention*; 2021. https://covid.cdc.gov/covid-data-tracker/#vaccinations. Published 2021. Accessed May 11.

31. Gaebler C, Wang Z, Lorenzi JCC, et al. Evolution of antibody immunity to SARS-CoV-2. *Nature.* 2021;591(7851):639–644. https://doi.org/10.1038/s41586-021-03207-w.

32. Li Q, Wu J, Nie J, et al. The impact of mutations in SARS-CoV-2 spike on viral infectivity and antigenicity. *Cell.* 2020;182(5):1284–1294. e9 https://doi.org/10.1016/j.cell.2020.07.012.

33. Lauring AS, Hodcroft EB. Genetic variants of SARS-CoV-2-What do they mean? *JAMA.* 2021;325(6):529–531. https://doi.org/10.1001/jama.2020.27124.

34. Wolff JA, Malone RW, Williams P, et al. Direct gene transfer into mouse muscle in vivo. *Science.* 1990;247(4949 Pt 1):1465–1468. https://doi.org/10.1126/science.1690918.

35. Zhang C, Maruggi G, Shan H, Li J. Advances in mRNA vaccines for infectious diseases. *Front Immunol.* 2019;10:594. Published 2019 Mar 27 https://doi.org/10.3389/fimmu.2019.00594.

36. Maruggi G, Zhang C, Li J, Ulmer JB, Yu D. mRNA as a transformative technology for vaccine development to control infectious diseases. *Mol Ther.* 2019;27(4):757–772. https://doi.org/10.1016/j.ymthe.2019.01.020.

37. Banerjee AK. 5′-terminal cap structure in eucaryotic messenger ribonucleic acids. *Microbiol Rev.* 1980;44(2):175–205.

38. Wickens M. How the messenger got its tail: addition of poly(A) in the nucleus. *Trends Biochem Sci.* 1990;15(7):277–281. https://doi.org/10.1016/0968-0004(90)90054-f.

39. Reichmuth AM, Oberli MA, Jaklenec A, Langer R, Blankschtein D. mRNA vaccine delivery using lipid nanoparticles [published correction appears in Ther Deliv. 2016 Jun;7(6):411]. *Ther Deliv.* 2016;7(5):319–334. https://doi.org/10.4155/tde-2016-0006.

40. Schlake T, Thess A, Fotin-Mleczek M, Kallen KJ. Developing mRNA-vaccine technologies. *RNA Biol.* 2012;9(11):1319–1330. https://doi.org/10.4161/rna.22269.

41. Tsui NB, Ng EK, Lo YM. Stability of endogenous and added RNA in blood specimens, serum, and plasma. *Clin Chem.* 2002;48(10):1647–1653.

42. Pardi N, Hogan MJ, Porter FW, Weissman D. mRNA vaccines - a new era in vaccinology. *Nat Rev Drug Discov.* 2018;17(4):261–279. https://doi.org/10.1038/nrd.2017.243.

43. de Vrieze J. *Suspicions grow that nanoparticles in Pfizer's COVID-19 vaccine trigger rare allergic reactions. Science*; 2021. https://www.sciencemag.org/news/2020/12/suspicions-grow-nanoparticles-pfizer-s-covid-19-vaccine-trigger-rare-allergic-reactions. Published 2021. Accessed May 11.

44. Polack FP, Thomas SJ, Kitchin N, et al. Safety and efficacy of the BNT162b2 mRNA Covid-19 vaccine. *N Engl J Med.* 2020;383(27):2603–2615. https://doi.org/10.1056/NEJMoa2034577.

45. Pfizer-BioNTech COVID-19 Vaccine. *U.S. Food and Drug Administration*; 2021. https://www.fda.gov/emergency-preparedness-and-response/coronavirus-disease-2019-covid-19/pfizer-biontech-covid-19-vaccine. Published 2021. Accessed May 11.

46. WHO issues its first emergency use validation for a COVID-19 vaccine and emphasizes need for equitable global access. *World Health Organization*; 2021. https://www.who.int/news/item/31-12-2020-who-issues-its-first-emergency-use-validation-for-a-covid-19-vaccine-and-emphasizes-need-for-equitable-global-access. Published 2021. Accessed May 11.

47. Liu Y, Liu J, Xia H, et al. Neutralizing activity of BNT162b2-elicited serum. *N Engl J Med.* 2021;384(15):1466–1468. https://doi.org/10.1056/NEJMc2102017.

48. Pfizer and BioNTech Initiate a Study as Part of Broad Development Plan to Evaluate COVID-19 Booster and New Vaccine Variants. *Pfizer*; 2021. https://www.pfizer.com/news/press-release/press-release-detail/pfizer-and-biontech-initiate-study-part-broad-development. Published 2021. Accessed May 11.

49. Shimabukuro TT, Kim SY, Myers TR, et al. Preliminary findings of mRNA Covid-19 vaccine safety in pregnant persons

[published online ahead of print, 2021 Apr 21]. *N Engl J Med.* 2021. https://doi.org/10.1056/NEJMoa2104983.

50. Coronavirus (COVID-19) Update: FDA Authorizes Pfizer-BioNTech COVID-19 Vaccine for Emergency Use in Adolescents in Another Important Action in Fight Against Pandemic. *U.S. Food and Drug Administration;* 2021. https://www.fda.gov/news-events/press-announcements/coronavirus-covid-19-update-fda-authorizes-pfizer-biontech-covid-19-vaccine-emergency-use. Published 2021. Accessed May 11.

51. Baden LR, El Sahly HM, Essink B, et al. Efficacy and safety of the mRNA-1273 SARS-CoV-2 vaccine. *N Engl J Med.* 2021;384(5):403–416. https://doi.org/10.1056/NEJMoa2035389.

52. Pfizer and BioNTech Submit COVID-19 Vaccine Stability Data at Standard Freezer Temperature to the U.S. FDA. *pfpfizeruscom. Pfizer.com;* 2021. https://www.pfizer.com/news/press-release/press-release-detail/pfizer-and-biontech-submit-covid-19-vaccine-stability-data. Published 2021. Accessed May 11.

53. Swissmedic Authorizes COVID-19 Vaccine Moderna for Use in Switzerland. *Moderna, Inc;* 2021. https://investors.modernatx.com/news-releases/news-release-details/swissmedic-authorizes-covid-19-vaccine-moderna-use-switzerland. Published 2021. Accessed May 8.

54. A Study to Evaluate the Safety, Reactogenicity, and Effectiveness of mRNA-1273 Vaccine in Adolescents 12 to <18 Years Old to Prevent COVID-19 - Full Text View - ClinicalTrials.gov. *Clinicaltrials.gov;* 2021. https://clinicaltrials.gov/ct2/show/NCT04649151. Published 2021. Accessed May 11.

55. Safety and Immunogenicity Study of a SARS-CoV-2 (COVID-19) Variant Vaccine (mRNA-1273.351) in Naïve and Previously Vaccinated Adults - Full Text View - ClinicalTrials.gov. *Clinicaltrials.gov;* 2021. https://clinicaltrials.gov/ct2/show/NCT04785144?term=covid-19+vaccine&draw=2. Published 2021. Accessed May 11.

56. Tatsis N, Ertl HC. Adenoviruses as vaccine vectors. *Mol Ther.* 2004;10(4):616–629. https://doi.org/10.1016/j.ymthe.2004.07.013.

57. Shiver JW, Fu TM, Chen L, et al. Replication-incompetent adenoviral vaccine vector elicits effective anti-immunodeficiency-virus immunity. *Nature.* 2002;415(6869):331–335. https://doi.org/10.1038/415331a.

58. Lasaro MO, Ertl HC. New insights on adenovirus as vaccine vectors. *Mol Ther.* 2009;17(8):1333–1339. https://doi.org/10.1038/mt.2009.130. Epub 2009 Jun 9 19513019. PMC2835230.

59. Ulmer JB, Wahren B, Liu MA. Gene-based vaccines: recent technical and clinical advances. *Trends Mol Med.* 2006;12(5):216–222. https://doi.org/10.1016/j.molmed.2006.03.007.

60. Sadoff J, Le Gars M, Shukarev G, et al. Interim results of a phase 1-2a trial of Ad26.COV2.S Covid-19 Vaccine [published online ahead of print, 2021 Jan 13]. *N Engl J Med.* 2021. https://doi.org/10.1056/NEJMoa2034201. NEJMoa2034201.

61. Livingston EH, Malani PN, Creech CB. The Johnson & Johnson Vaccine for COVID-19. *JAMA.* 2021;325(15):1575. https://doi.org/10.1001/jama.2021.2927.

62. A Study of Ad26.COV2.S in Healthy Pregnant Participants (COVID-19) - Full Text View - ClinicalTrials.gov. *Clinicaltrials.gov;* 2021. https://clinicaltrials.gov/ct2/show/NCT04765384?term=pregnancy+%2B+AD26&cond=covid-19&draw=2&rank=1. Published 2021. Accessed May 11.

63. Logunov DY, Dolzhikova IV, Shcheblyakov DV, et al. Safety and efficacy of an rAd26 and rAd5 vector-based heterologous prime-boost COVID-19 vaccine: an interim analysis of a randomised controlled phase 3 trial in Russia [published correction appears in lancet. 2021 Feb 20;397(10275):670]. *Lancet.* 2021;397(10275):671–681. https://doi.org/10.1016/S0140-6736(21)00234-8.

64. Voysey M, Costa Clemens SA, Madhi SA, et al. Single-dose administration and the influence of the timing of the booster dose on immunogenicity and efficacy of ChAdOx1 nCoV-19 (AZD1222) vaccine: a pooled analysis of four randomised trials [published correction appears in lancet. 2021 mar 6;397(10277):880]. *Lancet.* 2021;397(10277):881–891. https://doi.org/10.1016/S0140-6736(21)00432-3.

65. Dai L, Zheng T, Xu K, et al. A universal design of betacoronavirus vaccines against COVID-19, MERS, and SARS. *Cell.* 2020;182(3):722–733. e11 https://doi.org/10.1016/j.cell.2020.06.035.

66. Yang S, Li Y, Dai L, et al. Safety and immunogenicity of a recombinant tandem-repeat dimeric RBD-based protein subunit vaccine (ZF2001) against COVID-19 in adults: two randomised, double-blind, placebo-controlled, phase 1 and 2 trials [published online ahead of print, 2021 Mar 24]. *Lancet Infect Dis.* 2021. https://doi.org/10.1016/S1473-3099(21)00127-4.

67. Xia S, Zhang Y, Wang Y, et al. Safety and immunogenicity of an inactivated SARS-CoV-2 vaccine, BBIBP-CorV: a randomised, double-blind, placebo-controlled, phase 1/2 trial. *Lancet Infect Dis.* 2021;21(1):39–51. https://doi.org/10.1016/S1473-3099(20)30831-8.

68. Zhang Y, Zeng G, Pan H, et al. Safety, tolerability, and immunogenicity of an inactivated SARS-CoV-2 vaccine in healthy adults aged 18-59 years: a randomised, double-blind, placebo-controlled, phase 1/2 clinical trial. *Lancet Infect Dis.* 2021;21(2):181–192. https://doi.org/10.1016/S1473-3099(20)30843-4.

69. Ella R, Vadrevu KM, Jogdand H, et al. Safety and immunogenicity of an inactivated SARS-CoV-2 vaccine, BBV152: a double-blind, randomised, phase 1 trial [published correction appears in lancet infect dis. 2021 Apr;21(4):e81]. *Lancet Infect Dis.* 2021;21(5):637–646. https://doi.org/10.1016/S1473-3099(20)30942-7.

70. Falagas ME, Zarkadoulia E. Factors associated with suboptimal compliance to vaccinations in children in developed countries: a systematic review. *Curr Med Res Opin.* 2008;24(6):1719–1741. https://doi.org/10.1185/03007990802085692.

71. Leask J. Target the fence-sitters. *Nature.* 2011;473(7348):443–445. https://doi.org/10.1038/473443a.

72. François G, Duclos P, Margolis H, et al. Vaccine safety controversies and the future of vaccination programs. *Pediatr Infect Dis J.* 2005;24(11):953–961. https://doi.org/10.1097/01.inf.0000183853.16113.a6.

73. Stefanoff P, Mamelund SE, Robinson M, et al. Tracking parental attitudes on vaccination across European countries: the vaccine safety, attitudes, training and communication project (VACSATC). *Vaccine.* 2010;28(35):5731–5737. https://doi.org/10.1016/j.vaccine.2010.06.009.

74. Poland GA, Spier R. Fear, misinformation, and innumerates: how the Wakefield paper, the press, and advocacy groups damaged the public health. *Vaccine.* 2010;28(12):2361–2362. https://doi.org/10.1016/j.vaccine.2010.02.052.

75. COVID-19 Vaccination Considerations for Persons with Underlying Medica. *Centers for Disease Control and Prevention*; 2021. https://www.cdc.gov/coronavirus/2019-ncov/vaccines/recommendations/underlying-conditions.html. Published 2021. Accessed May 5.

76. American Academy of Neurology position statement on COVID-19 vaccination. *American Academy of Neurology*; 2021. https://www.aan.com/siteassets/home-page/policy-and-guidelines/policy/position-statements/21-positionstatement-covid-19-vaccination-v001.pdf. Published 2021. Accessed May 8.

77. Voysey M, Clemens SAC, Madhi SA, et al. Safety and efficacy of the ChAdOx1 nCoV-19 vaccine (AZD1222) against SARS-CoV-2: an interim analysis of four randomised controlled trials in Brazil, South Africa, and the UK. *Lancet.* 2020. https://doi.org/10.1016/S0140-6736(20)32661-1. published online Dec 8.

78. Renoud L, Khouri C, Revol B, et al. Association of facial paralysis with mRNA COVID-19 vaccines: a disproportionality analysis using the World Health Organization pharmacovigilance database [published online ahead of print, 2021 Apr 27]. [JAMA Intern Med].

79. Loza AMM, Holroyd KB, Johnson SA, Pilgrim DM, Amato AA. Guillain-Barré syndrome in the placebo and active arms of a COVID-19 vaccine clinical trial: temporal associations do not imply causality. *Neurology.* 2021. https://doi.org/10.1212/WNL.0000000000011881. Published April 6.

80. Advisory Committee on Immunization Practices April 23, 2021 Presentation Slides. *Centers for Disease Control and Prevention*; 2021. https://www.cdc.gov/vaccines/acip/meetings/slides-2021-04-23.html. Published 2021. Accessed May 7.

81. Cines DB, Bussel JB. SARS-CoV-2 vaccine-induced immune thrombotic thrombocytopenia [published online ahead of print, 2021 Apr 16]. *N Engl J Med.* 2021. https://doi.org/10.1056/NEJMe2106315. NEJMe2106315.

82. Taquet MHM, Geddes JR, Luciano S, Harrison PJ. *Cerebral venous thrombosis: a retrospective cohort study of 513,284 confirmed covid-19 cases and a comparison with 489,871 people receiving a covid mRNA vaccine*; 2021. https://osf.io/a9jdq/. osf.io. Preprint Version 2 posted online April 15.

83. Advisory Committee on Immunization Practices. *Reports of cerebral venous sinus thrombosis with thrombocytopenia after Janssen COVID-19 vaccine.* National Center for Immunization & Respiratory Diseases; 2021. https://www.cdc.gov/vaccines/acip/meetings/downloads/slides-2021-04/03-covid-shimabukuro-508.pdf. April 12, 2021. Accessed May 7.

84. American Heart Association/American Stroke Association Stroke Council Leadership. Diagnosis and Management of Cerebral Venous Sinus Thrombosis with Vaccine-Induced Thrombotic Thrombocytopenia [published online ahead of print, 2021 Apr 29]. *Stroke.* 2021. https://doi.org/10.1161/STROKEAHA.121.035564.

85. Thrombosis with Thrombocytopenia Syndrome (also termed Vaccine-induced Thrombotic Thrombocytopenia). *Hematology.org*; 2021. https://www.hematology.org/covid-19/vaccine-induced-immune-thrombotic-thrombocytopenia. Published 2021. Accessed May 7.

86. Volpicelli G. *They claimed the Covid vaccine made them sick—and went viral. Wired UK*; 2021. Published January 26, 2021. Accessed March 3 https://www.wired.com/story/they-claimed-the-covid-vaccine-made-them-sick-and-went-viral.

87. Functional Neurological Disorder Society. *Press release from the functional neurological disorder Society.* Published January 19, 2021; 2021. Accessed February 19 https://www.fndsociety.org/UserFiles/file/FNDSSocietyPressReleaseCOVIDVaccines.pdf.

88. Kim DD, Kung CS, Perez DL. Helping the public understand adverse events associated with COVID-19 vaccinations: lessons learned from functional neurological disorder [published online ahead of print, 2021 Apr 9]. *JAMA Neurol.* 2021. https://doi.org/10.1001/jamaneurol.2021.1042.

89. COVID-19 Vaccine Guidance for People Living with MS. *National Multiple Sclerosis Society*; 2021. https://www.nationalmssociety.org/coronavirus-covid-19-information/multiple-sclerosis-and-coronavirus/covid-19-vaccine-guidance. Published 2021. Accessed May 7.

90. Achiron A, Dolev M, Menascu S, et al. COVID-19 vaccination in patients with multiple sclerosis: What we have learnt by February 2021. *Mult Scler.* 2021;27(6):864–870. https://doi.org/10.1177/13524585211003476.

91. Ciotti JR, Valtcheva MV, Cross AH. Effects of MS disease-modifying therapies on responses to vaccinations: a review. *Mult Scler Relat Disord.* 2020;45:102439. https://doi.org/10.1016/j.msard.2020.102439.

92. Nasca TJ, Muder RR, Thomas DB, Schrecker JC, Ruben FL. Antibody response to pneumococcal polysaccharide vaccine in myasthenia gravis: effect of therapeutic plasmapheresis. *J Clin Apher.* 1990;5(3):133–139. https://doi.org/10.1002/jca.2920050304.

93. Heart disease and stroke medical experts urge the public to get COVID-19 vaccinations. *American Heart Association*; 2021. https://newsroom.heart.org/news/heart-disease-and-stroke-medical-experts-urge-public-to-get-covid-19-vaccinations. Published 2021. Accessed May 7.

94. COVID-19 vaccines and people with epilepsy. *International League Against Epilepsy*; 2021. https://www.ilae.org/patient-care/covid-19-and-epilepsy/covid-19-vaccines-and-people-with-epilepsy. Published 2021. Accessed May 7.

95. Donato MT, Guillén MI, Jover R, Castell JV, Gómez-Lechón MJ. Nitric oxide-mediated inhibition of cytochrome P450 by interferon-gamma in human hepatocytes. *J Pharmacol Exp Ther.* 1997;281(1):484–490.

96. Jackson LA, Anderson EJ, Rouphael NG. An mRNA vaccine against SARS-CoV-2 - preliminary report. *N Engl J Med.* 2020;383(20):1920–1931.

97. Sahin U, Muik A, Vogler I. BNT162b2 induces SARS-CoV-2-neutralising antibodies and T cells in humans. Preprint, *medRxiv.* 2020. https://doi.org/10.1101/2020.12.09.20245175.

98. Kow CS, Hasan SS. Potential interactions between COVID-19 vaccines and antiepileptic drugs. *Seizure.* 2021;86:80–81. https://doi.org/10.1016/j.seizure.2021.01.021.

CHAPTER 13

Response of the HealthCare Systems to the Pandemic

GREGORY L. BARKLEY[a,b] • ANGELOS KATRAMADOS[a,b]
[a]Department of Neurology, Henry Ford Hospital, Detroit, MI, United States, [b]Department of Neurology, Wayne State University, School of Medicine, Detroit, MI, United States

This chapter focuses on the changes made at Henry Ford Health System (HFHS) in response to the coronavirus disease 19 (COVID-19) pandemic. This has been described as a "low-chance, high-impact" event that has stressed health-care systems worldwide and has required that they take measures to maintain and improve their institutional resilience.[1] The discussion touches upon similar experiences undertaken at other health systems across the country.

The opening of the flagship hospital of HFHS, Henry Ford Hospital is associated with another pandemic: the 1918–1920 influenza pandemic. The unfinished Henry Ford Hospital (Fig. 13.1) had been temporarily transferred to the US Army during World War I and was renamed as the US Army General Hospital No. 36. The hospital was returned to Henry Ford by the government on January 1, 1920, and the original staff returned from their army service and again opened the hospital. It immediately became available to care for patients of the influenza pandemic. A total of 300 emergency beds were made available for the city.[2]

The COVID-19 pandemic, in a similar fashion, did not allow time for preparation. With the first reports of SARS-CoV-2 virus emerging in China in December 2019, there was recognition of its possible spread worldwide. The first two recognized patients with COVID-19 in Michigan were reported on March 10, 2020 which was also the day of the primary election in Michigan for candidates for the November 3, 2020 election. Following those two reports, there was a rapid rise in reported cases of COVID-19 and a consequent rise in hospitalizations and deaths. The first death from COVID-19 in Michigan was reported on March 18, 2020.

INTER/INTRADEPARTMENTAL COMMUNICATION

HFHS quickly recognized the need for an organized response. Incident command centers were developed in each of the five sister hospitals. There were daily discussions among hospital and unit leaders with the rapid exchange of information and ideas. Real-time decisions were made in a quickly changing environment. These were communicated to all system employees with daily communications and team meetings. Analytical dashboards were developed to facilitate situational and operational awareness.

The necessity of this (almost exclusively virtual) structure became apparent at a departmental level. This was especially the case during the pandemic surge because the entire Neurology department was being deployed in novel ways, the rules of social distancing and bans on in-person gatherings meant that social and communication networks were disrupted. With so many daily strategic changes, it was important to have a common touchpoint. Starting on March 15, 2020, every evening at 5 PM for 50 days, a voluntary huddle call was made, led by GLB, but with a planning call at 4 PM with the Clinical Vice Chair, Quality and Informatics Vice Chair, Residency Program Director, West Bloomfield Service Chief, and Administrative Manager. A call summary was sent out to each department member after the call. Each call featured open time for any questions. Most calls also had specific reports by department members. Each call included references to information on the state of the surge in Michigan, the HFHS, Ontario, Canada, and the USA as well as news items on the virus, research findings, information on PPE, economic support, etc.

Neurological Care and the COVID-19 Pandemic. https://doi.org/10.1016/B978-0-323-82691-4.00014-5

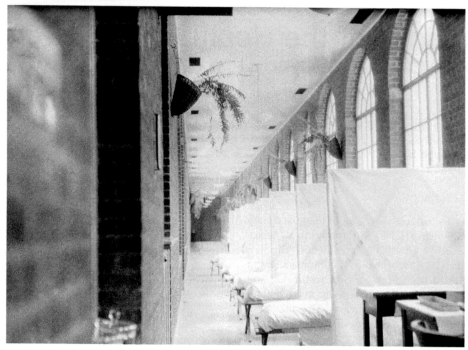

FIG. 13.1 Parallels between 1920 Influenza Pandemic and 2020 COVID-19 Pandemic at Henry Ford Hospital in Detroit, Michigan. Pictured here is the conversion of the Henry Ford Hospital M-Unit entrance into a makeshift influenza ward in 1920.

Similar incident command systems allowed for disaster preparedness in the setting of the COVID-19 pandemic. The Mayo Clinic has reported the need to activate an Incident Command Center early and maintain discipline in structure. This allows for coordination and improves preparedness, particularly in the context of a pandemic that threatens to overwhelm routine clinical operations.[3] This model was also followed at the Cleveland Clinic, a complex, integrated health-care system, that stressed the need to be proactive, clarify the model of governance, and act quickly.[4] Similar administrative structures were created worldwide and allowed for optimal pandemic response in the setting of limited resources.[5]

INFRASTRUCTURE TRANSFORMATION

At HFHS, it was soon realized that this pandemic would result in a "surge" that would require extreme measures to create capacity and allow for efficient care of large numbers of patients with COVID-19. In February 2020, GLB approached the Associate Medical Director (AMD) and told him that he realized that we would close the Epilepsy Monitoring Unit (EMU) once the virus had

spread to Detroit, since no patients would volunteer to come into a hospital where infected patients were being housed. The EMU was offered as a new source of patient rooms and was effectively converted to a COVID-19 unit a few weeks later.

Not only was the EMU turned into a COVID-19 ward, but the entire Henry Ford Hospital was rapidly transformed to care for almost exclusively patients with COVID-19. The number of patients admitted increased exponentially in March 2020, then showed a linear growth in the first week in April before declining (Fig. 13.2). All patients were placed in private rooms which greatly reduced total bed capacity since, prior to this, most general ward rooms were double occupancy rooms.

Our Neurology/Neurosurgery ICU, NICU, was maintained as a COVID-19-free unit, largely because of the fact that half of the beds in the NICU are in an open configuration, separated only by curtains. This arrangement is ideal from the point that a nurse, at a workstation can provide direct observation of several patients at one time but, in the face of a pandemic, this open arrangement is not adequate for the care of infected patients . As such, the NICU became a multipurpose ICU

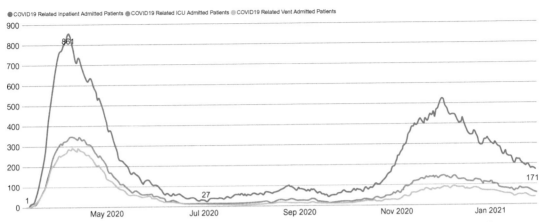

FIG. 13.2 March 2020 to February 2021 COVID-19 Admission run rate at the 5 Henry Ford Health System hospitals including total admissions, ICU admissions, and intubated patients. Note the initial rapid surge peaking on April 7, 2020, and a later, more gradual wave of admissions peaking on December 1, 2020.

for noninfected patients requiring ICU care and served as one of the places where ischemic stroke patients were housed for the first 24–48 h postthrombectomy.

Our Stroke Unit was transformed into a Medical ICU (MICU) ward under the direction of a MICU staff. The Neurology and Neurosurgery nurses remained on duty in the Stroke Unit . One of our Stroke Nurse Practitioners, who had previously been an ICU nurse, began a new assignment as a supplemental Nursing Educator for the unit. In addition, MICU nurses were also assigned to help supervise and assist in the care of these patients and provide training for the Stroke Unit nurses.

As the number of admitted patients began to rise, plans were made to convert outpatient rooms in the clinic tower to inpatient beds. There were two groups of patients being considered for such beds. The first group was patients who were recovering from COVID-19 but who needed inpatient rehabilitation. These patients were housed at the hospital because inpatient rehabilitation facilities were at capacity and/or were not accepting the transfer of patients with COVID-19. This was only put in place briefly in the K-13 Oncology Infusion clinic starting on 4/9/2020. Our departmental inpatient Physical Medicine and Rehabilitation specialist was one of those trained in caring for patients on 9 this ward. Very few patients were actually admitted to this unit. The second group of patients who were being considered for these beds if needed was COVID-19 infected patients who might be designated hospice patients. Fortunately, no such need arose.

An additional inpatient unit was developed at our Fairlane Medical Center. This ward was also assigned for convalescing patients with COVID-19 who were no longer infectious but who were too sick to be discharged home. A 15-bed ward was opened on April, 4, 2020, but by that time, hospital admissions had started to wane, and no patients were ever transferred there.

Another of our surge capacity methods was to utilize our five-hospital network to shift patients as needed. Intrahospital transfers are common between our hospitals but most of the transfers are from one of the other four hospitals to Henry Ford Hospital for quaternary care only provided at Henry Ford Hospital. HFH was at Triage Level 1 by April 1, 2020. On April 4, HFH transferred three patients to Allegiance Hospital in Jackson and two patients to UM Hospital in Ann Arbor due to escalation of triage level. The peak admission at HFH was on April 7, 2020 when 331 patients with COVID-19 were hospitalized at the 877-bed Henry Ford Hospital.

Similar measures to improve surge capacity were taken by the City of Detroit and State of Michigan governments in conjunction with Federal Emergency Management Agency (FEMA). The TCF Convention Center was mobilized in early April 2020. The center was prepared to house up to 1000 patients. It opened on April 10, 2020 and closed on May 7, 2020. A total of 39 patients were treated there with an average daily census of 15–20 patients for the first few weeks of operation but only a few patients were cared for in the last couple of weeks of operation. A 250-bed Suburban Collection Regional Care Center was also set up by FEMA and opened in April 2020. It had five patients admitted on May 7, 2020, its busiest day, and discharged its last patient on June 11, 2020. A total of 16 patients were cared for at this temporary field hospital.

The exponential rise of cases required modifications of clinical operations in health-care systems worldwide. Italy was one of the first countries to become severely affected by the pandemic. The Italian experience revealed the potential that entire health care systems could be overwhelmed and demonstrated the potential need to increase the number of ICU beds, in order to accommodate the increasing numbers of patients.[6] However, the uncertainty with regard to the course of the pandemic made resource planning challenging, particularly in early 2020. Complex predictive and planning models were developed in order to project surge capacity requirements over time, taking into account length of stay, occupancy, and ventilator capacity.[7]

TRAINEE REDEPLOYMENT

In the effort to treat acutely ill, hospitalized patients with COVID-19, medical residents-in-training of different subspecialties were rapidly trained, and redeployed in COVID-19 units. As the numbers of patients with COVID-19 surged, the HFH general neurology ward was converted to a COVID-19 ward. After a "general emergency" was declared by the Graduate Medical Education (GME) Department at HFH, five of our neurology residents were placed under the direction of an Internal Medicine staff. Nationwide, the Accreditation Council for Graduate Medical Education (ACGME) adapted its procedures and policies to allow for local decision-making that would enable effective care of patients by physicians-in-training. At the same time, it set a number of "inviolate" principles: Sponsoring institutions and their programs were required to ensure infection protection and safety for residents, adequate supervision, and compliance with work-hour requirements.[8] The impact of the pandemic on resident training, and the effects of redeployment continue to be evaluated and reported in the medical literature.[9,10]

CANCELATION OF ELECTIVE SURGERIES AND PROCEDURES

The redeployment also affected attending physicians at HFHS. Elective surgeries were canceled so that ICUs and general units could be converted to COVID-19 floors. In the Department of Neurology, all elective neurodiagnostics procedures (electroencephalograms—EEGs—and electromyograms—EMGs) were halted for almost 2 months. Redeployment was organized by the Incident Command Center, with the help of a Henry Ford Medical Group (HFMG) COVID-19 Redeployment shared, online, sign-up sheet. This began during the

week of March 16, 2020. The sign-up sheet had multiple tabs indicating the location of the need, shift times that workers were needed, and skill set/license needed in the volunteers.

Fortunately, within a few weeks, under the leadership of Henry Ford Medical Group CEA, Dr. Kalkanis, the backlog of elective surgical and diagnostic procedures had been eliminated.

However, this cessation of elective procedures, nationwide, has sparked a significant discussion with regard to the need to protect access to care, particularly for the most vulnerable and disadvantaged patients.[11] The disruption of standard surgical care resulted in a coordinated effort to prioritize access,[12] mitigate risk,[13] and create recommendations and guidelines for resuming safe surgeries for different specialties.[14,15]

PERSONAL PROTECTIVE EQUIPMENT PROVISION

Another early major challenge for HFHS was the need to find adequate personal protective equipment (PPEs) in order to prevent infection of health-care team members. Institutional efforts were quickly matched by offers from HFHS alumni and the general community of Metro Detroit. Strategic dashboards were created to track available supplies and consumption rates. Several policies were created to guide the rational and effective use of PPEs in aerosol-generating procedures and routine medical care.

Nationwide and worldwide, the PPE demand spike, in conjunction with panicked marketplace behavior and dysfunctional costing models resulted in supply chain disruptions and depletion of local and national inventories.[16] At the same time, export restrictions may have imperiled poorer countries' access to PPEs at a critical period of pandemic preparation.[17]

MENTAL HEALTH RESOURCES

All the above, unprecedented and unexpected, produced stressful working conditions and created a significant challenge to the mental health of health-care workers. At HFHS, the need for emotional support was quickly developed. A COVID-19 Emotional Response Team was developed with the scope to offer a variety of resources to help team members manage stress and anxiety: A "Stronger Together" Buddy Program was created. Team members could sign up with a buddy, or as an individual and be assigned a buddy to build an authentic and supportive relationship with a colleague through daily contact either by email, phone, or text.

Programs to promote a Good Night's Sleep (SleepWell/LiveWell) were offered through the institutional learning management system, HF University. Peer Processing Support Groups were created. These customized in-person or virtual interventions were intended for teams to discuss their experiences during the pandemic, provide peer support, and learn coping strategies. Finally, a COVID Stress and Anxiety Management Series was offered to employees. This three-module series aimed to teach improved focus, performance, and self-care during the pandemic.

At a national level, it was acknowledged that the COVID-19 pandemic raised mental health problems of public health significance. Stresses related to the uncertainty about the probability and severity of infection, together with fundamental changes in family, school, work, and social activities, resulted in an increased risk of psychological problems.[18] Addressing mental health needs has been identified as an integral part of COVID-19 response for health-care systems.[19]

TELEHEALTH BOOST

The need for infection control by social distancing also created unique challenges for patients, families, and health-care team members alike. Patients with COVID-19 would stay in the hospital for prolonged periods of time, unable to have family visits and with limited interaction with members of the treating team. HFHS committed significant resources in ensuring adequate and meaningful communication of patients with their families and treating clinicians. A large number of tablet devices was purchased. These were placed on stands, to remain in patient rooms and be available for use at any time. The Department of Information Technology (IT) supported this large-scale effort.

This effort was also combined with the wide-scale deployment of telemedicine in the ambulatory setting. Efforts had started 2 years prior to the beginning of the pandemic, but the surge helped jumpstart the process. On February, 4, 2020, it was announced that telemedicine visits had increased to more than 7500 video visits in a single week up from a prepandemic average of 150 per month (Fig. 13.3).

This feat was coordinated by the Department of Virtual Care, but it would not have been possible without a number of developments at a national level: On the evening of March 30, 2020, the Center for Medicare and Medicaid Services (CMS) issued an Interim Final Rule (IFR) to increase flexibility and access to health care in the setting of the pandemic. The rule covered emergency department visits, initial nursing facility and discharge visits, and home visits. It also included visits that were conducted through audio phone only. At the same time, the Office of Civil Rights (OCR) at the Department of Health and Human Services (HHS) announced that it would not impose penalties for using HIPAA-noncompliant private communications technologies to provide telehealth services during the COVID-19 pandemic. Similar efforts at a state level included expedited credentialing, approval of telemedicine privileges, enabling asynchronous communications, and ensuring reimbursement. Finally, modern technology has already solved the infrastructure problem on the patient side: smartphones are now ubiquitous, while the electronic health record is uniquely able to facilitate telemedicine visits compared to the paper medical records.[20]

Telemedicine has obvious benefits in a time of social distancing, including reduction of the infection risk, improvement of access, and increased patient and provider satisfaction. However, certain risks remain: lack of digital access may necessitate audio-phone-only consultations, and this may create problems in conditions that require visual monitoring or diagnosis. Older patients, or those with lower socioeconomic status, or in communities of color may be disproportionately affected by this lack of digital access.[21] Telemedicine also has significant limitations in the first-ever evaluation of neurological patients, as the ability to appreciate neurological signs, particularly in neuromuscular examination, is limited.[22]

FINANCIAL CONSIDERATIONS
HFHS Information
The COVID-19 pandemic has affected the financial health of health systems in the United States and worldwide. The cancellation of elective surgeries, the halting of outpatient, non-COVID 19 visits, and the guidance to minimize nonessential operations threaten the financial viability of health-care institutions.[23] Rural and safety-net hospitals and practices have been particularly affected.[24] For that reason, the Coronavirus Aid, Relief, and Economic Security (CARES) Act, and the Paycheck Protection Program and Health Care Enhancement Act have supported hospital operations and provided necessary revenue over the past months. However, future risks including the impending insurance coverage crisis, highlight the need for further health care reform.[25]

The public health science of infection control is well known: identification and isolation of infected individuals, early treatment, and contact tracing. The uncanny parallels of current public resistance to public lockdown

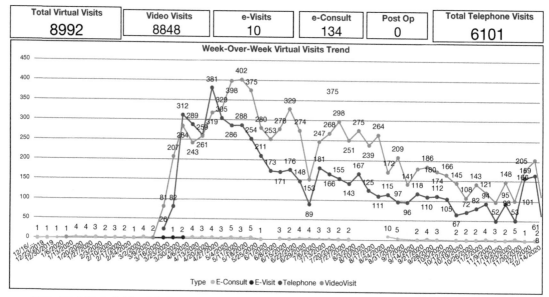

FIG. 13.3 Plot of video *(blue)* and telephone *(red)* office visits per week for 2020. Note that until late March 2020, there were almost no video/telephone visits performed. Then there was a dramatic rapid increase as all visits were done virtually for the next 6 weeks, followed by a gradual change to a mixture of virtual visits along with in-person visits as the pandemic infection rates declined and the clinics were reopened.

rules and mask ordinances during the COVID-19 pandemic to the same behaviors in San Francisco with the formation of the Antimask League during the 1918 influenza pandemic show the limits of public acceptance to sound public health measures.[26] The value of vaccination in the western world was demonstrated by Lister using cowpox inoculation as a method to protect against smallpox but his method was met with resistance from some quarters.[27] The scope of vaccine hesitancy has been broad enough that the World Health Organization established a Strategic Advisory Working Group (SAGE) on Vaccine Hesitancy in March 2012 and produced a number of publications in the pre-COVID-19 era including country-specific characteristics of vaccine resistance.[28] The world is now in a race between the implementation of public health measures supplemented by vaccinations and the inexorable mutation rate of this virus. Florence Nightingale, speaking of unsanitary conditions that fostered the infectious diseases that were killing more British soldiers in the Crimea than the battles themselves, said "Nature is the same everywhere, and never permit her laws to be disregarded with impunity." She went on to say "The three things which all but destroyed the army in Crimea were ignorance, incapacity, and useless rules".[29] The virus has been controlled without the vaccine in locations that strictly adhered to public health principles, but it has largely escaped control in most of the world because, as Paul Simon has said, "All lies and jest, a man hears what he wants to hear and disregards the rest".[30] With the worldwide pandemic now raging, we now face a future ahead of at least a number of years of cycling mutations of the COVID-19 virus, peaking during the winter months along with seasonal influenza, competing with control of the virus by vaccination programs.

REFERENCES

1. Lloyd-Smith M. The COVID-19 pandemic: resilient organisational response to a low-chance, high-impact event. *BMJ Leader.* 2020. https://doi.org/10.1136/leader-2020-000245, leader-2020-000245.
2. Rodengen JL. *Henry Ford Health System: A 100 Year Legacy.* 1st edition. Write Stuff Enterprises LLC; 2014.
3. Tosh PK, Bucks CM, O'Horo JC, DeMartino ES, Johnson JM, Callies Jr BI. Elements of an effective incident command center. *Mayo Clin Proc.* 2020;95(9S):S3–S7.
4. Stoller JK. Reflections on leadership in the time of COVID-19. *BMJ Leader.* 2020. https://doi.org/10.1136/leader-2020-000244, leader-2020-000244.
5. Adhikari S, Rijal S, Acharya PK, et al. Hospital incident command system, the pillar of COVID-19 outbreak response: an experience from Patan Hospital, Nepal. *J Patan Acad Health Sci.* 2020;7:80–84.
6. Remuzzi A, Remuzzi G. COVID-19 and Italy: what next? *Lancet.* 2020;395:1225–1228.

7. Klein MG, Cheng CJ, Lii E, et al. COVID-19 models for hospital surge capacity planning: a systematic review. *Disaster Med Public Health Prep.* 2020;1–17.

8. Nasca TJ. *ACGME's Early Adaptation to the COVID-19 Pandemic: Principles and Lessons Learned.* The Accreditation Council for Graduate Medical Education; 2020.

9. Faria G, Tadros BJ, Holmes N, et al. Redeployment of the trainee orthopaedic surgeon during COVID-19: a fish out of water? *Acta Orthop.* 2020;1–4.

10. Villarin JM, Gao YN, McCann RF. Frontline redeployment of psychiatry residents during the COVID-19 pandemic. *Psychiatr Serv.* 2020;71:1207.

11. Fu SJ, George EL, Maggio PM, Hawn M, Nazerali R. The consequences of delaying elective surgery: surgical perspective. *Ann Surg.* 2020;272, e79.

12. Carlson GL. Prioritizing access to surgical care during the coronavirus pandemic. *Dis Colon Rectum.* 2020;63:879–880.

13. Myles PS, Maswime S. Mitigating the risks of surgery during the COVID-19 pandemic. *Lancet.* 2020;396:2–3.

14. Mouton C, Hirschmann MT, Ollivier M, Seil R, Menetrey J. COVID-19-ESSKA guidelines and recommendations for resuming elective surgery. *J Exp Orthop.* 2020;7:1–7.

15. Parvizi J, Gehrke T, Krueger C, et al. Resuming elective orthopaedic surgery during the COVID-19 pandemic: guidelines developed by the International Consensus Group (ICM). *J Bone Joint Surg Am.* 2020;102:1205.

16. Cohen J, van der Meulen Rodgers Y. Contributing factors to personal protective equipment shortages during the COVID-19 pandemic. *Prev Med.* 2020;141. https://doi.org/10.1016/j.ypmed.2020.106263, 106263.

17. Bown CP. COVID-19: demand spikes, export restrictions, and quality concerns imperil poor country access to medical supplies. COVID-19 and trade policy: why turning inward won't. *Work.* 2020;31.

18. Pfefferbaum B, North CS. Mental health and the Covid-19 pandemic. *N Engl J Med.* 2020;383:510–512.

19. Ghebreyesus TA. Addressing mental health needs: an integral part of COVID-19 response. *World Psychiatry.* 2020;19:129.

20. Bashshur R, Doarn CR, Frenk JM, Kvedar JC, Woolliscroft JO. Telemedicine and the COVID-19 Pandemic, lessons for the future. *Telemed J E Health.* 2020;26:571–573.

21. Roberts ET, Mehrotra A. Assessment of disparities in digital access among Medicare beneficiaries and implications for telemedicine. *JAMA Intern Med.* 2020;180:1386–1389.

22. Garibaldi M, Siciliano G, Antonini G. Telemedicine for neuromuscular disorders during the COVID-19 outbreak. *J Neurol.* 2020;268(1):1–4.

23. Khullar D, Bond AM, Schpero WL. COVID-19 and the financial health of US hospitals. *JAMA.* 2020;323:2127–2128.

24. Barnett ML, Mehrotra A, Landon BE. Covid-19 and the upcoming financial crisis in health care. *NEJM Catal Innov Care Deliv.* 2020;1.

25. King JS. Covid-19 and the need for health care reform. *N Engl J Med.* 2020;382, e104.

26. *San Francisco, California and the 1918–1919 Influenza Epidemic. The American Influenza Epidemic of 1918: A Digital Encyclopedia;* 1918. influenzaarchive.org.

27. Conis E. *Vaccination Resistance in Historical Perspective.* The American Historian; 2015. August.

28. Dube E, et al. Mapping vaccine hesitancy – country-specific characteristics of a global phenomenon. *Vaccine.* 2014;32(49):6649–6654.

29. Nightingale F. *A Contribution to the Sanitary History of the British Army During the Late War with Russia, London 1859, quoted in Kucharski A, The Rules of Contagion: Why Things Spread – And Why They Stop.* UK: Profile Books; 2020. 352 pages; p. 132.

30. Simon P, The Boxer. *Columbia Records;* 1969.

COVID-19-Directed Medications

QUINTON J. TAFOYA
Department of Pharmacy, Veterans Affairs, San Antonio, TX, United States

BAMLANIVIMAB WITH ETESEVIMAB AND CASIRIVIMAB WITH IMDEVIMAB

Monoclonal antibodies were first conceived as a target for disease-causing pathogens in the early 1900s by Elie Metchnikoff. This idea led to the developmental theory of immunology, in which Metchnikoff was awarded the Nobel Prize for Physiology or Medicine in 1908. Additional discoveries and techniques through the 1990s led to the progressive improvement in using monoclonal antibodies, ultimately leading to multiple therapeutic uses in various diseases.

During the COVID-19 pandemic, renewed interest surrounded the use of monoclonal antibodies for treatment. After the SARS-CoV-2 genome was decoded, of the four major structural proteins identified, the surface spike protein was targeted to inhibit viral attachment and entry into human cells with the expectation of neutralizing the viral infection.[1, 2]

Two combination products—bamlanivimab with etesevimab, and casirivimab with imdevimab—are experimental monoclonal antibodies developed specifically to inhibit the SARS-CoV-2 coronavirus by binding to different but overlapping receptors (bamlanivimab/etesevimab) or nonoverlapping regions (casirivimab/imdevimab), thereby inhibiting the spike protein of the virus from attaching and gaining entry to the human cell.[3, 4] Both are administered intravenously, ideally within days of infection for maximum therapeutic benefit. With the relatively long half-life between 17 and 26 days, one dose administration is expected to be sufficient for COVID-19 treatment.

There are several ongoing clinical trials evaluating the safety and efficacy of these monoclonal antibodies. While many are providing initial results, none have yet established the safety and efficacy of SARS-CovC-2-specific monoclonal antibodies.[5–11] Because of the variability and heterogeneity of the primary and secondary outcomes between all the trials, including four randomized controlled trials (RCTs), a metaanalysis was not performed. However, the most up-to-date data from the casirivimab/imdevimab studies suggest efficacy in reducing mortality and hospitalization.[12–16]

As a result of the initial data gathered, all have received Emergency Use Authorizations from the FDA. However, the safety and efficacy of these therapeutics against COVID-19 has not been established, requiring further studies. The NIH COVID-19 Treatment Guidelines Panel and the Infectious Diseases Society of America (IDSA) recommend utilizing bamlanivimab/etesevimab or casirivimab/imdevimab to treat outpatients with mild-to-moderate COVID-19, who may be at a higher risk of developing more severe disease. The panel recommends against their use in hospitalized patients except in the context of a clinical trial.[16, 17]

BARICITINIB

Baricitinib is a nonbiologic, small-molecule medication approved by the FDA in May 2018 for moderately to severely active rheumatoid arthritis (RA) after having an inadequate response to other RA treatments.[18, 19] The initial FDA application of baricitinib in April 2017 was declined due to safety concerns regarding thrombosis in the higher 4 mg dose, which ultimately led to only the 2-mg dose being approved the following year. As a disease-modifying antirheumatic drug (DMARD), it inhibits the intracellular Janus kinase (JAK) enzymes that modulate downstream cellular processes which are believed to be responsible for activation of inflammatory mediators in RA. With 80% bioavailability, baricitinib is an oral medication dosed at 2 mg daily in RA.[20] About 50% of baricitinib is bound to plasma proteins, is hepatically metabolized via CYP3A4, and has a half-life of about 12 h. About 75% is excreted in the urine (69% as unchanged drug) and around 20% excreted in the feces (15% as unchanged drug). Baricitinib is not recommended in patients with severe hepatic impairment or moderate-to-severe renal impairment. As an immunomodulator, some potential side effects include upper respiratory tract infection, hypercholesterolemia, and other potential infection reactivations including herpes zoster, herpes simplex, urinary tract infections, and gastroenteritis.[20]

As a JAK enzyme inhibitor, it is believed to help reduce viral entry while interfering with viral assembly completed within the host cell. This along with the ability of inhibiting various proinflammatory cytokines, thereby potentially reducing cytokine release syndrome in severely ill patients, made baricitinib an attractive study medication for COVID-19 infections. With 18 studies identified on https://ClinicalTrials.gov evaluating the use of baricitinib in COVID-19 infections, one of the higher impact clinical studies to date is the Adaptive COVID-19 Treatment Trial 2 (ACTT-2).[21–25] The ACTT-2 trial is a multinational, randomized, placebo-controlled trial evaluating the time-to-clinical recovery in hospitalized patients who are administered baricitinib and remdesivir. Of the 1033 participants, half of those who received baricitinib had a shorter clinical recovery time versus placebo, specifically in patients requiring high-flow oxygen or noninvasive ventilation. There were no statistically significant differences in mortality between those who received baricitinib and remdesivir versus remdesivir alone.[26–28] On November 19, 2020, the FDA issued an EUA for the use of baricitinib.[29] The NIH COVID-19 Treatment Guidelines have specific recommendations regarding baricitinib's use, stating there are insufficient data to recommend either for or against the use of baricitinib in combination with remdesivir for hospitalized patients, when corticosteroids can be used.[16] Both NIH and IDSA guidelines suggest that baricitinib may be used in conjunction with remdesivir when corticosteroids cannot be used. Otherwise, baricitinib should only be used in the context of a clinical trial.[16, 17]

Convalescent Plasma

Convalescent plasma is a serum product derived from human or nonhuman donors containing monoclonal or polyclonal antibodies that can provide passive immunity in many diseases. First developed by Emil Behring in the late 1800s, the first serum was produced using Guinea pigs, then began utilizing horses, which were believed then to not carry diseases that humans could contract.[30] The first known antiserum developed and injected into a human by Emil Behring was used in 1891 to treat a young girl suffering from diphtheria, which led him to be the recipient of the first Nobel Prize in Medicine for his research in diphtheria.

The accepted mechanism of action is believed to be the neutralization of pathogens with antibodies that bind to the infectious agent or antigen.[30] However, donated antibodies to develop an antiserum to a pathogen must come from an initial survivor who was able to produce the initial immunological response leading to the body's development of antibodies. With the development of effective antimicrobial agents over the last several decades, the development of convalescent plasma was not deemed a viable approach given the constraints of producing the serum.[31–33] However, with the emergence of Ebola, SARS-1, and MERS, there was a renewed interest in developing convalescent plasma.[34, 35]

At the start of the COVID-19 pandemic, there were few known effective and reliable treatment options. The use of convalescent plasma was considered as a potential avenue in the most severe cases. Among 56 studies noted on https://ClinicalTrials.gov, 11 of the higher-impact RCTs and a single-arm registry study with over 20,000 registrants led to the current recommendations for convalescent plasma's use in patients with COVID-19.[36] In one arm of the preliminary (nonpeer-reviewed) data of the Randomized Evaluation of COVID-19 Therapy (RECOVERY) trial, convalescent plasma plus standard of care did not achieve a significant reduction in 28-day mortality compared to standard of care alone. Two other systematic reviews had conflicting conclusions.[37, 38] The Cochrane review found low-to-very low confidence in the safety and efficacy of convalescent plasma while a nonpeer-reviewed systematic review found evidence of its therapeutic efficacy in reducing mortality.[39–42] However, the latter study had great data variability across the study populations.[42] As a result, the NIH guidelines recommend the use of convalescent plasma depending on varying disease severity and patient characteristics such as impaired immunity. The IDSA guidelines do not recommend convalescent plasma use in hospitalized patients and state it can be considered in ambulatory patients with mild-to-moderate disease in the context of a clinical trial.[16, 17]

DEXAMETHASONE

Dexamethasone is a small molecule, potent glucocorticoid with minimal sodium-retaining potential. While it is a long-acting corticosteroid, the mineralocorticoid activity is negligible.[43] As a result of binding to the glucocorticoid receptor, neutrophil migration is suppressed, lymphocyte colony proliferation is decreased, and capillary permeability is reduced. Gene expression changes take place when corticosteroids bind to the glucocorticoid receptor, leading to several downstream effects including neutrophil apoptosis and demargination that ultimately lead to changes in other inflammatory transcription factors that promote antiinflammatory genes like interleukin-10. When administered intravenously, dexamethasone's onset of action is rapid. It is hepatically metabolized and has a half-life elimination of approximately 1–5 h in adults. Dexamethasone IV/oral dosing for the treatment of COVID-19 is 6 mg, once daily for up to 10 days or until hospital discharge (or equivalent dose of an alternative glucocorticoid if dexamethasone is unavailable). There are no dose adjustments provided by manufacturer's labeling in adult patients with renal or hepatic impairment but are advised to use with caution. Monitoring parameters include blood glucose, blood pressure, and signs/symptoms of new infection. It is recommended before use to screen patients for *Strongyloides* hyperinfection or fulminant HBV reactivation. Dexamethasone is a moderate CYP3A4 inducer as well as a CYP3A4 substrate.[43]

In the RECOVERY Trial, over 11,500 patients were enrolled in more than 175 National Health Service hospital organizations in the United Kingdom in which patients were randomized to usual care, usual care plus either lopinavir/ritonavir, dexamethasone, hydroxychloroquine, or azithromycin.[44, 45] In the dexamethasone arm, lower mortality was associated with those receiving oxygen or invasive mechanical ventilation, but not in the arm of patients on no oxygen supplementation. A metaanalysis of seven trials led to the recommendation by the NIH and IDSA to use systemic corticosteroids in patients with severe and critical disease.[16, 17, 46]

HYDROXYCHLOROQUINE

Hydroxychloroquine was first approved for medical use in the United States in 1955 and is currently used in rheumatic disorders and as an antimalarial agent.[47] Hydroxychloroquine is a 4-aminoquinoline derivative, which is hepatically metabolized to *N*-desethyl hydroxychloroquine and excreted by the kidneys as both unchanged drug and metabolites.[48] With a large volume of distribution and roughly 40% binding primarily to albumin, hydroxychloroquine's half-life is about 40 h.[48] It has demonstrated both antiviral and some immunomodulatory properties, with in vitro activity against several coronaviruses.[49, 50] As a result, an emergency use authorization (EAU) was issued for hydroxychloroquine on March 28, 2020 by the FDA for the treatment use of COVID-19.

Dozens of studies have evaluated the safety and efficacy of hydroxychloroquine, with variable dosing strategies and endpoints. One of the largest studies, the RECOVERY Trial, was an open-label RCT with a control arm and multiple treatment arms, evaluating the safety and efficacy of hydroxychloroquine with the primary endpoint of all-cause mortality at day 28 after randomization.[51] Study enrollment was stopped early after it was concluded that there was no benefit of hydroxychloroquine compared to standard of care.[51] As a result of this study and several others reporting the lack of efficacy of hydroxychloroquine in improving all-cause mortality or decreasing hospitalization, in addition to the increased incidence of dangerous adverse events, the FDA revoked the EUA it had issued.[51–55] Both the NIH COVID-19 Treatment Guidelines Panel and IDSA currently recommend against the use of hydroxychloroquine regardless of disease severity.[16, 17]

IVERMECTIN

Ivermectin is a semisynthetic compound derived from the macrocyclic lactone, avermectin, which was first discovered in the 1970s by a Japanese microbiologist after stumbling upon a then unknown bacterium, *Streptomyces avermitilis*. Approved by the FDA in 1981, this antiparasitic agent is the drug of choice for several treatments and has become an important medication in both veterinary practice and in human use.[56, 57] Ivermectin, dosed generally at 150–200 µg/kg, is widely distributed in the body and is highly protein bound.[58, 59] By selectively binding with strong affinity to the glutamate-gated chloride ion channels of invertebrate nerve and muscle cells, the hyperpolarization causes paralysis of the affected tissue, resulting in death.[58] With a half-life of about 18 h, it is hepatically metabolized via the CYP4A4, CYP2D6, and CYP2E1, causing concerns for drug interactions, and is excreted in the feces.[58] Ivermectin has demonstrated in vitro activity against several human and animal viruses, including against SARS-CoV-2 at high drug concentrations.[60, 61]

As a result, several studies have evaluated the efficacy and safety of ivermectin against SARS-CoV-2.[62–64] There has been no adequately powered and well-designed RCT to provide sufficient evidence for the major medical governing bodies to recommend its use. Studies that have been published to date have significant methodological limitations with incomplete data regarding the participants and results. Those studies demonstrating potential promising data are also limited by the design of the studies, lack of information regarding the safety and efficacy of the drug, and had small samples.[65–69]

The WHO, the European Medicines Agency, and the IDSA all recommend against the use of ivermectin for treatment of COVID-19, with the NIH stating that there is insufficient data to recommend for or against its use outside the context of a clinical trial.[16, 17]

LOPINAVIR AND RITONAVIR

Lopinavir and ritonavir are antiviral medications initially developed to inhibit a step in the replication cycle of the human immunodeficiency virus (HIV).[70] While both compounds have antiviral activity against HIV, a subtherapeutic ritonavir dose, acting as a pharmacokinetic booster, is paired with lopinavir to increase lopinavir's bioavailability. The FDA approved the combination tablet for HIV treatment in 2000 and was once recommended as a first-line agent in conjunction with other antiretroviral medications, to suppress HIV replication and prevent disease progression. The active antiretroviral agent, lopinavir, targets the HIV protease, which is responsible for cleaving polyprotein precursors to functioning proteins, resulting in immature, noninfectious viral particles.[70] Lopinavir and ritonavir are both hepatically metabolized via the CYP3A4 enzyme, leading to significant drug interactions.[70] Being mostly protein bound, lopinavir's half-life is approximately 5–6 h, and is mainly excreted in the feces.[70]

Lopinavir was previously discovered to have in vitro activity against SARS-CoV and MERS-CoV, with observed benefit in animal studies infected with MERS-CoV, and reduced rates of ARDS and mortality in those infected by SARS-CoV.[71–74] Lopinavir also exhibited some in vitro activity against SARS-CoV-2, which resulted in over 90 clinical studies evaluating the use of lopinavir in COVID-19 infections.[72] Some of the more significant studies did not reveal clinical benefits in patients with COVID-19.[72, 75–79] The WHO Solidarity trial and the UK RECOVERY trial did not demonstrate significant differences in 28-day mortality, ventilation use, or duration of hospitalization.[80] In a metaanalysis and a systematic review, no significant clinical advantage over the standard of care was noted.[71] As a result, the WHO, the NIH, and IDSA all recommend against the use of lopinavir/ritonavir for the treatment of COVID-19.[16, 17]

REMDESIVIR

Remdesivir is an adenosine analog that has broad-spectrum antiviral activity. Originally developed to treat Ebola hemorrhagic fever, the antiviral demonstrates activity against several other RNA viruses. Remdesivir is a prodrug of the parent molecule GS-441524, which is subsequently metabolized by the host into an active nucleoside triphosphate (NTP).[81] GS-441524 and NTP exhibit antiviral activity both in vitro and in vivo in various animal models.[81] Remdesivir is administered intravenously and interrupts the viral replication process by binding to the viral RNA polymerase, leading to delayed chain termination.[82] Remdesivir is moderately protein bound (free fraction: 12.1%) compared to GS-441524, which has low protein binding (free fraction $\geq$ 85%).[82] The half-life of the prodrug is approximately 1 h while GS-441524 is 24.5 h with the majority of the metabolites excreted in the urine (74%).[82]

Remdesivir was approved by the FDA in October of 2020 for COVID-19. Dosing requires a loading dose of 200 mg on day 1, followed by 100-mg once daily for 4–10 days depending on disease severity and clinical course.[82, 83] To date, there is no formal safety or pharmacokinetic data available in patients with renal impairment. However, it is not recommended to use remdesivir for eGFR < 30 mL/min, unless it is determined that the benefit outweighs the risk.[82] Remdesivir has not been evaluated in hepatic impairment, but its use is not recommended in patients with baseline ALT elevation of greater than 5 times the upper limit of normal (ULN). If hepatotoxicity develops while on remdesivir with ALT $\geq$ 5 times the ULN, increasing conjugated bilirubin, alkaline phosphatase, or INR, it is recommended to discontinue its use. Remdesivir may be resumed once ALT is < 5 times the ULN.[82]

Several high impact clinical studies have contributed to the FDA approval of remdesivir.[79, 84–91] The Adaptive COVID-19 treatment Trial (ACTT-1) was a multinational, placebo-controlled, double-blinded RCT comparing remdesivir versus placebo in 1062 hospitalized patients with primary endpoint of time-to-clinical recovery.[84] Recovery time was reduced in the remdesivir arm for patients with severe COVID-19. However, there was no observed benefit in patients with mild or moderate disease.[84] Another important study, the WHO SOLIDARITY Trial, was an adaptive, open-label, randomized phase III trial conducted in 405 hospitals in 30 countries, comparing five repurposed medications, including remdesivir.[92] The primary endpoint was 28-day mortality with secondary endpoints of ventilation and duration of hospitalization. Interestingly, this study did not demonstrate accelerated recovery with remdesivir. Overall, remdesivir appears to have benefit in patients who are hospitalized on low-flow oxygen.[93] As a result, the NIH and IDSA guidelines make their recommendations for the use of remdesivir based on disease severity.[16, 17]

TOCILIZUMAB

Tocilizumab is a recombinant human monoclonal antibody against the interleukin-6 receptor.[94] Interleukin 6 is a proinflammatory cytokine that contributes to the immune response, and is believed to be central in the pathogenesis of many autoimmune diseases. Developed as an immunosuppressant drug for the treatment of RA, tocilizumab is the first Interleukin-6 receptor inhibitor approved by the FDA in January 2010.

Patients who are severely ill with COVID-19 are at a higher risk of cytokine release syndrome and pulmonary symptoms.[95] As an antagonist, tocilizumab is thought to minimize cytokine release by binding the interleukin-6 receptor.[95, 96] To date, there are 84 studies that have evaluated or are currently evaluating the efficacy of tocilizumab in COVID-19.[97-101] One of the high impact clinical trials, the REMAP-CAP trial, is a multicenter, open label, international trial using a randomized, embedded multifactorial adaptive platform.[102] Following confirmation of COVID-19 infection and subsequent ICU admission, patients were randomized to receive either an IV dose of tocilizumab 8 mg/kg or standard care. Tocilizumab decreased in-hospital mortality (28%) compared to standard care (36%) while also showing more organ support-free days.[102] In the RECOVERY Trial, patients hospitalized with hypoxia and systemic inflammation who received tocilizumab had improved survival and other clinical outcomes compared to those who received standard care.[103] While additional research is needed, based on the collective studies thus far collected, the NIH and IDSA recommend the combined use of tocilizumab and dexamethasone in specific patient populations, stratified based on disease severity and inflammatory laboratory markers.[16, 17]

REFERENCES

1. Zost SJ, Gilchuk P, Case JB, et al. Potently neutralizing and protective human antibodies against SARS-CoV-2. *Nature.* 2020;584:443–449. https://doi.org/10.1038/s41586-020-2548-6. 32668443.
2. Marovich M, Mascola JR, Cohen MS. Monoclonal antibodies for prevention and treatment of COVID-19. *JAMA.* 2020;324:131–132. https://doi.org/10.1001/jama.2020.10245. 32539093.
3. US Food and Drug Administration. *Fact Sheet for Health Care Providers: Emergency Use Authorization (EUA) of Bamlanivimab and Etesevimab.* Available from: https://www.fda.gov/media/145802/download. Accessed 8 May 2021.
4. US Food and Drug Administration. *Fact Sheet for Health Care Providers: Emergency Use Authorization (EUA) of Casirivimab and Imdevimab*; 2020. Available from: https://www.fda.gov/media/143892/download. Accessed 8 May 2021.
5. *US National Library of Medicine.* ClinicalTrials.gov; 2021. Available from: https://clinicaltrials.gov. Accessed 28 April 2021.
6. *A Study of LY3819253 (LY-CoV555) and LY3832479 (LY-CoV016) in Participants With Mild to Moderate COVID-19 Illness (BLAZE-1).* NCT04427501. Update posted 2021 April 20 https://www.clinicaltrials.gov/ct2/show/study/NCT04427501.
7. *Lilly Announces Proof of Concept Data for Neutralizing Antibody LY-CoV555 in the COVID-19 Outpatient Setting;* 2020. Press Release. September 16. Available from: https://investor.lilly.com/newsreleases/news-release-details/lilly-announces-proof-concept-data-neutralizing-antibody-ly.
8. *VIR-7831 for the Early Treatment of COVID-19 in Outpatients (COMET-ICE).* NCT04545060. Update posted 2021 March 29 https://www.clinicaltrials.gov/ct2/show/study/NCT0455060.
9. *Safety, Tolerability, and Efficacy of Anti-Spike (S) SARS-CoV-2 Monoclonal Antibodies for the Treatment of Ambulatory Adult and Pediatric Patients With COVID-19.* NCT04425629. Update posted 2021 April 5 https://www.clinicaltrials.gov/ct2/show/study/NCT04425629.
10. *COVID-19 Study Assessing the Efficacy and Safety of Anti-Spike SARS CoV-2 Monoclonal Antibodies for Prevention of SARS CoV-2 Infection Asymptomatic in Healthy Adults and Adolescents Who Are Household Contacts to an Individual With a Positive SARS-CoV-2 RT-PCR Assay.* NCT04452318. Update posted 2021 April 8 https://www.clinicaltrials.gov/ct2/show/study/NCT04452318.
11. Regeneron. *RECOVERY COVID-19 Phase 3 Trial to Evaluate Regeneron's REGN-COV2 Investigational Antibody Cocktail in the UK.* Press Release. 2020 September 29. Available from: https://newsroom.regeneron.com/news-releases/news-release-details/recovery-covid-19-phase-3-trial-evaluate-regenerons-regn-cov2.
12. *Lilly Provides Comprehensive Update on Progress of SARS-CoV-2 Neutralizing Antibody Programs.* Press Release. 2020 October 7. Available from: https://investor.lilly.com/news-releases/news-releasedetails/lilly-provides-comprehensive-update-progress-sars-cov-2.
13. *ACTIV-2: A Study for Outpatients With COVID-19.* NCT04518410. Update posted 2021 April 23 https://www.clinicaltrials.gov/ct2/show/NCT04518410.
14. US Food and Drug Administration. *Letter of Authorization: Emergency Use Authorization for Use of REGEN-COV® (Casirivimab and Imdevimab) for the Treatment of Mild to Moderate Coronavirus Disease 2019 (COVID-19);* 2021 February 25. Reissued https://www.regeneron.com/sites/default/files/treatment-covid19-eua-fda-letter.pdf.
15. Regeneron. *Fact Sheet for Health Care Providers: Emergency Use Authorization (EUA) of REGEN-COV® (Casirivimab and Imdevimab).* FDA Website; 2021 March. https://www.fda.gov/media/145611/download.
16. Therapeutic Management. *COVID-19 Treatment Guidelines;* 2021. https://www.covid19treatmentguidelines.nih.gov/therapeutic-management/. Accessed 11 May 2021.

17. *COVID-19 Guideline, Part 1: Treatment and Management;* 2021. Idsociety.org https://www.idsociety.org/practice-guideline/covid-19-guideline-treatment-and-management/. Accessed 11 May 2021.

18. Richardson P, Griffin I, Tucker C, et al. Baricitinib as potential treatment for 2019-nCoV acute respiratory disease. *Lancet.* 2020;395:e30–e31. https://doi.org/10.1016/S0140-6736(20) 30304-4. PMID: 32032529.

19. Ceribelli A, Motta F, De Santis M, et al. Recommendations for coronavirus infection in rheumatic diseases treated with biologic therapy. *J Autoimmun.* 2020;109:102442.

20. *Bariicitnib.* Lexicomp. https://online-lexi-com.va.proxy.liblynxgateway.com/lco/action/Bariicitnib; https://online-lexi-com.va.proxy.liblynxgateway.com/lco/action/doc/retrieve/docid/dental_f/6653509?cesid=3vrcGfsd-v54&searchUrl=%2Flco%2Faction%2Fsearch%3Fq%3D-baricitinib%26t%3Dname%26va%3Dbaricitinib; 2021 Accessed 10 May 2021.

21. *Lilly Begins Clinical Testing of Therapies for COVID-19;* 2020. Press Release. Lilly. April 10. Available from: https://investor.lilly.com/news-releases/news-release-details/lilly-begins-clinicaltesting-therapies-covid-19.

22. Stebbing J, Phelan A, Griffin I, et al. COVID-19: combining antiviral and anti-inflammatory treatments. *Lancet Infect Dis.* 2020;20:400–402.

23. Zhang W, Zhao Y, Zhang F, et al. The use of anti-inflammatory drugs in the treatment of people with severe coronavirus disease 2019 (COVID-19): the perspectives of clinical immunologists from China. *Clin Immunol.* 2020;214:108393. https://doi.org/10.1016/j.clim.2020.108393. PMID: 32222466.

24. National Institutes of Health. *NIH Clinical Trial Testing Antiviral Remdesivir Plus Anti-Inflammatory Drug Baricitinib for COVID-19 Begins;* 2020 May 8. NIH Website https://www.nih.gov/news-events/news-releases/nih-clinical-trial-testing-antiviral-remdesivir-plus-anti-inflammatory-drug-baricitinib-covid-19-begins. Accessed 11 May 2020.

25. Cantini F, Niccoli L, Matarrese D, et al. Baricitinib therapy in COVID-19: a pilot study on safety and clinical impact. *J Infect.* 2020;(April 23). https://doi.org/10.1016/j.jinf.2020.04.017 [Epub ahead of print] 32333918.

26. *Lilly Begins a Phase 3 Clinical Trial With Baricitinib for Hospitalized COVID-19 Patients.* Press Release. Lilly: 2020 June 15. Available from: https://investor.lilly.com/node/43351/pdf.

27. Lilly E. *Baricitinib Has Significant Effect on Recovery Time, Most Impactful in COVID-19 Patients Requiring Oxygen.* Press Release 2020 October 8. Available from: https://investor.lilly.com/newsreleases/news-release-details/baricitinib-has-significant-effect-recovery-time-most-impactful.

28. Kalil AC, Patterson TF, Mehta AK, et al. Baricitinib plus remdesivir for hospitalized adults with COVID-19. *N Engl J Med.* 2020;(December 11). https://doi.org/10.1056/NEJMoa2031994 [published online ahead of print] PMID: 33306283.

29. US Food and Drug Administration. *Letter of Authorization: Emergency Use Authorization (EUA) for Emergency Use of Baricitinib, in Combination With Remdesivir, for Treatment of Suspected or Laboratory Confirmed Coronavirus Disease 2019 (COVID-19) in Hospitalized Adults and Pediatric Patients 2 Years of Age or Older, Requiring Supplemental Oxygen, Invasive Mechanical Ventilation, or Extracorporeal Membrane Oxygenation (ECMO).* FDA Website; 2020 November 19. https://www.fda.gov/media/143822/download. Accessed 30 November 2020.

30. Cunningham AC, Goh HP, Koh D. Treatment of COVID-19: old tricks for new challenges. *Crit Care.* 2020;24:91. https://doi.org/10.1186/s13054-020-2818-6. PMID: 32178711.

31. Bloch EM, Bailey JA, Tobian AAR. Deployment of convalescent plasma for the prevention and treatment of COVID-19. *J Clin Invest.* 2020;130:2757–2765. https://doi.org/10.1172/JCI138745. PMID: 32254064.

32. Tiberghien P, de Lambalarie X, Morel P, et al. Collecting and evaluating convalescent plasma for COVID-19 treatment: why and how. *Vox Sang.* 2020;115:488–494. https://doi.org/10.1111/vox.12926. PMID: 32240545.

33. Roback JD, Guarner J. Convalescent plasma to treat COVID-19: possibilities and challenges. Editorial. *JAMA.* 2020;323:1561–1562. https://doi.org/10.1001/jama.2020.4940. PMID: 32219429.

34. Cheng Y, Wong R, Soo YOY, et al. Use of convalescent plasma therapy in SARS patients in Hong Kong. *Eur J Clin Microbiol Infect Dis.* 2005;24:44–46. https://doi.org/10.1007/s10096-004-1271-9. PMID: 15616839.

35. Rubin R. Testing an old therapy against a new disease: convalescent plasma for COVID-19. *JAMA.* 2020;323:214–2117. https://doi.org/10.1001/jama.2020.7456. PMID: 32352484.

36. Joyner MJ, Bruno KA, Klassen SA, et al. Safety update: COVID-19 convalescent plasma in 20,000 hospitalized patients. *Mayo Clin Proc.* 2020;95:1888–1897. https://doi.org/10.1016/j.mayocp.2020.06.028. PMID: 32861333. PMCID: PMC7368917.

37. RECOVERY Collaborative Group. Convalescent plasma in patients admitted to hospital with COVID-19 (RECOVERY): a randomised, controlled, open-label, platform trial. *medRxiv.* 2021. Posted March 10. Preprint (not peer reviewed).

38. Rajendran K, Narayanasamy K, Rangarajan J, et al. Convalescent plasma transfusion for the treatment of COVID-19: systematic review. *J Med Virol.* 2020;92:1475–1483. https://doi.org/10.1002/jmv.25961. PMID: 32356910.

39. Piechotta V, Chai KL, Valk SJ, et al. Convalescent plasma or hyperimmune immunoglobulin for people with COVID-19: a living systematic review. *Cochrane Database Syst Rev.* 2020;7(7):CD013600. https://doi.org/10.1002/14651858.CD013600.pub2. PMID: 32648959.

40. Joyner MJ, Carter RE, Senefeld JW, et al. Convalescent plasma antibody levels and the risk of death from Covid-19. *N Engl J Med.* 2021;384(11):1015–1027. https://doi.org/10.1056/NEJMoa2031893. PMID: 33523609.

41. Valk SJ, Piechotta V, Chai KL, et al. Convalescent plasma or hyperimmune immunoglobulin for people with COVID-19: a rapid review. *Cochrane Database Syst Rev.* 2020;5:CD013600. https://doi.org/10.1002/14651858.CD013600. PMID: 32406927.

42. Salazar E, Christensen PA, Graviss EA, et al. Treatment of coronavirus disease 2019 patients with convalescent plasma reveals a signal of significantly decreased mortality. *Am J Pathol*. 2020;190:2290–2303. https://doi.org/10.1016/j.ajpath.2020.08.001. PMID: 32795424.

43. *Dexamethasone*. www.lexicomp.com. https://online-lexi-com.va.proxy.liblynxgateway.com/lco/action/doc/retrieve/docid/dental_f/2074521?cesid=4GeIFTT5mu2&searchUrl=%2Flco%2Faction%2Fsearch%3Fq%3Ddexamethasone%26t%3Dname%26va%3Ddexamethasone; 2021 Accessed 14 May 2021.

44. US National Library of Medicine. *Randomised Evaluation of COVID-19 Therapy (RECOVERY)*. ClinicalTrials.gov; 2021. Available from: https://clinicaltrials.gov/ct2/show/NCT04381936. Accessed 16 June 2020.

45. RECOVERY Collaborative Group, Horby P, Lim WS, Emberson JR, et al. Dexamethasone in hospitalized patients with COVID-19. *N Engl J Med*. 2021;384:693–704. https://doi.org/10.1056/NEJMoa2021436. PMID: 32678530.

46. Halpin DMG, Singh D, Hadfield RM. Inhaled corticosteroids and COVID-19: a systematic review and clinical perspective. *Eur Respir J*. 2020;55:2001009. Editorial https://doi.org/10.1183/13993003.01009-2020. PMID: 32341100.

47. Barber BE. Chloroquine and hydroxychloroquine. In: Grayson ML, ed. *Kucers' the Use of Antibiotics: A Clinical Review of Antibacterial, Antifungal, Antiparasitic, and Antiviral Drugs*. 7th ed. Boca Raton, FL: CRC Press; 2018:3030–3048.

48. *Hydroxychloroquine*. www.lexicomp.com. https://online-lexi-com.va.proxy.liblynxgateway.com/lco/action/doc/retrieve/docid/dental_f/46891?cesid=aEOCIc5OHbW&searchUrl=%2Flco%2Faction%2Fsearch%3Fq%3Dhydoxychloroquine%26t%3Dname%26va%3Dhydoxychloroquine; 2021 Accessed May 1, 2021.

49. Devaux CA, Rolain JM, Colson P, et al. New insights on the antiviral effects of chloroquine against coronavirus: what to expect for COVID-19? *Int J Antimicrob Agents*. 2020;105938. PubMed:32171740 https://doi.org/10.1016/j.ijantimicag.2020.105938.

50. Gao J, Tian Z, Yang X. Breakthrough: chloroquine phosphate has shown apparent efficacy in treatment of COVID-19 associated pneumonia in clinical studies. *Biosci Trends*. 2020;14:72–73. PubMed:32074550 https://doi.org/10.5582/bst.2020.01047.

51. RECOVERY Collaborative Group. Effect of hydroxychloroquine in hospitalized patients with COVID-19. *N Engl J Med*. 2020;(October 8). https://doi.org/10.1056/NEJMoa2022926. NEJMoa2022926 [Epub ahead of print] PMID: 33031652.

52. Cortegiani A, Ingoglia G, Ippolito M, et al. A systematic review on the efficacy and safety of chloroquine for the treatment of COVID-19. *J Crit Care*. 2020. https://doi.org/10.1016/j.jcrc.2020.03.005. PubMed: 32173110.

53. Gautret P, Lagier JC, Parola P, et al. Hydroxychloroquine and azithromycin as a treatment of COVID-19: results of an open-label non-randomized clinical trial. *Int J Antimicrob Agents*. 2020;56:105949. PubMed: 32205204 https://doi.org/10.1016/jantimicag.2020.105949.

54. Wang M, Cao R, Zhang L, et al. Remdesivir and chloroquine effectively inhibit the recently emerged novel coronavirus (2019-nCoV) in vitro. *Cell Res*. 2020;30:269–271. PubMed: 32020029 https://doi.org/10.1038/s41422-020-0282-0.

55. Keyaerts E, Vijgen L, Maes P, et al. In vitro inhibition of severe acute respiratory syndrome coronavirus by chloroquine. *Biochem Biophys Res Commun*. 2004;323:264–268. PubMed: 15351731 https://doi.org/10.1016/j.bbrc.2004.08.085. Huang M, Tang T, Pang P, et al. Treating COVID-19 with chloroquine. *J Mol Cell Biol*. 2020;(April 1). https://doi.org/10.1093/jmcb/mjaa014. PubMed: 32236562.

56. Yang SNY, Atkinson SC, Wang C, et al. The broad spectrum antiviral ivermectin targets the host nuclear transport importin α/β1 heterodimer. *Antivir Res*. 2020;177:104760. https://doi.org/10.1016/j.antiviral.2020.104760. PMID: 32134219.

57. Azeem S, Ashraf M, Rasheed MA, et al. Evaluation of cytotoxicity and antiviral activity of ivermectin against Newcastle disease virus. *Pak J Pharm Sci*. 2015;28:597–602. PMID: 25730813.

58. *Ivermectin*. www.lexicomp.com. https://online-lexi-com.va.proxy.liblynxgateway.com/lco/action/doc/retrieve/docid/dental_f/2074521?cesid=4GeIFTT5mu2&searchUrl=%2Flco%2Faction%2Fsearch%3Fq%3Divermectin%26t%3Dname%26va%3Divermectin; 2021 Accessed 10 May 2021.

59. Schmith VD, Zhou JJ, Lohmer LR. The approved dose of ivermectin alone is not the ideal dose for the treatment of COVID-19. *Clin Pharmacol Ther*. 2020;108:762–765. https://doi.org/10.1002/cpt.1889. PMID: 32378737.

60. Caly L, Druce JD, Catton MG, et al. The FDA-approved drug ivermectin inhibits the replication of SARS-CoV-2 in vitro. *Antivir Res*. 2020;178:104787 [Epub] https://doi.org/10.1016/j.antiviral.2020.104787. PMID: 32251768.

61. Momekov G, Momekova D. Ivermectin as a potential COVID-19 treatment from the pharmacokinetic point of view: antiviral levels are not likely attainable with known dosing regimens. *Biotechnol Biotechnol Equip*. 2020;34:469–474. https://doi.org/10.1080/13102818.2020. PMID: 1775118.

62. *US National Library of Medicine*. ClinicalTrials.gov. Available from: https://clinicaltrials.gov. Accessed 23 April 2021.

63. Gorial FI, Mashhadani S, Sayaly HM, et al. Effectiveness of ivermectin as add-on therapy in COVID-19 management (pilot trial). *medRxiv*. 2020. Posted July 8. Preprint (not peer reviewed) https://www.medrxiv.org/content/10.1101/2020.07.07.20145979v1.

64. Ahmed S, Karim MM, Ross AG, et al. A five-day course of ivermectin for the treatment of COVID-19 may reduce the duration of illness. *Int J Infect Dis*. 2020;103:214–216. https://doi.org/10.1016/j.ijid.2020.11.191. PMID: 33278625.

65. Rajter JC, Sherman MS, Fatteh N, et al. Use of ivermectin is associated with lower mortality in hospitalized patients with coronavirus disease 2019: the ivermectin in COVID nineteen study. *Chest*. 2021;159:85–92. https://doi.org/10.1016/j.chest.2020.10.009. PMID: 33065103.

66. Chaccour C, Casellas A, Blanco-Di Matteo A, et al. The effect of early treatment with ivermectin on viral load, symptoms and humoral response in patients with non-severe COVID-19: a pilot, double-blind, placebo-controlled, randomized clinical trial. *EClinicalMedicine.* 2021;32:100720.

67. Behera P, Patro BK, Singh AK, et al. Role of ivermectin in the prevention of SARS-CoV-2 infection among healthcare workers in India: a matched case-control study. *PLoS One.* 2021;16(2):e0247163. https://doi.org/10.1371/journal.pone.0247163. PMID: 33592050.

68. Elgazzar A, Eltaweel A, Youssef SA, et al. *Efficacy and Safety of Ivermectin for Treatment and Prophylaxis of COVID-19 Pandemic.* Research Square; 2020. (preprint not peer reviewed). Available from: https://www.researchsquare.com/article/rs-100956/v3.

69. López-Medina E, López P, Hurtado IC, et al. Effect of ivermectin on time to resolution of symptoms among adults with mild COVID-19: a randomized clinical trial. *JAMA.* 2021;325:1426–1435. https://doi.org/10.1001/jama.2021.3071. PMID: 33662102.

70. *Lopinavir/ritonavir.* www.lexicomp.com. https://online-lexi-com.va.proxy.liblynxgateway.com/lco/action/doc/retrieve/docid/dental_f/46977?cesid=2nDktyS31N0&searchUrl=%2Flco%2Faction%2Fsearch%3Fq%3Dkaletra%26t%3Dname%26va%3Dkaletra; 2021 Accessed 5 May 2021.

71. Yao TT, Qian JD, Zhu WY, et al. A systematic review of lopinavir therapy for SARS coronavirus and MERS coronavirus—a possible reference for coronavirus disease-19 treatment option. *J Med Virol.* 2020;92:556–563. PubMed:32104907 https://doi.org/10.1002/jmv.25729.

72. Chu CM, Cheng VC, Hung IF, et al. Role of lopinavir/ritonavir in the treatment of SARS: initial virological and clinical findings. *Thorax.* 2004;59:252–256. PubMed:14985565 https://doi.org/10.1136/thorax.2003.012658.

73. Chen F, Chan KH, Jiang Y, et al. In vitro susceptibility of 10 clinical isolates of SARS coronavirus to selected antiviral compounds. *J Clin Virol.* 2004;31:69–75. PubMed:15288617 https://doi.org/10.1016/j.jcv.2004.03.003.

74. Kim UJ, Won EJ, Kee SJ, et al. Combination therapy with lopinavir/ritonavir, ribavirin and interferon-α for Middle East respiratory syndrome. *Antivir Ther.* 2016;21:455–459. PubMed:26492219 https://doi.org/10.3851/IMP3002.

75. Cao B, Wang Y, Wen D, et al. A trial of lopinavir-ritonavir in adults hospitalized with severe covid-19. *N Engl J Med.* 2020;382:1787–1799. PubMed:32187464 https://doi.org/10.1056/NEJMoa2001282.

76. Arabi YM, Alothman A, Balkhy HH, et al. Treatment of Middle East Respiratory Syndrome with a combination of LOPINAVIR-ritonavir and interferon-β1b (MIRACLE trial): study protocol for a randomized controlled trial. *Trials.* 2018;19:81. PubMed:29382391 https://doi.org/10.1186/s13063-017-2427-0.

77. Liu F, Xu A, Zhang Y, et al. Patients of COVID-19 may benefit from sustained lopinavir-combined regimen and the increase of eosinophil may predict the outcome of COVID-19 progression. *Int J Infect Dis.* 2020;95:183–191. PubMed:32173576 https://doi.org/10.1016/j.ijid.2020.03.013.

78. Deng L, Li C, Zeng Q, et al. Arbidol combined with LPV/r versus LPV/r alone against Corona Virus Disease 2019: a retrospective cohort study. *J Infect.* 2020;81:e1–e5. PubMed:32171872 https://doi.org/10.1016/j.jinf.2020.03.002.

79. Martinez MA. Compounds with therapeutic potential against novel respiratory 2019 coronavirus. *Antimicrob Agents Chemother.* 2020;64. https://doi.org/10.1128/AAC.00399-20. e00399-20. PubMed:32152082.

80. RECOVERY Collaborative Group. Lopinavir-ritonavir in patients admitted to hospital with COVID-19 (RECOVERY): a randomized, controlled, open-label, platform trial. *Lancet.* 2020;396:1345–1352. https://doi.org/10.1016/S0140-6736(20)32013-4. PMID: 33031764.

81. Sheahan TP, Sims AC, Graham RL, et al. Broad-spectrum antiviral GS-5734 inhibits both epidemic and zoonotic coronaviruses. *Sci Transl Med.* 2017;9. https://doi.org/10.1126/scitranslmed.aal3653. PubMed: 28659436.

82. *Remdesivir.* www.lexicompcom. https://online-lexi-com.va.proxy.liblynxgateway.com/lco/action/doc/retrieve/docid/dental_f/6925326?cesid=2RNQQ3o6mZS&searchUrl=%2Flco%2Faction%2Fsearch%3Fq%3Dremdesivir%26t%3Dname%26va%3Dremdesivir; 2021 Accessed 20 February 2021.

83. Gilead Sciences. *Veklury® (Remdesivir) for Injection and Injection Prescribing Information.* Foster City, CA; 2021 February.

84. *Adaptive COVID-19 Treatment Trial (ACTT).* NCT04280705 https://clinicaltrials.gov/ct2/show/NCT04280705.

85. Sheahan TP, Sims AC, Leist SR, et al. Comparative therapeutic efficacy of remdesivir and combination lopinavir, ritonavir, and interferon beta against MERS-CoV. *Nat Commun.* 2020;11:222. PubMed:31924756 https://doi.org/10.1038/s41467-019-13940-6.

86. *Study to Evaluate the Safety and Antiviral Activity of Remdesivir (GS-5734) in Participants With Severe Coronavirus Disease (COVID-19).* NCT04292899 https://www.clinicaltrials.gov/ct2/show/NCT04292899.

87. *Study to Evaluate the Safety and Antiviral Activity of Remdesivir (GS-5734) in Participants With Moderate Coronavirus Disease (COVID-19) Compared to Standard of Care Treatment.* NCT04292730. https://www.clinicaltrials.gov/ct2/show/NCT04292730.

88. Wang Y, Zhang D, Du G, et al. Remdesivir in adults with severe COVID-19: a randomized, double-blind, placebo-controlled, multicentre trial. *Lancet.* 2020;395:1569–1578. https://doi.org/10.1016/S0140-6736(20)31022-9. PMID: 32423584.

89. Goldman JD, Lye DCB, Hui DS, et al. Remdesivir for 5 or 10 days in patients with severe covid-19. *N Engl J Med.* 2020;383:1827–1837. https://doi.org/10.1056/NEJMoa2015301. PMID: 32459919.

90. Spinner CD, Gottlieb RL, Criner GJ, et al. Effect of remdesivir vs standard care on clinical status at 11 days in patients with moderate COVID-19: a randomized clinical trial. *JAMA.* 2020;324:1048–1057. https://doi.org/10.1001/jama.2020.16349. PMID: 32821939.

91. *Study to Evaluate the Safety and Efficacy of Remdesivir (GS-5734) Treatment of Coronavirus Disease 2019 (COVID-19) in an Outpatient Setting.* NCT04501952. Update posted 2020 November 4 https://clinicaltrials.gov/ct2/show/NCT04501952.

92. World Health Organization. *Public Health Emergency SOLIDARITY Trial: World Health Organization COVID-19 Core Protocol, Version 10.0.* WHO Website; 2020 March 22. https://www.who.int/publications/m/item/an-international-randomised-trial-of-additional-treatments-for-covid-19-in-hospitalised-patients-who-are-all-receiving-the-local-standard-ofcare. Accessed 7 December 2020.

93. WHO Solidarity Trial Consortium. Repurposed antiviral drugs for COVID-19—interim WHO Solidarity Trial results. *N Engl J Med.* 2021;384:497–511. https://doi.org/10.1056/NEJMoa2023184. PMID: 33264556.

94. *Tocilizumab.* www.lexicomp.com. https://online-lexicom.va.proxy.liblynxgateway.com/lco/action/doc/retrieve/docid/dental_f/2138405?cesid=7lqItj3ClkK&searchUrl=%2Flco%2Faction%2Fsearch%3Fq%3Dtocilizumab%26t%3Dname%26va%3Dtocilizumab; 2021 Accessed 8 May 2021.

95. Mehta P, McAuley DF, Brown M, et al. COVID-19: consider cytokine storm syndromes and immunosuppression. *Lancet.* 2020 March 16. https://doi.org/10.1016/S0140-6736(20)30628-0. pii:S0140-6736(20)30628-0 [Epub ahead of print] 32192578.

96. Liu B, Li M, Zhou Z, et al. Can we use interleukin-6 (IL-6) blockade for coronavirus disease 2019 (COVID-19)-induced cytokine release syndrome (CRS)? *J Autoimmun.* 2020;102452. https://doi.org/10.1016/j.jaut.2020.102452. [Epub ahead of print]. Available from: doi:10.1016/j.kint.2020.04.002.

97. Xu X, Han M, Li T, et al.. *Effective Treatment of Severe COVID-19 Patients With Tocilizumab* chinaXiv Website; 2020 Accessed 19 March 2020.

98. Luo P, Liu Y, Qiu L, et al. Tocilizumab treatment in COVID-19: a single center experience. *J Med Virol.* 2020. April 6. [Epub ahead of print.] Updated 04-30-2021. The current version of this document can be found on the ASHP COVID-19 Resource Center. PubMed:32253759 https://doi.org/10.1002/jmv.25801. Available from: https://onlinelibrary.wiley.com/doi/epdf/10.1002/jmv.25801.

99. *Tocilizumab Improves Significantly Clinical Outcomes of Patients With Moderate or Severe COVID-19 Pneumonia.* Press Release. Paris; Assistance Publique—Hôpitaux de Paris; April 27, 2020 Accessed 22 June 2020.

100. Sciascia S, Apra F, Baffa A, et al. Pilot prospective open, single-arm multicentre study on off-label use of tocilizumab in patients with severe COVID-19. *Clin Exp Rheumatol.* 2020;38:529–532. PubMed:32359035.

101. Stone JH, Frigault MJ, Serling-Boyd NJ, et al, For the BACC Bay Tocilizumab Trial Investigators. Efficacy of tocilizumab in patients hospitalized with Covid-19. *N Engl J Med.* 2020;(October 21). https://doi.org/10.1056/NEJMoa2028836. [Online ahead of print]. PubMed:33085857.

102. REMAP-CAP Investigators, Gordon AC, Mouncey PR, et al. Interleukin-6 receptor antagonists in critically ill patients with Covid-19. *N Engl J Med.* 2021. February 25. [Epub ahead of print] https://doi.org/10.1056/NEJMoa2100433. PMID: 33631065.

103. RECOVERY Collaborative Group, Hornby PW, Campbell M, Staplin N, et al. Tocilizumab in patients admitted to hospital with COVID-19 (RECOVERY): preliminary results of a randomised, controlled, open-label, platform trial. *medRxiv.* 2021. Posted February 11 Preprint (not peer reviewed) https://www.medrxiv.org/content/10.1101/2021.02.11.21249258v1.

FURTHER READING

104. Renn A, Fu Y, Hu X, et al. Fruitful neutralizing antibody pipeline brings hope to defeat SARS-Cov-2. *Trends Pharmacol Sci.* 2020;(July 31). https://doi.org/10.1016/j.tips.2020.07.004. S0165-6147(20)30166-8. PMID: 32829936.

Index

Note: Page numbers followed by *f* indicate figures and *t* indicate tables.